Praise for
"So Hard to Die"

"An essential book for anyone who is interested in Meriwether Lewis. Written by a physician and a psychologist/psychoanalyst, it combines a thoroughly researched history of Lewis's life with, for the first time, a very detailed psychological profile of Lewis, using available material to reconstruct his developmental history and emotional state during the difficult adult years leading to his mysterious death."

    Calvin A. Colarusso, M.D.
    Clinical Professor of Psychiatry
    University of California at San Diego
    Training and Supervising Analyst in Adult and Child
        Psychoanalysis
    San Diego Center for Psychoanalysis

"Join the authors as they delve into the life and times of Meriwether Lewis in a new and fascinating approach using forensics of the cultural, medical, and psychological aspects of his life and times up to and including the untimely demise of this true American hero. What and how did aspects of the society and culture of the colonial life preceding and present during this period of the American experience affect Lewis? This book presents an excellent discussion of the diseases present in Lewis's America and how they could have affected him. How did the medications used by the doctors of that era affect Lewis and his party? Did diseases, medications, and alcohol contribute to his demise? This book presents a most fascinating virtual psychoanalysis of Lewis and is presented in an unprecedented form. For any reader with an interest in the life and times of Meriwether Lewis, this is a must-read!"

    Dale Carrison, D.O., M.S., FACEP, FACOEP
    Professor Emeritus, Emergency Medicine
    University of Nevada at Reno

"In *So Hard to Die,* David and Marti Peck place the reader in the world of Meriwether Lewis. The cultural, medical, and other practices of the day place Lewis in the context of his time to best understand his life and its influences and challenges. As trained and experienced medical and clinical psychology professionals, the Pecks thoroughly explore the motivations and the demons that drove Lewis and, in the end, contributed to his death. This is a must-read for those interested in the life and death of Meriwether Lewis and the America of the late 18th and early 19th centuries."

    James J. Holmberg, Historian
    The Filson Historical Society, Louisville, Kentucky
    Editor of *Dear Brother: Letters of William Clark to Jonathan Clark*

"This fascinating account makes a unique contribution to scholarship on Meriwether Lewis and the circumstances of his death. Because no experts in contemporary psychoanalytic assessment, a skill that takes years to master, have previously weighed in on Lewis's possible personality structure, the book is groundbreaking. Without resorting to professional jargon, the authors apply relevant concepts with sensitivity and discipline, appreciating the formidable problem of diagnosing the personality of a man born long before the age of psychological assessment. The result is a brilliant engagement with Lewis's probable mental state and with the psychological world of men of his era, culture, and class. I recommend it to all readers interested in Lewis and Clark and the time in which they lived."

    Nancy McWilliams, Ph.D.
    Psychologist/Psychoanalyst
    Rutgers Graduate School of Applied and Professional Psychology
    New Brunswick, New Jersey
    Co-Editor of the *Psychodynamic Diagnostic Manual* (2nd ed.)

"This is a most welcome book in which Drs. David and Marti Peck bring all of their expertise to bear upon the enigma of the life and death of Meriwether Lewis. In this thoroughly researched volume, these clinicians use their trained minds to review the literature to date, interrogate the source materials about Lewis's last days, and, using medical and psychological tools at their disposal, create a "patient" named Meriwether Lewis whom they can newly interview and assess.

The kind of critical thinking involved in their study can only be achieved by those who possess these kinds of professional credentials. I would draw your attention to the work in this book of Dr. Marti Peck from my discipline. She is as careful to make the distinction between original materials from her imaginative filling in of gaps to construct the person of Lewis as she is in laying out the rationale for the diagnostic tools she makes use of and the systematic manner in which she arrives at her conclusions. It was a pleasure for me to follow the working of her mind as she interviewed the patient she had so astutely created. From my background in medicine, I can say the same about the level of expertise I found in the sections researched and written by Dr. David Peck. His analysis of the various medical arguments put forth by others that may have been part of the equation in Lewis's end-of-life issues is both in-depth and understandable.

Each of these clinicians possesses a special talent for translating technical concepts into understandable language so that they retain the authoritative voice earned from their training while never losing the reader in confusing jargon that obscures more than it reveals. This is a must-read for Lewis scholars, for other lifelong devotees of Lewis and Clark, and for those curious enough to enter this subject beginning with this informative and delightful book."

    Fred L. Griffin, M.D.
    Clinical Professor of Psychiatry
    University of Texas, Southwestern Medical School
    Training and Supervising Analyst, Dallas Psychoanalytic
       Center

"Friends of Lewis and Clark will delight in accompanying the Drs. Peck on a bold and daring new adventure as they explore the mysteries and suppositions about the too-early death of a great American hero, Meriwether Lewis. Their knowledge and love of their subject, along with their medical and psychological expertise accompanied by humor, create a satisfying, plausible theory of how Lewis died at the young age of 35 after becoming one of the greatest explorers of all time.

"Lewis and Clark enthusiasts will be enthralled as the authors take them on a scintillating expedition of discovery into the heart, mind, and psyche of Meriwether Lewis in the time leading up to his mysterious death in 1809. The Pecks are knowledgeable sleuths who share his medical and psychological history while discussing the sociocultural, political, philosophical, and religious thought of the time in which he lived that impacted his manner of dying. With humor and expertise, the authors delve into the people and places of Lewis's life, uncovering facts and turning over previous suppositions, encouraging readers to become co-theorists as they explore possible answers to the question of what led to the early demise of this iconic personality in American history."

    Rev. Rebecca Cole-Turner, Ph.D., M.Div.
    Clinical Psychologist/Minister
    Gibsonville, North Carolina

"The authors combine medicine, psychology, and a thorough review of the actual historical record to bring an undistorted Meriwether Lewis fully to life for the modern reader. A brilliant illustration of how we can understand historical figures in an imaginary but fact-based interview between Lewis and a psychologist (one of the authors). The interview could have been constructed only after complete immersion in Lewis's life. The authors have created a compelling account which illuminate the roles of Lewis's era, his upbringing, his personality, and his drinking to help us appreciate his accomplishments, his suffering, and why he merits our compassion."

    Tom Horvath, Ph.D.
    American Board of Professional Psychology, Certified
        Substance Abuse Psychologist
    Founder, Practical Recovery, La Jolla, California

"Previous Lewis biographers and authors have speculated about the numerous illnesses that may have marked Lewis's final days. Dr. Dave Peck addresses the medical issues in question with an understanding not seen in other works, and Dr. Marti Peck's analysis of Lewis's psyche is groundbreaking. From disease to gunshots, alcohol abuse to mental illness—it is all here! This book will be the authoritative treatment of Lewis's death for years to come."
    Keith D. Bortnem, D.O.
    Orthopedic Surgeon, FACOS
    Great Falls, Montana

"This book provides a convincing account of the demise of one of the key figures in the pivotal American story of the opening of the West. Who was Captain Meriwether Lewis as a personality, and what exactly were the social and personal circumstances of his life leading up to his death? Adding to the rich Lewis and Clark scholarship, the authors bring their medical knowledge and psychoanalytic clinical experience together to form a unique and long-missing perspective on Lewis's controversial end. Deeply informed by decades of clinical experience and a firm, clear understanding of psychopathology communicated in a straightforward, accessible style, history, medicine, and psychoanalysis are brought together in this fascinating chronicle."
    Harry Polkinhorn, Ph.D.
    Professor Emeritus of English and Comparative Literature
    San Diego State University
    Supervising and Training Analyst
    San Diego Psychoanalytic Center

"This book changed my mind about the fate of Meriwether Lewis. The Drs. Peck provide a logical and convincing analysis of the many factors that may have contributed to Lewis's death in a thoroughly compelling manner. Not only are medical and psychological issues explored, but a groundbreaking analysis of the key issues such as alcoholism in early America and the probable religious beliefs of

Lewis's mother Lucy are thoroughly explained and tied into the narrative."
    C. Dwayne Shafer, M.D. Ph.D.
    Family Medicine (Retired)
    Stephenville, Texas

"An excellent syntopical work! Full of historical facts and reasoned extrapolation, all while reading like a friendly summer's eve chat on the porch. Intriguing . . . informative . . . delightful!"
    Ty Hutchins, M.D.
    Anesthesiology
    Clovis, California

"This book is a challenging, in-depth analysis of the times and the state of mind of Meriwether Lewis in the final years of his most interesting life. It is a must-read for anyone hoping to really understand this incredibly important historic figure."
    Larry Epstein, J.D.
    Past President of the Lewis and Clark Trail Heritage
       Foundation
    Essex, Montana

"This book presents an authoritative, insightful, well referenced review of the murder/suicide debate surrounding the causes of Meriwether Lewis's death. Multiple basic and detailed explanations of life and of medical and mental health care during the late 18th and early 19th centuries provide interest for the novice or scholar with discussion and analysis from the view point of a physician and a clinical psychologist. The authors leave the reader with a good understanding of life and society two hundred years ago and discuss many causes not frequently mentioned, especially in regard to the effects of mental illness and alcohol and substance abuse in that era. A complex personality, Lewis encountered difficulty and stress upon his reentry into civilian life after the expedition. Multiple contributing factors such as family history, upbringing, and social standing are included in the Pecks' thorough analysis of the life and death of this American hero."

>Anthony L. Kovac, M.D.
>Kasumi Arakawa Professor of Anesthesiology
>Affiliate Professor, Dept. of History and Philosophy of Medicine
>University of Kansas Medical Center
>Kansas City, Kansas

"The Drs. Peck shed new light on the controversial nature of the life and death of one of America's greatest . . . Meriwether Lewis. The issues contributing to his untimely death are thoroughly covered with their compelling style and logic which address the analysis of previous authors with a no-holds-barred honesty. This book will create new controversy, but the truth often does. This is a masterful book and a necessary academic source for all those interested in Lewis's life, times, and mysterious death."

>Chandler Gunning, D.O., M.S.
>Diplomate, American Board of Psychiatry and Neurology
>Scottsdale, Arizona

"Weaving an ornate tapestry of rich historical detail and unparalleled expertise in the discipline of frontier medicine, forensics, and psychoanalysis, this dedicated pair of 'Lewis and Clark-ologists' will elegantly transport readers two centuries back in time to discover insights into the nebulous enigma that was Meriwether Lewis. The authors invite you to come along on this compelling journey and to explore the many complexities of his life and the long-disputed nature of his mysterious, solitary, and untimely death."

>Anthony Leo, M.D., FACS
>Board Certified General/Vascular Surgeon
>Oelwein, Iowa

"So Hard to Die"

"So Hard to Die"

A PHYSICIAN AND A PSYCHOLOGIST EXPLORE THE MYSTERY OF MERIWETHER LEWIS'S DEATH

DAVID J. PECK   MARTI E. PECK

Copyright © 2021 by The Marti and David Peck Family Trust of 1992

All rights reserved. No part of this book may be reproduced in any form or by any electronic or mechanical means including information storage and retrieval systems without permission in writing from the author. The only exception is by a reviewer, who may quote short excerpts in a review.

Scripture quotations marked (NLT) are taken from the Holy Bible, New Living Translation, copyright ©1996, 2004, 2015 by Tyndale House Foundation. Used by permission of Tyndale House Publishers, Carol Stream, Illinois 60188. All rights reserved.

Scripture quotations marked (GNT) are from the Good News Translation in Today's English Version - Second Edition Copyright © 1992 by American Bible Society. Used by Permission.

ISBN Paperback: 978-1-7378114-1-1
ISBN Hardcover: 978-1-7378114-0-4
ISBN eBook: 978-1-7378114-2-8

Printed in the United States of America

Cover Art: *The Missouri River at Dearborn, Montana*, oil on canvas by David J. Peck 2019

Portrait on Cover: *Meriwether Lewis* by Charles Saint-Mémin (1803, American Philosophical Society)

Title Page Artwork: Todd Conner, *Ft. Benton, Montana, Captain Lewis and Seaman*, oil on canvas.

Cover and Interior Design: Creative Publishing Book Design

For our parents,

*Alexander Smuszkiewicz and Anne Triumpho Smuszkiewicz
and
Leonard E. Peck, Sr., and Ann Beniger Peck*

*They gave up much so that we might have good lives . . .
and their love allowed us to thrive.*

Contents

Acknowledgments xvii

Introduction 1

Chapter 1—Life in Early America 13

Chapter 2—Family Background and Biography
of Meriwether Lewis 31

Chapter 3—Philosophical Influences on Meriwether Lewis:
Thomas Jefferson and the Enlightenment 79

Chapter 4—Intoxication Nation: Meriwether Lewis
and Alcohol 89

Chapter 5—Pleasures and Poisons: Medicine in the
World of Meriwether Lewis 121

Chapter 6—Meriwether Lewis: Mental Derangement
and Syphilis 143

Chapter 7—A Collision of Worldviews: Christianity,
the Enlightenment, and Freemasonry 157

Chapter 8—Meriwether Lewis and Malaria: Truth
and Fiction 187

Chapter 9—Bullets and How They Kill 207

Chapter 10—Understanding Mental Health and
Meriwether Lewis 223

Chapter 11—A Psychological Interview of Meriwether Lewis 245

Chapter 12—A Psychological Profile of Meriwether Lewis 281

Chapter 13—Meriwether Lewis and the Second Man
  on the Moon 317

Chapter 14—Murder or Suicide? 337

Appendix—A Conversation with Dr. Glenn Wagner. 377

Bibliography. 389

About the Authors 397

Endnotes 401

Index 431

List of Figures

Figure 1. Family Tree of Meriwether Lewis 38

Figure 2. Diagramatic Lateral Views of Possible Bullet Path 218

Figure 3. The Fatal Gunshot of Meriwether Lewis 220

Photo Section. 239–243

Acknowledgments

Our most sincere gratitude goes to the following people who have contributed to the completion of this book as well as to the fullness of our lives. In many ways, this short section of our book has been the most difficult to write as we wish to acknowledge those people who are important to us in so many ways . . . . our friends and family.

Leonard Peck Jr. and Randy Peck for their examples as older brothers.

David's aunt, Elsie Beniger Magennis, who passed away at the age of ninety-five as we finished this book. I grew up a block away from her and her husband Ernie and shared many great times with them in Santa Barbara, California, and in Montana as well. She was the very best aunt any kid could hope for.

Our sister-in-law, Jan Peck, for her production and editing assistance.

Our nieces and nephews, Deborah Peck Tillson, Jerome and Jessica Peck and their daughter Allie Marie, Joseph and Holly Peck, and Benjamin and Chelsea Peck.

Our copy editor, Kathy McKay, for her excellent work in polishing up our manuscript. Any errors in the text are ours alone.

Mike Bischetsrieder, whose photographic and computer skills helped in multiple areas of this book. He and his wife Irene have been great friends for fifty-plus years.

Keith Bortnem, D.O. (orthopedic surgeon), and his wife Becky of Great Falls, Montana, who have listened to our rants about Lewis and Clark for twenty-plus years—always with good humor. Keith's late parents, Al and Janet, were among the best people on earth. I (David) shared some exhilarating "Lewis and Clark moments" with Al on our motorcycles in the backcountry of the Little Belt and Highwood Mountains in Montana.

Stephen and Moira Ambrose for their kindness and encouragement of David's writing *Or Perish in the Attempt: The Hardship and Medicine of the Lewis and Clark Expedition.* This book has changed our lives for the better.

Those who have read our manuscript and offered suggestions and encouragement, including Dave Cogley, J.D., Fred Dickey, Arend Flick, Ph.D., Jim Magrane, Suzanna Morgenstern, Ph.D., Mary McKenzie, Benjamin Peck, Jim Riley, Dan Sturdevant, J.D., and Emilie Sfregola, Psy.D.

The physicians who allowed David to interview them and tap into their vast medical experience: Dale Carrison, D.O. (emergency medicine), Anthony Leo, M.D. (general/vascular surgery/forensics), Dale Mortenson, M.D. (general/vascular surgery), and Glenn Wagner, D.O. (forensic pathology).

Introduction

Don't believe everything you think!
—Anonymous

In the mid-1990s, Marti gave me (David) the book *Undaunted Courage: Meriwether Lewis, Thomas Jefferson, and the Opening of the American West* by Stephen Ambrose as a birthday gift. This was the beginning of my deep interest in the Lewis and Clark Expedition and the Corps of Discovery. Marti also enthusiastically voted in favor of building a Montana log cabin within a few miles of the farm where my grandparents, Frank and Anna Beniger, had labored and raised my mother Ann and her four siblings just outside of Helena. Although I am a born-and-raised southern Californian, Montana, with its amazing beauty and history, has long been a main strand of my DNA. Ambrose's book, our log cabin, and my love for Montana provided a critical mass for my embryonic interest in the adventure of the Lewis and Clark story.

Our cabin was a team effort. While the logs were being milled and finished, Marti and I spent the winter months of '98 building window cornices, a log coffee table, and other furnishings and watched the plans for our Lewis and Clark Room take shape. The coming summer promised to be the adventure of a lifetime—seeing our dream of a Montana cabin come to fruition with the added element of a small, vicarious twentieth-century Lewis and Clark adventure for a guy who, in my moments of unrealistic fantasy, could have gone along on the expedition.

Before taking two months off that summer from my job as a physician in a San Diego medical group in order to help build the cabin, I had written a letter to Stephen Ambrose in Helena. I told him about my upcoming hiatus in Montana and my love for everything Lewis and Clark, and I invited him to "come up to my building site for a cup of campfire coffee and a talk about Lewis and Clark." I felt like I already knew Ambrose due to my love of World War II history; I had read his books and seen him on numerous World War II documentaries. Needless to say, I was flabbergasted to receive a handwritten note from Steve that included his home phone number—and a message to call him when our cabin construction was underway.

On a brutally hot and dry June day in western Montana, Steve and Moira drove up our dirt driveway to our log cabin in its early stages. The Ambroses were particularly excited to see our cabin as they were in the process of building their own cabin on the North Fork of the Blackfoot River some eighty miles to the northwest. Steve, appropriately, was wearing a Lewis and Clark T-shirt. I brought over several sawn logs to use as stools, and we sat in the shade of the pine trees and talked a bit about our motives for building such places. I showed them around the cabin and then offered up a question to Steve. His response would reveal one reason why I immediately liked him. I referred to the Battle of Normandy in the Second World War and teasingly goaded him a bit, questioning his marked difference of opinion from the noted British military historian John Keegan concerning the military capabilities of General Bernard Montgomery during the battle for Caen, France, in June and July of 1944. Keegan thought that Monty was a military genius, but Ambrose was not quite so complimentary. In a playful manner, I provoked Ambrose a bit more and with a smile pointedly asked him, "What's up with that?" He paused a few seconds and finally said, "John has to look at himself in the mirror in the morning, and John is *just wrong!*" I burst out laughing. My medical career has permanently set my truth meter to a high rating, and hearing this internationally acclaimed author and historian being completely honest was refreshing to me in the extreme!

When I (Marti) witnessed my husband David's growing enthusiasm for the story of the Lewis and Clark Expedition, I encouraged him to write about the medicine of the expedition as he had presented a number of lectures to various groups about this fascinating topic. David's first book, *Or Perish in the Attempt: The Hardship and Medicine of the Lewis and Clark Expedition*, opened the door for my participation in his adventure as well. During a day trip with Steve and Moira Ambrose driving around western Montana, I discussed with them the various psychological issues involved in the story, particularly in regard to the personality and end-of-life issues with Meriwether Lewis. I found the Ambroses' comments fascinating since I knew of all the difficult moments experienced by the Corps during the twenty-eight months of their trip. Steve told us that he thought the toughest moment psychologically for the men was when they ran out of tobacco. We traded stories and opinions about a number of issues, and this furthered my own interest in Lewis. Through the years, as I read various books on Lewis and the expedition as well as numerous articles in *We Proceeded On*, the quarterly journal of the Lewis and Clark Trail Heritage Foundation, I found that my ideas concerning the psyche of Meriwether Lewis are not always reflected in the writings of many Lewis and Clark scholars. This in part is why David and I have decided to contribute our knowledge and experience to challenge what we see as some inaccuracies in the scholarship based on misunderstandings of both medical and psychological principles.

As you process the title of this book on the life, times, and death of Captain Meriwether Lewis, your own truth meter may well be sounding an alarm. Perhaps you are thinking, "I believe I've heard it all regarding the death of Lewis." Numerous articles in past issues of *We Proceeded On* have covered various issues concerning both the life and the death of Lewis. No consensus has been reached as to whether Lewis, who died of gunshot wounds in 1809 in an inn on the Natchez Trace, was murdered or killed himself. Historian David Nicandri expressed his opinion in a recent article in the journal that as far as future topics with regard to Lewis and Clark literature are concerned, "The murder/suicide debate would seem to be a good candidate for an interpretive cease-fire. At this point, it should only be reopened if we discover new sources."[1] Several books have explored various death scenarios that are filled with conspiracy theories, mysterious interpretations of diseases, armchair psychological interpretations, and questions without answers. John Guice, historian and editor of the book *By His Own Hand?*, made the dramatic claim that his book about the final days of Lewis "should serve as the authoritative treatment of the topic for the foreseeable future."[2] Guice considered the suicide theory completely unbelievable.

During the years prior to the Lewis and Clark bicentennial in 2003–06, a mock public coroner's jury took up the subject of Lewis's death and heard "testimony" from several noted experts in forensic anthropology, pathology, medicine, and history. Various physicians, mental health clinicians, historians, and aficionados weighed in on a wide array of issues concerning Lewis's mysterious and early death. Given the great amount of attention paid to how Lewis died, should we "call a truce," as Nicandri suggests, in the murder/suicide debate?

We believe that although many issues have already been covered regarding the demise of Meriwether Lewis, a great deal of value has never been brought into the light of day. Much is still poorly understood by many of those who love this story, and much, as Steve Ambrose would have said, is *just wrong*. Understanding the final days of Lewis involves a complex calculus of medical and psychological issues that are often too elusive to allow modern-day clinicians to make an ironclad diagnosis of his medical state and the condition of his mental functioning over two hundred years ago. At the same time, a great deal of wildly erroneous information has been published in past years that does not agree with established medical and mental health knowledge or accepted historical fact. Also, a significant amount of information not related to Lewis's physical and mental health has been inadequately explored, yet these topics undoubtedly influenced Lewis's fate. This book addresses some of these issues.

Because of the many medical and psychological issues in this story, we are forced to weigh the evidence for the various diagnoses of Lewis's physical and mental condition. If a diagnosis is possible but highly improbable, we will point that out in our discussion. It is an easy task to provide diagnostic critiques of the opinions that others have written, both medical and psychological. Many of the conclusions reached by other writers, including key points of their arguments concerning Lewis's last days, are untrue. This is our opinion, but we can back it up with both our clinical experience and academic sources. Authors, publishers, and reviewers of books and journal articles are full of confidence in their opinions: "This book proves that Lewis was murdered" or "This book sheds new light on the death of Lewis, proving that he killed himself, not because he was depressed but because he had _____ " (fill in the blank with whatever medical or psychological condition you choose). Gary E. Moulton, arguably the best informed professional historian concerning the Lewis and Clark Expedition and editor of the *Journals of the Lewis and Clark Expedition*, in the afterword of his excellent volume *The Lewis and Clark Expedition Day by Day*, writes in reference to Lewis, "His eventual fate inevitably attracts the attention of amateur psychoanalysts seeking the roots of his emotional problems."[3] Dr. Moulton might have included amateur physicians and psychologists among those eager to examine Lewis's death.

In their contributions to *By His Own Hand?*, James J. Holmberg and Clay Jenkinson, both supporters of the suicide theory, covered many of the arguments for and against Lewis's reported suicide. As a historian, Holmberg covered not only some of the same clinical topics we cover in this work but also others that pertain more directly to historical issues. He did excellent work in his analysis of the various historical issues involved and came to the conclusion that "the evidence strongly supports suicide."[4] We have written about many of these same historical issues, but not as well as Holmberg. Much to his credit, he reported and discussed some of the clinical medical and psychological issues as described by clinicians within the appropriate specialties and thus avoided becoming one of Moulton's "armchair psychoanalysts." We are throwing our hats into this ring as a physician (David) and a psychologist/psychoanalyst (Marti), each of us with something unique and hopefully authoritative to add to the discussion. As medical and psychological clinicians, we spotlight the issues relevant to our professions and both dissect and explain many of the claims that have been made by other authors.

Clay Jenkinson analyzed many of these issues in both *By His Own Hand?* and his excellent work *The Character of Meriwether Lewis: Explorer in the Wilderness*. Jenkinson does a wonderful job of analyzing multiple areas of Lewis's personality and touches on some of the same areas of Lewis's life and death that we address. Many of the misconceptions concerning the death of Lewis set off Jenkinson's truth meter (our characterization). Jenkinson wrote, regarding the various claims about Lewis's end, that "conjecture is piled on wild speculation on top of improbability to create a story that appears much more solid than in fact it is."[5] We believe Jenkinson's comment applies to many of the opinions that have been written regarding Lewis, even those that are not conspiratorial in nature but are erroneously presented as factual analyses of the many medical and psychological topics involved in this mystery. This situation has resulted because some Lewis and Clark authors lack knowledge in medical and psychological areas yet state their personal theories on these subjects as if they were authorities.

A nonmedically trained person's opinion may be true—and some Lewis and Clark authors who are not physicians or psychologists, as we have already noted, have done exemplary work. But the books they wrote are valuable because, in spite of their lack of training in medicine or psychology, many of their claims agree with known medical and psychological facts. If opinions regarding Lewis's fate are factually erroneous, regardless of how attractively novel they may seem as new "historical interpretations," these opinions misrepresent reality. They do nothing to further our knowledge about a true American hero and only serve to further muddy the already murky waters of the story of Meriwether Lewis. In short, it is a mistake to unquestioningly believe a medical or psychological opinion based solely on an individual's perceived credibility lent only by their academic or professional credentials unrelated to medicine or psychology. At the same time, it is a philosophically risky position for historians and others to offer their opinions on medical and psychological issues or the opinions of physicians without the support of qualified authorities—even given today's cultural acceptance of the postmodernist confusion over what is and is not reality.

In our attempts to address several factors that heavily influenced both Lewis's life and the culture in which he lived, we admit we have stepped into the philosophical trap we have set for ourselves in the previous paragraph. In order to give a more complete view of Lewis's worldview as well as of his spiritual/religious training and beliefs, we wade into the subjects of theology and cultural history—areas in which we may be knowledgeable but are not experts. We have therefore called on experts in these fields for their insights and judgments on our thoughts. No study of the life and death of Lewis would be complete without exploring these subjects, and we believe that these areas have been shortchanged in previous works on Lewis. In order to make our view more comprehensive, we examine numerous cultural and religious issues of interest that were unique to the times in which Lewis lived and should weigh heavily in any analysis of his death.

We have made an honest attempt to read nearly everything that has been written about Lewis and his untimely and tragic early death by multiple gunshot wounds in a lonely cabin along the Natchez Trace in Tennessee. The death of Lewis is a complex puzzle. One may justifiably challenge our positions by noting that it is impossible to accurately and reliably assess Lewis since we have no living patient to examine, test, or interview and, up to this point in history, no forensic pathological evaluation of his remains. To provide an authoritative assessment of the physical and mental health of Lewis, we would need to perform a physical and mental health exam, take imaging studies, draw labs for body chemistries, run a toxicology screen to determine the presence of any medicinal or poisonous substances, and administer a set of psychological tests as well as conduct an in-depth psychological interview. Of course, much of this desired clinical information is forever unobtainable. But if a picture puzzle of a horse is fairly complete, lacking only a few pieces around his head, it is fairly easy to deduce the pieces that are missing. Multiple pieces of valuable historical information are at our disposal that we believe allow us to assemble a great deal of the picture puzzle of Lewis's final days and thus give excellent evidence as to what may be contained in the missing pieces. We examine the historical evidence of Lewis's death, provide accurate medical and psychological opinions regarding previously written work, and include new factors that we believe played a significant role in his death.

Our education as a physician and a doctoral-level psychologist has involved exposure to a myriad of topics. Physicians study physiology, anatomy, pharmacology, pathology, microbiology, and many other subjects. Clinical psychologists master various theories of mental illness, abnormal psychology and pathology, research methods, statistics, and therapeutic interventions. All this academic training is then put into practice through years of clinical training and the practical experience of caring for people with a thousand different illnesses. Much of what we know today about medicine and psychology is not the result of reading about it in a book. One cannot become a physician or psychologist simply by reading. That approach was tried during the Middle Ages and even into the Enlightenment—and it failed miserably. Our decades of clinical experience give us an advantage in evaluating many issues in both medical science and psychology that other scholars of Lewis have not had. That is not being grandiose. We know our limitations. For example, I (David) would never argue with my brothers about an aspect of engineering. I know almost nothing about their field of expertise. Such is not the situation in regard to the death of Lewis. Not only do we know facts about alcohol and drug abuse, infectious disease, depression, and suicide, we have seen them all too often in our professional practices.

Even though we have significant academic and clinical backgrounds, this does not make us the oracles of truth. David was board certified in family medicine and worked in an emergency medicine setting in San Diego for twenty-one years. This gives him some expertise in his field but by no means in everything medical. Despite Marti's years of academic training and thirty-plus years of clinical experience with hundreds of patients, she continues to consult with her mentors in the mental health field regarding clinical cases. When we cover topics of medicine or psychology outside our areas of expertise, we have made concerted efforts to consult with experts in those fields.

All authors hope their work and thoughts will have a beneficial effect on their readers' lives and society as a whole. Whether or not Lewis was addicted to or abused drugs and/or alcohol, we believe that the ongoing abuse of opioids, alcohol, and other substances in our country that kills thousands of people annually has not improved at all since 1809, the year Lewis died. Our relative state of scientific enlightenment has not solved the problem. In fact, the epidemic of opioid abuse is likely worse today than it was in 1809. The same human factors that lead to substance abuse today were also present in the early nineteenth century and in some ways were more pronounced during Lewis's time than in our day. Although our focus in this book is on Meriwether Lewis, the parallel factors involved in addiction and other mental health issues in our own time are both alarming and tragically sad.

It is important to note that the title and themes of our work may suggest to some readers that we are approaching this subject with the attitude that the legitimate answers to the problems we identify in the mystery of Lewis's life and death come by way of the hard sciences available to modern medicine. That conclusion would be wrong. We criticize the philosophy-based practice of medicine by Benjamin Rush and other physicians of long ago because philosophy alone was incapable of producing solid answers to the physical causes of disease. Medical problems require a data-driven, experimental model to provide answers, and that model was not available to the physicians of that era. One may philosophize about the *reasons* that living things exist, but their behavior, molecular makeup, and physiology are better handled via the scientific method. If you want to discuss *life's meaning*, *morality*, or *love*, that is best handled through a philosophical discussion. Hard data and a well-designed scientific study would most likely fall flat with such topics. The truth is that philosophy undergirds the entire world of modern science and is the only method of answering many questions we raise in life. We believe there is ample evidence that there is more truth in the universe than a purely mechanistic or naturalistic view of reality provides. We know that Thomas Jefferson would probably disagree with us on that note, and that is fine with us. We wish he were still around to discuss it. We agree with the noted scientist, mathematician, and philosopher Blaise Pascal, who stated, "Reason's last step is the recognition that there are an infinite number of things which are beyond it. It is merely feeble if it does not go as far as to realize that."[6]

Meriwether Lewis had a great deal of interaction with Native Americans. Numerous journal entries by Lewis reflect his blatant racism and the sense of superiority that he felt toward many of the tribes. In our own writing, we sometimes refer to Native Americans as "Indians." In my (David's) writing and speaking career, I have had the honor of consulting with various tribal leaders who assured me that they were fine with the use of the word "Indian." We cannot speak for every Native American in this country, but it is definitely not our intent to be racist in our work. We do not take any responsibility for the historical terms and attitudes portrayed by members of the Corps of Discovery, nor do we engage in politically correct censorship of their writings.

Our work follows two parallel paths through this book. Some chapters address very specific topics that are medically or psychologically oriented, such as topics that some authors have cited as major factors in Lewis's health. Our other path involves a historical narrative that describes the world in which Lewis lived in order to, we hope, give a panoramic view of his life and times. We have appreciated the opportunities to consult with Jane Lewis Henley and Guy Meriwether Benson, descendants of the Lewis and Meriwether families, in our attempt to publish as historically accurate information about Lewis's genealogy as possible. In the chapters that by necessity address medical and mental health issues, we have made special efforts to express ourselves with as little "doctor talk" and "psychobabble" as possible while still covering the issues sufficiently. There is no escape from presenting these issues with a degree of content-specific information that some readers may find challenging. But, we are convinced that readers who make the effort to understand our presentation will finish our book with an informed and comprehensive view of the life and death of Meriwether Lewis.

We do not need to wait until the end of the book to note in all humility that we do not pretend to know the *absolute truth* of what happened to Lewis during the early-morning hours of October 11, 1809, although we believe the evidence overwhelmingly supports our opinions. We hope that, through the material presented, readers will examine their own conclusions about Lewis. Even if you finish this work and disagree with our conclusions, your view will at least be more complete and better informed. We fully realize that many people believe as they do concerning the death of Lewis based not on factual evidence but on what they wish had happened. These folks have their stories, and they are sticking to them. It is their right to do so.

Despite all the great adventures experienced, maps made of the virgin territory, Native American tribes who first had contact with White Americans, and the over three hundred new biological species discovered by Lewis and the Corps of Discovery during their journey across North America, the end of Captain Meriwether Lewis's life is an unhappy story. In our years of involvement with the amazing adventure of the Lewis and Clark Expedition, we have yet to meet a single individual who enjoys the sad narrative of the ending of Captain Lewis's life. Lewis was an accomplished naturalist; in some ways, he was an excellent commander of a small military group; and he was a hard-working governor, loyal friend, and, according to many reports, an honorable and trustworthy man. His personality contained both positive and negative traits, which is true of all of us. His ability to keep a cool head in the most dangerous circumstances suggests remarkable strength of character, but his anger and reactions to perceived slights to his sense of honor often worked against him. He deserves his reputation as an American legend of the highest order. He was the talented co-leader of a small army on an amazingly adventurous and dangerous trip of roughly eight thousand miles that in our opinion is, quite simply, the greatest story in American history.

The title of our book is taken from the words that witnesses reported Meriwether Lewis said while he lay dying from two reported gunshot wounds: "I am no coward; but I am so strong, [it is] so hard to die."[7] Whoever fired the fatal shots that ended the life of Meriwether Lewis, he deserved better. Nothing that occurred in his life after his return to civilization in September of 1806 can erase or even tarnish what he and the other expedition members accomplished. In our final judgment, this is what we choose to emphasize and remember as most important in our thoughts about Meriwether Lewis. We consider it a privilege to be able to contribute our ideas to this discussion.

Proceed On!

Drs. David and Marti Peck
July 2, 2021

Chapter 1

Life in Early America

When you think of the good old days, think one word: dentistry.
—P. J. O'Rourke

It seems likely that children in every generation hear their parents tell tales about the difficulties they had to overcome during their childhoods as the parents attempt to portray the rough-and-tumble world they endured growing up. These parental tales of woe have the hoped-for effect of instilling an appreciation for how soft children's lives are today. My father (Leonard Peck Sr.) told me about his boyhood chores, which included milking goats early in the morning in Santa Barbara, California. Marti and I both heard stories from our mothers about growing up on farms (in upstate New York and western Montana, respectively), getting up before the crack of dawn and doing chores before breakfast and then walking two miles to school in the snow in below-zero temperatures. These stories of our mothers were undoubtedly true, and I think the implication that their children had it relatively easy as kids in the America of the 1950s and '60s was equally true. Present-day parents now tell their kids that when they were young they only had three TV channels to watch that were free and they had to go out and play with their friends all day because they did not have any computer games to entertain them indoors. Children of the '50s and '60s had to attend public health events where we received polio immunization injections to ward off that potentially fatal infectious disease. If those hardships are not sufficient, when we were old enough to drive, we had to learn to drive with a manual transmission. How did we survive such hardships?

Much of this book is our attempt to not only comment on medical and psychological aspects of the life of Meriwether Lewis but to also give the reader a feel for what everyday life was like for most people in early America. Our topics vary widely, but all have the intended hope of putting the reader, at least for a few brief moments, into the world of early America.

For Meriwether Lewis's generation, and the generation of some of the key players in our story of the mid-eighteenth to early nineteenth centuries, the circumstances of their lives were greatly different and in many ways vastly more difficult than what many of us have experienced. For many Americans alive during the lifetime of Meriwether Lewis (August 18, 1774–October 11, 1809), life was filled with physical demands. Their daily lives often included back-breaking manual labor necessary to grow crops and raise animals with which to keep their families alive and healthy. The majority of Americans who lived outside of cities also hunted to augment their diet of plants and farm-raised animals. People arose early, often before dawn, in order to fix their breakfast, and then they spent hours in the fields tilling, planting, hoeing, weeding, watering, and warding off insects and other pests who tried to steal their crops. Without indoor plumbing, wells needed to be dug or nearby streams had to be tapped to provide water for cooking and occasional bathing. Our ancestors often worked until dusk or until they were so exhausted they could work no more. After the sun went down, they generally would eat something and go to sleep, only to get up again the next day and start the demanding routine all over again.

Threats to these early Americans came from a variety of sources. Infectious diseases were misunderstood by the medical community, and the treatments provided were more often than not either ineffective or outright dangerous. Any disease manifested by a fever might have been treated with a variety of injurious therapies, including but not limited to bleeding, purging, or poisonous medications such as mercury. As an example of another type of challenge encountered by early Americans, in 1778 my (David's) six-times-great-grandfather Patrick Magee signed a letter from his Pennsylvania militia unit in which he begged the American revolutionary government for more weapons and ammunition to provide for the defense of their lives from the local "Indians and Tories who are skulking in the mountains" around their community in Path Valley, Pennsylvania.

With numerous threats coming from both the biological and political worlds, life was quite different at the turn of the eighteenth century from the life of modern-day Americans. Modern cultural concepts such as equal rights for females were not part of early America. This cultural reality was expressed in numerous ways. Women could not vote or hold elected office. Any wealth obtained by a woman during Lewis's day was passed along to her husband after marriage. Following the death of Lewis's father when Lewis was five years old, he (not his mother) inherited the bulk of the estate, with his mother Lucy receiving only a small percentage of it. Many young women's entire education took place at home, with an emphasis on mastering the household duties of managing a budget, cooking, child care, and perhaps learning how to brew beer and distill ardent spirits.[1]

It was not uncommon during the early days of this country for men in their twenties and thirties to marry women in their mid-teens. One figure in our story, Sergeant Patrick Gass of the Corps of Discovery, was well into his sixties when he married a woman in her twenties. First cousins were considered appropriate marriage partners. Women were expected to have children and raise families. Unlike many contemporary unmarried women who pursue careers, a practice that most people today view as normal behavior, unmarried women in their late twenties were considered suspect in early American society. During the years 1721–1800, American teenagers between the ages of fifteen and nineteen married at twice the rate of women between twenty and twenty-nine.

A suitable marriage was initially often as much a business transaction as a romantic affiliation in early America. It was believed that love would follow the ceremony, even though love was not necessarily the reason for the marriage. Marriage often meant the difference between survival and death, wealth and poverty. If death took one's spouse, one might remarry within months, as did Lucy Meriwether Lewis, who reportedly remarried and became Lucy Marks within six months of the death of

Meriwether's father, William Lewis, in 1779. Marriages among the social elite, particularly in the South, were often under the direct influence of and perhaps were arranged by the parents of the brides and grooms.[2]

Most well-established American families raised their children in typically European ways. A well-provided-for gentleman's son would get a good early education in a private academy or with a private tutor and would prepare himself for university study in one of the three broad areas of respected higher education; medicine, theology, or the law. If there were a local school available, such as one run by James Waddell or the "atrabilious" Matthew Maury, both teachers of Meriwether Lewis, the son would be educated in the finer things of life. Some of the better private schools taught their students Latin and Greek. Latin was at that time the universal language of the learned and was often a requirement for admission to an American college. Such was the education of one of the key players in our story of the Lewis and Clark Expedition, Benjamin Rush (1745–1813), whose medical beliefs and treatments are an important part of the story of Lewis's death.[3]

A significant cultural aspect of the raising of boys in the southern colonies and states in the eighteenth and nineteenth centuries is illustrated by a story presented by historian Darren Stoloff. A young boy who was a member of the gentry in the South was discovered by his mother to have hacked a goose to death with his toy sword. When the boy's father witnessed the bloody mess, he asked about the incident. His young son replied that the gander had attacked and bitten him. Rather than scolding his son for killing the goose, the father praised the boy for defending his honor against the goose's insult.[4] Although this boy was not Meriwether Lewis, Lewis was undoubtedly raised in a similar southern family of means, as evidenced by his personality characteristic of being self-assertive and extremely sensitive to any perceived slights to his honor throughout his lifetime. We trace this common thread of his personality throughout this book.

Unmarried young girls needed to become good cooks for their future families as most women in early America spent hours laboring over an open fireplace to provide their families with a few pleasant moments spent eating together in an otherwise labor-intensive day. Apple pastries and gingerbread were among the favorite foods that were cooked for Christmas celebrations in early America. Other dishes appear in the historical record that might appeal to modern taste. A Harvard graduate of 1755, John Wentworth, the future governor of New Hampshire, wrote the recipe for his favorite Christmas dish of onion soup:

> Cut a plate full of thin slices of Bread, and sett them before ye fire to Crisp. Then cutt about half a Dozen of Middle Size Onions into bits, boyle half a pound of Butter Stiring it well till it be very red and have done frothing and then put ye Onions to it, and boyle them till they begin to turn Blackish, Still stiring of them, to this put about 2 quarts of water, and thicken it with 2 yolk of Eggs, then break ye Bread into small pieces and put it in with Some Spice & a little Salt, when it is ready pour in some Lemon Juce, or a Spoonfull or two of Vinegar if ye like it.[5]

Several of the favorite dishes of early Americans would be disgusting to many modern Americans' taste and culinary sensibility. John Adams loved calf hearts stuffed with chopped onions, green peppers, bread crumbs, celery, and bacon drippings. Betsy Ross preferred her "Bacon Liver Loaf," made of ground liver, bacon, onions, eggs, and bread crumbs. The liver and bacon were simmered in water, then mixed with the other items and baked for about forty minutes in a medium-hot oven. The boiling water was then poured over the loaf, and it was served immediately.[6]

William Clark's family favorite was "sour Cream biscuits," made with flour, salt, baking powder, baking soda, and sour cream.[7] And who can forget the evening when Lewis was unable to partake of his beloved elk marrowbone dinner because he was suffering a bout of intestinal troubles while camping by himself along the Missouri River, just a day's hike from the Great Falls of the Missouri River? We laugh out loud to imagine what Betsy Ross, John Adams, William Clark, or Meriwether Lewis might think of an In-N-Out burger, a taco, or guacamole and tortilla chips.

Many Protestant denominations underwent remarkable growth in the years of Meriwether Lewis's life, and during this period their belief in sex as permissible only within marriage became much stronger. Early American society was not influenced solely by pietistic Puritan sexuality; in fact, the premarital pregnancy rate in the latter half of the 1700s was about 30 percent.[8]

In addition to premarital sexual relations in early America, sexual relations between slave-owning masters and their female slaves were not uncommon. Slave women often became the sex toys of their masters. Thomas Jefferson, according to his biographer Jon Meacham, wrote to a friend in 1764, during his college days in Williamsburg, Virginia, and made an apparent reference to prostitution or sexual activity with enslaved women or with women in the servant class. Meacham's view is that Jefferson was discreetly challenging the topic of marriage as the only legitimate vehicle for the expression of one's sexuality when he wrote,

> Many and great are the comforts of a single state, and neither of the reasons you urge can have any influence with an inhabitant and a young inhabitant too of Williamsburg. For St. Paul only says that it is better to be married than to burn. Now I presume that if that apostle had known that providence would at an after day be so kind to any particular set of people as to furnish them with other means of extinguishing their fire than those of matrimony, he would have earnestly recommended them to their practice.[9]

Jefferson apparently was including himself, a slaveholder, within the "particular set of people" who were furnished with some other means of "extinguishing the fire" in nonmarital relations. Modern-day genetic analysis would support Jefferson's implication of himself as a participant in such behavior; genes from the Jefferson family are common among African American descendants of his slaves.

Many of the children born in early America lived past infancy, but infant mortality in early America was probably somewhere between 25 and 35 percent. A significant percentage of young people met an early death before they turned fifteen, the victims of numerous infectious diseases. Not only did these diseases lack effective treatments during this period, but the physicians who plied their trades had no idea what they were doing and more often than not killed the patient sooner than the disease would have. Mortality statistics for Sweden, Japan, West Indies, and Poland reveal that during this same period at least 50 percent of children died by the age of fifteen.[10] Meriwether Lewis lost a sister at an early age, and his father died when Meriwether was but five years old.

Many financially healthy early American families owned African American slaves or perhaps benefitted from the labor of a White indentured servant. The slaves, of course, had no say in their situation. An indentured servant paid for the right to come and work for a period of years for the sponsoring family, after which time they would be given their freedom to pursue their life as they saw fit. Both of these classes of people would have been considered culturally inferior to men such as Meriwether Lewis, a member of the land-holding gentry. There were winners and losers in the cultural hierarchy of early America, and baby Meriwether was declared a winner on the day he was born. American egalitarianism had its limits, even in those days.

As discussed in chapter 4, by the time many boys reached their adolescent years, they were familiar with the taste of hard alcohol. Its perceived health benefits were a "fact" that was accepted by nearly all members of society. By the time many young men were in their mid-teens, they were going with their father and uncles to a nearby tavern to enjoy a drink of hard liquor. Perhaps this tradition was considered early American male bonding at its best.

One of the most culturally fortunate people associated with the Lewis and Clark Expedition was Benjamin Rush (1745–1813). Young Benjamin showed great academic promise under the tutelage of his headmaster and uncle, Rev. Dr. Finley. Learning Greek and Latin, English, mathematics, and other classical subjects, in addition to an extensive amount of Christian (Presbyterian) training, Benjamin was well prepared to attend the Presbyterian-sponsored College of New Jersey (which later became Princeton), and he received his bachelor's degree at the age of fourteen in 1760. Rush, as did most American physicians-in-training at that time, prepared for his practice by serving a six-year apprenticeship with an established physician, who in Rush's case was the Philadelphia physician Dr. John Redmond. Rush, sensing the need for more formal medical education after his six years of practical training, enrolled in the University of Edinburgh in Scotland to finish his formal medical studies.

Modern physicians find it simply incredible that most young doctors of the late eighteenth and early nineteenth centuries, when they began their practice, lacked any experience whatsoever in clinical medicine—interaction with a real patient. In contrast, physicians today spend years in supervised clinical patient care, beginning in their first year of medical school. At Oxford and Cambridge Universities in Rush's time, one became a physician by reading books and discussing the medical theories popular during that period and perhaps attending a human body dissection. Edinburgh's medical program had the great advantage of maintaining an associated hospital where students could see living (and deceased) patients and attend lectures about the patients and their diseases. The fact that Edinburgh had clinical facilities was only valuable in theory, however, as the actual value of such clinical education was nearly worthless since the teaching professors held many erroneous beliefs concerning the causes of diseases. Students in Edinburgh were allowed to choose their own course of medical study from the following classes: Logic, Moral Philosophy, Institutes of Medicine, Anatomy, Midwifery, Materia Medica, and Chemistry.[11] Some class lectures were conducted in Latin, the language of the learned in those times. Once a physician became established in his practice, he might receive large payments for consultations from a distance. This could be accomplished (if he were sufficiently famous) via mail with a colleague in another city, discussing the patient without the need or the bother of ever seeing, talking to, or examining the patient.

The living conditions in Edinburgh were probably not remarkably different than those in American cities of that same era. When Rush arrived for his studies in Scotland in 1766, he was in for a rude awakening about at least one aspect of Edinburgh culture. Lest we take our modern sanitation for granted, we should note that before indoor plumbing, human waste was collected in bowls and emptied outside the house on the city streets at night. In Edinburgh, if a family lived on a second floor, it was routine for them to take the bowls full of human waste collected during the day and throw the contents down to the street below. These Scottish folks, at least the more polite ones, warned anyone down below with a shouted "Gardy loo!" If one were unlucky enough to be beneath this promised foul downpour, the response of "Haud yer haun" might get the person above to hold back their bowl for a few seconds. In a letter home, Rush noted that he had escaped one such shower but that "my unfortunate friend Potts had gained the honour before me."[12]

Rush finished his course of professional study and returned to Philadelphia in 1769 as one of America's best-trained doctors. He also entered into the American Revolutionary scene and signed the Declaration of Independence in 1776. By 1803, his professional standing would be near its zenith. Jefferson wrote to Rush and asked him to become Meriwether Lewis's medical tutor in 1803.

In rural areas, sewage was the source of many of the pathogenic bacteria and viruses that cause many human diseases, including various types of dysentery (caused by the bacteria *Salmonella, E. coli, Campylobacter,* and *Shigella* and by viruses such as rotavirus, Norwalk virus, and poliovirus). The sewage was often sent either into local streams or into cesspools that leaked into groundwater and potentially into wells supplying drinking water. In urban areas, city sewers and storm drains carried much human waste as recently as the early 1800s. Sewage-polluted river water, which served as drinking water for the public, continued to cause serious human disease for Americans for decades to come. Philadelphia's pollution via sewage of the Schuylkill River laid the foundation for a deadly typhoid epidemic as late as the 1880s. It was not until a series of steam-powered pumping stations were finished in 1812 that water was pumped from the Schuylkill River to a conduit that delivered water to the center city via hollowed-out wooden logs. Hydrants were located along the distribution system, and people could get water for free if they carried it away. In the late nineteenth century, the concept that invisible small microbes in the drinking water, food supply, and environment could cause disease, promoted by legendary men of medical science such as Louis Pasteur (France), Joseph Lister (England), and Robert Koch (Germany), became accepted thinking. Filtration, boiling, or chlorination to kill these microscopic pathogens allowed for a safe drinking water supply in major cities by around 1907.

A young American man who was privileged enough to become a college student during the late eighteenth century would likely attend one of the well-known centers of higher learning such as Harvard (founded in 1636), the College of William and Mary (1693), St. John's (1696), Yale (1701), the University of Pennsylvania (founded in 1740 as the College of Philadelphia), or Princeton (1746). If the young man had a family that would be leaving him a sizable amount of land and property, he needed to receive an informal and practical education that would cover the management of every aspect of the plantation or farm—planting crops and caring for animals, selling products, and managing the slaves or other laborers.

The two main population centers of the early nation in 1790 were New York City (population 60,514) and Philadelphia (41,220). In 1790, the year that Lewis started his studies in Virginia, Virginia was the most populous state with 692,000 citizens. New York came in a distant fifth with 340,000 citizens. Immigrants from across the Atlantic continued to stream into America in the post-American Revolution years. The possibility of becoming a landowner with the right to vote for one's political leadership was a new opportunity for many coming from European countries.

When Lewis rode into Philadelphia in 1803 as an unknown explorer-in-waiting, the city's population was around sixty-three thousand. When he returned to Philadelphia in 1807 as the conqueror of the West and co-commander of the Corps of Discovery, Philadelphia had grown to over sixty-seven thousand residents and the bridges to Trenton, New Jersey, and over the Schuylkill had been completed.[13] Its streets were paved with cobblestones and, according to a writer in *The Port Folio*, were

> bordered with ample footways, raised one foot above the carriageway, for the ease and safety of passengers. They are kept cleaner than those of any city in Europe, excepting the towns of Holland. . . . London is the only capital in the world that is better lighted at night. Many of the New Streets have been latterly planted with Poplars. . . . Their introduction has already given to some sections the air of Public Walks, for ornament of which nothing is wanting but Fountains and Statuary.[14]

When Lewis arrived in Philadelphia in 1803, the first medical school at the University of Pennsylvania was already well established and had a forty-year history of producing American physicians. The leading Penn professors were products of the medical training at the University of Edinburgh. Medical students at the College of Philadelphia (it was renamed the University of Pennsylvania in 1791) could earn either a bachelor's or doctor's degree in medicine. The first M.D. degrees were granted in 1771. Prior to graduation, a student had to

a. attend at least one course of lectures in the following subjects: anatomy, materia medica, chemistry, and the theory and practice of physick (the art of healing, or medicine);
b. attend one course of clinical lectures;
c. attend the practice of the Pennsylvania Hospital for one year;
d. be examined privately by medical trustees and professors and other trustees and professors who wished to attend; and
e. be examined publicly.

The young man (no young women were allowed) had to be at least twenty-four years of age and have a knowledge of Latin, mathematics, and relevant areas of natural philosophy (physics, chemistry, biology).[15]

Today, attending the theater and viewing a play is a popular form of entertainment. This was not uniformly true during America's colonial period and early nationhood. Theater troupes who performed a number of Shakespeare's plays in Williamsburg were warmly greeted but met significant opposition in 1753 in New York and also faced Quaker-led opposition in Philadelphia. Historian Louis B. Wright noted, "To convince doubting New Yorkers that drama was not harmful, they [the Hallam company] opened with the highly moralized play by Richard Steele, *The Conscious Lovers*." Steele was a playwright "whose reputation for good morality was so great that any work of [his] would take the taint off theatrical entertainment and lull the audience into accepting less-edifying plays."[16] Another theater troop gained acceptance for productions in Newport, Rhode Island, in 1761 by presenting a letter of support from the governor of Virginia declaring that the actors behaved "with prudence and discretion" and were "capable of entertaining a sensible and polite audience."[17]

The rapidity of modern-day communications and travel, when we can use our cell phones to "FaceTime" with our foreign-based friends and relatives and can fly around the world in one day, represents the most remarkable difference between our culture and that of the era of Meriwether Lewis. As Stephen Ambrose noted in *Undaunted Courage*, nothing moved faster than a horse or a boat on a river in the world of Lewis.[18] Many of our ancestors put their lives at risk by spending six to eight weeks crossing the Atlantic to immigrate to the United States. At best, that perilous trip would take a month. During this period, a letter mailed in Philadelphia and sent to Boston took six days, with even longer delivery times for letters headed into the southern and western areas of the new nation. Meriwether Lewis's letter asking William Clark to co-command the expedition took a month to reach Clark.[19]

Native American populations, who had not been exposed to White populations and their endemic diseases, paid a terrible price for their communication with White Europeans. The Native American population began to suffer devastating mortality from the European-introduced smallpox virus in the 1770s along the northwest coast of what is now the United States. Repeated smallpox epidemics also decimated many tribes along the future path of the Corps of Discovery on the Missouri River, often wiping out entire villages.[20]

Many of the tribes that battled these diseases also battled with one another. Various Native American political and military factions formed during the decades prior to the arrival of Europeans. The Sioux and the Arikara became allies and, farther north, the Mandan and the Hidatsa did the same to defend themselves against each other during the 1780s and 1790s. Farther west, the Blackfeet dominated the eastern edge of the Rocky Mountains into Canada with help from horses obtained from the Spanish and, somewhat later, modern firearms obtained from other European traders based in present-day Canada. The Teton Sioux exerted control over the middle Missouri and muscled their way to the top of American Indian politics on the Missouri River in the late eighteenth and early nineteenth centuries.[21]

During Lewis's lifetime, America underwent a myriad of changes, with some important historical landmarks occurring in Europe as well. When Lewis turned seventeen and was living the life of a young member of the gentry in Albemarle County, Virginia, the still-young Wolfgang Mozart died in 1791 at the age of thirty-five, the victim of an infectious disease referred to in history as "severe military fever." Some modern medical commentators believe his death was the result of kidney failure brought on by a streptococcal infection.[22]

In 1790, the population of the United States was remarkably young, and the young nation showed many characteristics of its youthful makeup. The median age in the nation was only sixteen, and the life expectancy at birth was about forty-four years. The average man was 5'8" tall. Over 80 percent of the population had an English, Irish, or Scots-Irish background.[23]

During Lewis's teenage years, the young nation was rife with political turmoil. Contentious disagreements about the nature and extent of the national government played out in both houses of Congress as well as the press. Disagreements between the Federalists, whose ideas of government primarily echoed the country's previous English-based ideals, were forcefully opposed by Jefferson and his support of the common person and the disillusionment with any influence of English-based government and many of the old world's aristocracy-based class distinctions. In spite of these remarkable differences in philosophy, the young nation adopted the U.S. Constitution in 1787, with George Washington serving two terms and firmly establishing the authority of the federal government. Washington, without concern for varying political opinions, appointed Jefferson, a political rival, as his secretary of state in 1790.

With frequent wars occurring between France and England during the following twenty-plus years, American presidents, from Washington, Adams, and Jefferson to Madison, attempted with varying degrees of success to avoid entangling America in these conflicts. Sometimes their legislative attempts to accomplish U.S. neutrality resulted in hostility from both France and Great Britain directed at American shipping in the Mediterranean and Atlantic.

The French Revolution, during its reign of terror in 1793–94, not only overthrew the French monarchy and the Catholic clerical authority of France but was also responsible for murdering seventeen thousand French citizens.[24] This bloodbath occurred when Lewis was a budding young plantation owner in Virginia.

In the year before Jefferson's election to the presidency in 1800, while Lewis was serving in western Pennsylvania in the U.S. Army, Napoleon Bonaparte seized political power in France in a coup d'état, crowning himself emperor in 1804. He exercised his arrogance and love of military conquest for the next decade and was responsible for the deaths of thousands across both Europe and Asia.

Napoleon's military fortunes were thwarted on October 21, 1805, when his French and Spanish forces lost the pivotal naval Battle of Trafalgar, which ended his plans to invade Britain. Napoleon lost that battle on the same day that Meriwether Lewis and the Corps of Discovery were unable to find enough wood to cook their breakfast and endured a cold, windy morning while descending the Columbia River. That night, they ate boiled dogs and fish purchased from the local tribes.

The reality of Napoleon's unenlightened persona created conflicts with Jefferson's idealistic view of human nature and his support of the French revolution and its ideals of personal liberty, equality, and fraternity as well as his profound dislike of the English government and its sociocultural structure. Although he did not support Napoleon's warlike acts, Jefferson was hardly one to take sides with Napoleon's enemy, England. After the Battle of Trafalgar, continued British-French conflict that threatened America's shipping industry led to the passage by America of the Non-Importation Act in April 1806, when Lewis and the Corps were making their way eastward up the western slopes of the Rockies. The result of this ill-advised law was a disaster for American shipping and greatly angered the British government, leading to armed conflicts between the British and American navies that culminated in the British HMS *Leopard* searching American ships for deserters just offshore of Norfolk, Virginia, and the subsequent hanging of an American seaman. According to historian Paul Johnson, "[N]either he [Jefferson] nor Madison knew how to steer the United States through the troubled waters of the Napoleonic Wars. The truth is, they were emotionally involved, a fatal propensity in geopolitics."[25] Americans viewed this act, justifiably, as an international outrage. Many were in favor of war with Britain. Jefferson's anti-British sentiments did not allow him to pursue a diplomatic solution with England's constitutional monarchy, which might have ended the ongoing controversy.

In 1807, with Lewis basking in his fame during his return tour of America, the European war led Jefferson to push through the Embargo Act, which prohibited U.S. ships from sailing for foreign ports. This resulted in great economic hardship for American shipping interests and accusations that "the American government was being run in the interest of the 'Virginia Dynasty' and its slave-owning planters by a pack of pro-French ultra-republican ideologues."[26] Letters of condemnation poured into Washington, leading to Congress passing the Non-Intercourse Act in 1809, effectively ending the previous legislative nightmare. But during some of the darkest days of Meriwether Lewis's life, in the spring of 1809, Jefferson, "who had been an optimist up to the turn of the century, was now gloomy, shaken and demoralized . . . and left office a beaten man."[27] Lewis's inability to finish his journals of the expedition may have been but one of the discouragements affecting Jefferson at this time.

Shortly after the triumphant return of the Corps of Discovery to civilization in 1806, and in the midst of Lewis's post-expedition glory, Jefferson "rewarded" Lewis with an appointment as the governor of Upper Louisiana Territory. This appointment and Lewis's acceptance would ultimately spell disaster for the young hero. It would seem that, once again, Jefferson's idealism had blinded him to the realities of how such a demanding appointment would affect the life of his young protégé, who still had his expedition's journals to complete. Clay Jenkinson, in *The Character of Meriwether Lewis*, is more understanding in his assessment of this act of Jefferson. Jenkinson writes that "Jefferson believed that Lewis would have no trouble finding time to engage in his literary pursuits and serve as a frontier governor. Jefferson could not have foreseen that Lewis would be a disastrous governor."[28] That may be true in part as the ultimate performance of anyone cannot be known before it occurs, but what Jefferson should have been able to foresee was that the job he gave Lewis placed a significant demand on his time. We agree more with Stephen Ambrose, who commented that the appointment represented a "big mistake, easily seen and easily avoidable."[29]

Thomas Jefferson, despite all of his abilities, interests, and profoundly great contributions to America, seemed at times to be naive about a number of issues. His judgment on several occasions reflected his Enlightenment philosophy of believing the very best of human nature. At times, Jefferson displayed behaviors that leave us and many others mystified at his lack of consistency and apparent lack of wisdom. His instructions and his poor knowledge of existing Indian political structure gave Lewis and Clark the impossible task of convincing native tribes such as the Lakota Sioux that they should be at peace with their neighbors and obey the new "great father" of the seventeen "great nations" back in Washington, D.C. Some Jefferson supporters might justly push the argument that it is easy for modern-day people to realize this more than two hundred years later, after reading excellent books such as James Ronda's *Lewis and Clark among the Indians* that help us understand the political and social situation along the middle Missouri River in the early nineteenth century. We, however, would counter that

Jefferson knew about the warlike behavior of the Teton Sioux and their desire to control the middle Missouri River area. He should have realized it was unlikely that these Native Americans would want to become his idealized yeoman farmers and cooperate in any way with the new American government. Some historians have noted Jefferson's dismay at the warlike behavior of Napoleon during the many wars he perpetrated on Europe during the opening years of the nineteenth century, which led to his administration's passage of the Embargo Act and other ill-fated legislation that profoundly failed to address the targeted problems in Europe and instead damaged American commerce. Again, Jefferson seems to have been naive in his overly benevolent assessment of human nature, the result of his personality and his wholesale buy-in to aspects of Enlightenment philosophy.

During the spring of 1809, the political disaster that was to encompass Lewis began with the election and ascent to power of James Madison as the fourth president of the United States. Madison's effectiveness as president is, not surprisingly, controversial. Some historians have noted that in spite of his sharp mind and grasp of politics, his abilities in writing and political theory in many ways did not translate into effective political leadership. Historian Paul Johnson, notes that as bad as things were at the end of Jefferson's presidency, "[W]orse was yet to come." Madison "proved a classic illustration of Tacitus' maxim 'omnium consensu capax imperii nisi imperasset ["universally seen as capable of ruling, had he never ruled"]. He was no good."[30] Certainly, his appointment of some members of his cabinet, specifically William Eustis as secretary of war, would prove to be a disaster for Lewis. Both Jefferson and Madison were spectacularly gifted political theorists and writers whose practical leadership abilities seemed to lag behind their remarkable gifts.

England's King George III, under whose reign the young Lewis grew up and came to manhood, continued to rule over England until 1810, the year after Lewis's death. King George's health was beginning to fail him when Lewis assumed his duties as Jefferson's secretary, and this continued into the years of the journey of the Corps of Discovery. King George's last decade of life was characterized by a slide into mental illness and loss of health, perhaps as the result of porphyria (a group of illnesses caused by liver dysfunction), which in the early nineteenth century was an unknown and therefore untreatable disease.

Following the revolutions in both America and France, former slaves declared the island of Haiti an independent republic in 1804. This temporary mood of human freedom from slavery in Haiti quickly devolved, in the few months prior to Lewis's departure on the expedition, to genocide against several thousand White and Creole French still living in Haiti. In 1806, the leader of Haiti's revolution and self-declared emperor, Jean-Jacques Dessalines, was murdered by his generals and hacked to pieces by machetes.[31] It seems that the self-proclaimed status of emperor of both Napoleon and Dessalines did not work out well for them.

While Meriwether Lewis was enjoying his first year of U.S. Army life as an officer, as well as the "mountains of beef and oceans of whiskey"[32] supplied by the U.S. government, far across the Atlantic Ocean the young Ludwig van Beethoven gave his first public performance in Vienna, at which he played one of his first piano concertos. Ten years later, as Lewis prepared to depart with the Corps of Discovery from its winter camp at Wood River, Beethoven, in disgust and anger, scratched out the dedication to Napoleon on his third symphony (*Eroica*) after hearing the news of Napoleon proclaiming himself emperor of France. With words born from the Enlightenment, Beethoven said, "So he is no more than a common mortal! Now he, too, will tread underfoot all the rights of man [and] indulge only his ambition; now he will think himself superior to all men [and] become a tyrant!"[33]

Rapid industrialization was beginning to occur in the young United States in the last decade of the eighteenth century. Processing cotton became much faster with the invention of the cotton gin by Eli Whitney in 1794. In 1807, the first steamship puffed its way up the Hudson River. Scientific progress and the useful knowledge supplied by practical machines were rapidly increasing.

By the time Lewis was born in 1774, the world of science, particularly in the fields of math and physics, had made spectacular advances courtesy of such men as Galileo, Kepler, Descartes, Pascal, Leibniz, and Newton. Newton's theory of gravitation had been established, although it was not entirely accepted as its explanation of unseen forces acting through millions of miles of empty space violated the human reason so revered by some Enlightenment figures. Modern chemistry had advanced with the discovery of various elements (oxygen in 1774, hydrogen in 1766) during the last decades of the 1700s. Various chemical reactions had been under investigation for hundreds of years through the work of a worldwide network of alchemists. The spectacularly talented French chemist Antoine Lavoisier discovered important chemical reactions, such as oxygen's important role in combustion as well as within the human body. His genius was rewarded by the revolutionary French government with a trip to the guillotine in 1794. Lavoisier, during the French monarchy, had been involved in tax collection, which infuriated the radical French revolutionaries. He was sent to the guillotine on May 8, 1794, for "conspiracy against the people of France." The following day, the French mathematician Joseph Lagrange sadly summed up the tragedy of his execution by stating, "[I]t took them only an instant to cut off that head, and a hundred years may not produce another like it."[34] Modern-day chemical theory took a giant leap forward with John Dalton's introduction in the first decade of the nineteenth century of various modern chemical principles.

The world of biology lacked any understanding of cell theory or biochemistry. Its study revolved chiefly around the collection of biological specimens in museums and the classification of new species discovered by naturalists such as Meriwether Lewis and Thomas Jefferson, who were talented and active naturalists. Medicine, which suffered from the poor understanding of biological and chemical processes, in 1806 was a pathetic combination of philosophical logic and false beliefs about the human body. Perhaps the most amazing thing about this medical framework is that many patients did get well in spite of the treatment they received.

Lewis lived in a time filled with significant changes in nearly every area of American life as well as significant changes in the culture of much of Europe. The manner in which the "old world" operated with the authority of kings and queens, the influence of the Catholic church, and the presence of aristocratic social distinctions were slowly losing ground in Europe and had already been overturned in the young United States of America.

In the next two chapters, we examine in more detail some of the cultural circumstances that directly and profoundly influenced Lewis's life. Through the lenses of culture and philosophy, we hope to increase readers' appreciation of Lewis and his times and provide a focused view of Lewis's life and the world in which he lived.

Chapter 2

Family Background and Biography of Meriwether Lewis

*In all of us there is a hunger, marrow-deep, to know our heritage—
to know who we are and where we have come from.*
—Alex Haley

Although the day we are born is the first day of our life, both our unique existence and our individuality are the products of the generations of our family that preceded us back to the dawn of human history. The 20,000–25,000 genes each of us has on our forty-six chromosomes, each coding for a specific protein, are ultimately responsible for our physical appearance and, to a significant degree, our health and behavior. Today, commercial DNA testing companies enable people to trace their ancestry and identify the regional and ethnic sources of their DNA. For many, this is a fascinating pastime. If you do not share this interest quite so strongly, you may want to skip over the details of Meriwether Lewis's genealogy that we provide in this chapter.

Our parents influence our lives, and our parents themselves have ancestors whose lives influenced them. This was true as well for Meriwether Lewis, born on August 18, 1774, at Locust Hill Plantation, in Albemarle County, Virginia. The context of his birth was colonial America at the beginning of the Revolutionary War.

One challenge in writing about the life of this famed co-captain of the Lewis and Clark Expedition is that a number of biographies have already been written about this noteworthy figure in America's history. Some reading this book may have read many accounts of Lewis's life and are familiar with the details; others may know very little or nothing about him. In an attempt to address both audiences and everyone in between, we summarize in this chapter what others have written as well as add new information not previously published.

Meriwether Lewis was never married, nor is he reported to have had any children. He does have indirect descendants through his sister Jane Lewis Anderson and his uncle Francis Meriwether. We feel privileged to have been able to consult with three descendants of Jane and Francis to help ensure the accuracy of the information in this chapter: Jane Lewis Henley (Meriwether's four-times-great-grandniece), her brother Andy Sale (Meriwether's four-times-great-grandnephew), and Guy Meriwether Benson (Meriwether's first cousin, five times removed, through Lewis's uncle Francis Meriwether).

Lewis Family Lineage

The privileged social position enjoyed by Meriwether Lewis becomes clear with a review of his distinguished ancestry. Previous biographies of Lewis describe his ancestors as originating in Wales and England. Of significant note, his paternal ancestors have been reliably traced back as far as 1548 to the birth of Sir Edmund Lewis, who married Lady Anne (born 1552), daughter of the Earl of Dorset in Brecon, Wales.

Genealogical researchers disagree over whether Robert Lewis (1605–55) was the first individual from the Lewis family to immigrate to the colony of Virginia in 1635, as historian Steven Ambrose reported.[1] Some Lewis family members believe that a different Lewis family member, John "the Immigrant" Lewis (1592–1657), was actually the first family member to arrive in the colonies, and that he came from Monmouthshire, England.[2] Monmouthshire is today a county located in the southeastern region of Wales, but this region was very close to the border of England, and boundary disputes sometimes placed this area in

Wales and sometimes in England. This explains why Monmouthshire is referred to as in Wales or England, depending on the date and context.

One source of the difficulty in correctly identifying who the first Lewis immigrant was to emigrate from Wales stems from the fact that so many of Meriwether Lewis's ancestors were named either Robert or John because of the tradition of parents naming their children after their parents and grandparents. Thus, it can be challenging to know which John or Robert is being referred to when tracing the ancestral lines. The many intermarriages among the most prominent landholding families in Virginia from 1650–1850 also complicate the story, including the Warner, Washington, Jefferson, Meriwether, and Lewis families. Even within families, it was not uncommon for first or second cousins to marry. In addition, due to the occasional early deaths of spouses, it was also not uncommon for one spouse to remarry two, three, or even four times after their partner met an early death due to illness or accident.[3]

Both the Meriwether and Lewis families emigrated from England and Wales and arrived in Virginia well after the founding of Jamestown. They received large land grants—these families were among the most land-rich families in early colonial Virginia—that they passed down to their descendants. Meriwether Lewis was preceded by several generations on both sides of his family who lived in the colony of Virginia (see figure 1). According to Arend Flick, most historians would dispute Ambrose's claim that Robert Lewis arrived with a land grant from the British king for 33,333 1/3 acres. Flick notes that Ambrose's position was based on an essay titled "The Colonial Childhood of Meriwether Lewis," which he stated "is replete with errors."[4]

Concerning the question of who can be most reliably identified as the first Lewis family immigrant to the Virginia colony, Lewis's four-times-great-grandniece Jane Lewis Sale Henley believes that John Lewis of Monmouthshire, England, was the first immigrant and is the ancestor through whom current descendants can most reliably trace their relation to Meriwether Lewis.[5] Henley wrote to us,

> In 1948 a grave of John Lewis of Monmouthshire, England, appeared in what was then New Kent County. My family's book *Lewises, Meriwethers, and Their Kin,* by my great-grandmother, was published in the early 1930s before his grave was found. It

names Robert Lewis as the first Lewis emigrant. The evidence that John is the emigrant of our line seems stronger. The book *The Meriwethers and Their Connections*, by Heath Meriwether, and updated by his son, in 1964 and 1991 have provided new information. I am inclined to go with the John Lewis information because . . . the grave of his wife Isabelle is also found. She is the connection to the Warner family. . . . [W]hen folks tell me they have Lewis family members, I say that if they can trace back their lineage to the 'Warner Hall' Lewises, they are indeed kin to Meriwether Lewis.[6]

On another topic related to these complicated family dynamics, Henley reported:

Robert, grandfather of Meriwether, was born there [Warner Hall]. He then married Jane Meriwether, eldest daughter of Nicholas Meriwether II, and moved to Albemarle County onto the Nicholas Meriwether Grant which was divided into twelve parcels. . . . Robert was the first to take up land within this grant. In the unusual circumstances of those years of family intermarriages, when Robert's first wife died in 1765, he married Lucy Meriwether's mother. So Lucy and William may have lived in the same household for a period of time, although William was much older than Lucy.[7]

In April 2017, we visited Warner Hall in Gloucester County, Virginia, with Jane Lewis Henley, who explained to us the fascinating history of this site and elaborated on the background of some of its inhabitants. This estate has been completely renovated and now operates as a very elegant bed-and-breakfast establishment. Across a grassy field from the house lies a wrought-iron-gated cemetery that contains thirteen large, flat, rectangular gravestones, including those of Col. Augustine Warner (1611–74), who founded the plantation in 1642, and his wife, Mary Towneley (1614–62); they were great-great-grandparents of George Washington (1732–99). Their son, Augustine II (1642–81), married Mildred Reade Warner (1641?–94), whose grave also rests in this cemetery. Around 1690, their daughter Elizabeth (1672–1720) married John "the Councilor" Lewis (1669–1725), thus uniting these two prominent families of early Virginia. John and Elizabeth are the great-grandparents of Meriwether Lewis and are also buried in this graveyard. Elizabeth and John had fourteen children, one of whom was Robert Lewis "of Belvoir" (Meriwether Lewis's grandfather).

The inscription on Elizabeth's gravestone reads:

Here Lyeth Interr'd ye Body of Elizabeth Lewis the daughter of Col Augustine Warner and Mildred his wife and late wife of John Lewis Esq. She was born at Chesake [Chesapeake, Virginia] the 24th of November 1672. Aged 47 years 2 Months and 12 Days, and was a tender Mother of 14 Children. She Departed this Life the 5th Day of February 1719/20.

The grave of Elizabeth's husband John is situated beside hers, and its inscription reads:

Here Lyeth Interred the Body of Collo John Lewis son of John and Isabella Lewis, and one of his Majestys Honble Council for this colony who was born ye 30th of November 1669 and departed this Life on ye 14th of November 1725.

This information definitively places the ancestry of Meriwether Lewis with the "Warner Hall Lewises." It has been well documented that John "the Councilor" and his wife Elizabeth Warner, buried in this cemetery at Warner Hall, were the parents of Lewis's grandfather, Col. Robert "of Belvoir" Lewis, whose son William Lewis married Lewis's mother Lucy Meriwether. Thus, we can be certain that Lewis's ancestry in Virginia can be traced back to his great-great-grandparents, Major John Lewis and Isabella Miller, whose graves were identified in 1948 in New Kent County (now King and Queen County), Virginia.

Col. Robert Lewis's first marriage to Jane Meriwether is the first point of convergence of the Lewis and Meriwether families. Their son William was Meriwether Lewis's father. William married a grandniece of his mother, Lucy Meriwether. William and Lucy Lewis lived on the 1,896-acre portion of his father's land grant in Albemarle County that William inherited in 1757, which became known as Locust Hill plantation. This was the birthplace of Meriwether Lewis in 1774.

Meriwether Family Lineage

Nicholas Meriwether (1631–78) immigrated to Virginia from Norfolk, England, and by 1730 King George II had granted his son, Nicholas Meriwether II (1665–1744; Meriwether Lewis's maternal great-great-grandfather) two land patents totaling nearly 18,000 acres in Albemarle County, Virginia, near Charlottesville. This combined grant was divided into twelve parcels.

Nicholas II and his wife Elizabeth Crawford Meriwether had nine children. Their oldest daughter, Jane Meriwether (1705–53), married Robert "of Belvoir" Lewis (1702–65); these were the grandparents of Meriwether Lewis. Nicholas Meriwether II gave his daughter Jane and son-in-law Robert a parcel from his grant that was named Cloverfields, and this became the Meriwether family's ancestral home.[8] Meriwether Lewis's mother Lucy (1752–1837), was the fifth generation of Meriwethers to live in colonial Virginia (see figure 1).

One of the fascinating aspects of the lineage of Meriwether Lewis's mother Lucy is that her great-aunt Jane (1705–57) was married to her future father-in-law, Robert Lewis. This resulted from her great-aunt Jane's death in 1757 and her husband Robert marrying his late wife's niece (see figure 1). In other words, the intermarriages that took place between the Lewis and Meriwether families resulted in Lucy Meriwether's father-in-law becoming her stepfather and her mother, once she married Robert Lewis in 1761, becoming her stepmother-in-law. Another interesting relationship was that between Lewis's parents. William and Lucy were first cousins once removed, but they also became step-siblings following the marriage of Robert "of Belvoir" and Elizabeth Thornton, which took place when Lucy (Lewis's mother), was nine years old.

Many aspects of this story reflect the great cultural differences between colonial America and today. At the time of the marriage of Meriwether Lewis's parents, his father William was thirty-four years old and Lucy was sixteen. It was not uncommon in that era for there to be such a large age difference between marital partners (we revisit this cultural practice during our discussion of the adulthood of both Lewis and Clark). Their firstborn child was a daughter born about two years after their marriage, whom they named Jane (1770–1844), followed by a second daughter, Lucinda, in 1772, who died as an infant. Meriwether was born in 1774; his brother Reuben (1777–1844) was the last child from their union.

The Importance of Class

It is important to note that when the ancestors of Meriwether Lewis arrived in Virginia, they were members of a high socioeconomic class and were granted patents of land that they later added to and developed. Arend Flick has proposed that it is possible that the Lewis family came from the merchant class and had some wealth but were not titled nobility.[9] They were likely considered among the most affluent families in their area of colonial America, and they served in high political positions within the government as well as officers in the military. They were people of ambition, befitting the mottos of both the Lewis family's coat of arms, which can be translated as "Everything the Brave Man Does Is for His Country," and of the Meriwether family's coat of arms, "Force and Counsel."[10] In essence, certain elements of Lewis's personality were no doubt acquired through the role models and the culture in which he grew up, characterized by male authority figures who exhibited a strong sense of duty to their country and immense pride in both their families and their landholdings. Members of this family would have believed themselves to be special and worthy of respect. These principles, when fused with the cultural phenomenon of young southern male gentry being raised to be both assertive and cognizant of their sense of honor, would yield a personality such as that of Meriwether Lewis (see chapter 10).

What were the activities in which some of Meriwether's ancestors participated that contributed to their sense of being elite? Besides being a significant landowner and enjoying the social status of such a position, Meriwether Lewis's grandfather Robert (of Warner Hall) served as a representative in the Virginia House of Burgesses. His paternal uncle Charles served as a captain of the Minutemen in one of the first regiments of Virginia when the Revolutionary War began, and he died while guarding British prisoners in 1779, having achieved the rank of colonel. And his father, William Lewis, served as a patriot during the Revolutionary War (family narratives passed down through the generations have identified him as possessing the rank of a lieutenant; official

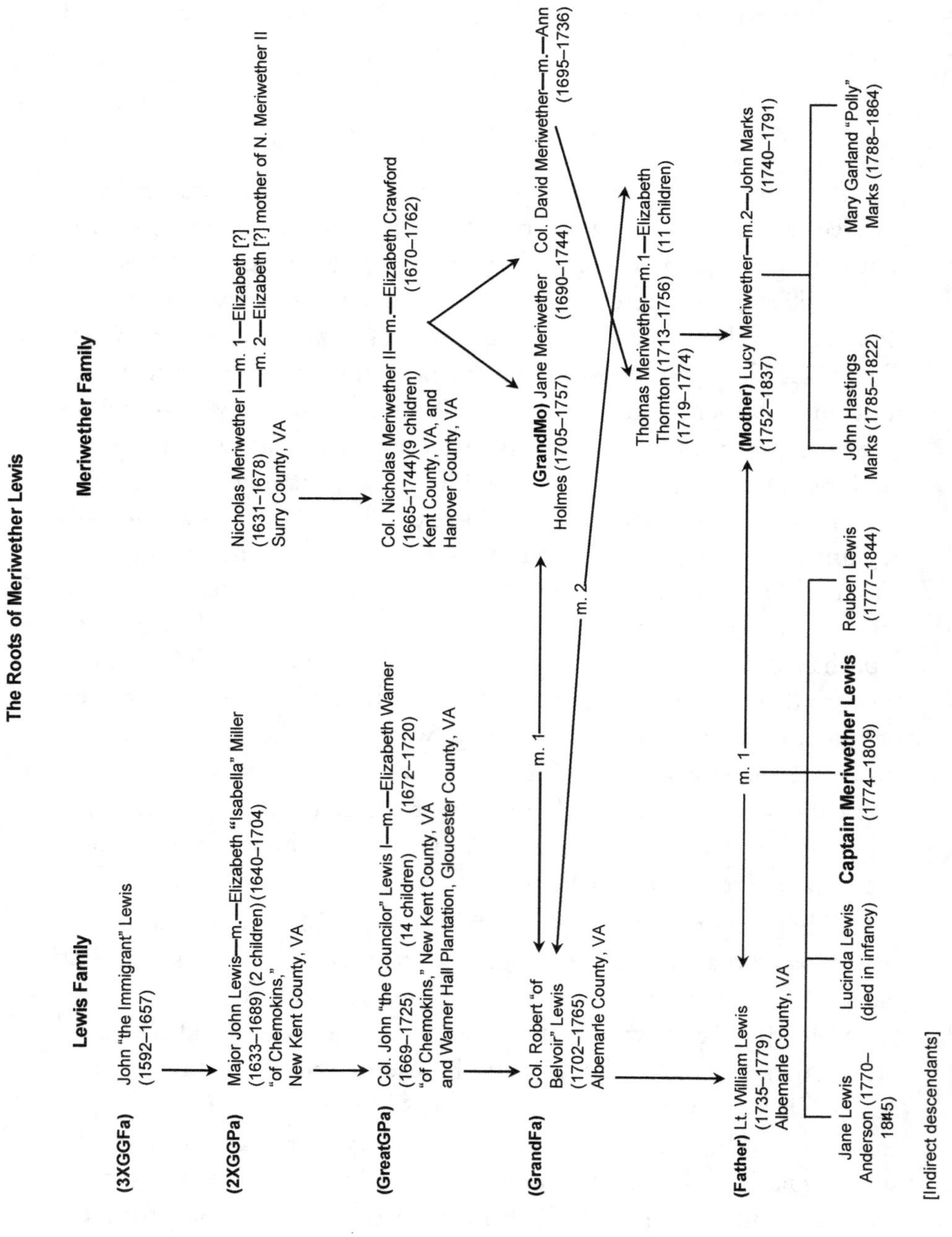

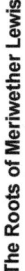

Figure 1. Family tree of Meriwether Lewis. Note that some birth and death dates are best approximations (prepared by Marti E. Peck).

documentation of this has yet to be discovered, but documentation does exist that William did serve as a private in the Albemarle militia in the period 1775–76).[11]

Meriwether Lewis lived in the same region as the most influential founding members of the United States, and knew that some of these people were related to him by blood or marriage (e.g., George Washington was Meriwether Lewis's second cousin once removed through Colonel Augustine Warner II; Thomas Jefferson's sister Lucy married Charles Lilburn Lewis, Meriwether's second cousin). Arend Flick notes that "Charles Lilburn Lewis was himself related to Jefferson—his mother was Mary Randolph, the younger sister of Jefferson's mother. So, while I am not persuaded that Jefferson and Meriwether Lewis were related by blood, they were definitely related by marriage. Throw in the fact that Jefferson's sister, Ann Scott Jefferson, married the brother of Meriwether's stepfather, a man named Hastings Marks, and you have a pretty tight connection."[12]

This would have led Meriwether Lewis to believe that he too should strive to attain greatness in whatever endeavor he undertook. Flick, who is currently conducting extensive research into the backgrounds and genealogies of the fathers of Lewis and Clark, states, "I am pretty certain that Meriwether Lewis knew he was related to Washington. Virginians were pretty obsessed with their family connections even then. Fielding Lewis, Meriwether Lewis's first cousin once removed, was married to Washington's sister Elizabeth (Betty). Certainly by the time he got to the position of Jefferson's secretary he must have known they had a common ancestor, and knew that his stepfather's brother was married to Jefferson's sister."[13]

Childhood, 1774–86 (Birth through Age Twelve)

Although we cannot know for certain what effects particular events might have had on Lewis, we can speculate that his mother Lucy would have been grieving the death of her second child Lucinda at the time she became pregnant with Meriwether, which was most likely within a year or so of the loss of her infant daughter. It is reasonable to expect that she may have felt ambivalent over her new pregnancy—happy to have the opportunity to conceive another child while at the same time sad to have lost a life that on some level she knew could never be replaced.

Previous interpretation of the historical record of Meriwether's father, William Lewis, has traditionally placed him in the Continental army, where he served as an officer during the Revolution and then until his death in either 1779 or 1781. Family lore about his death has it that William was home in Virginia on leave in November 1779. Upon his departure to return to duty with his unit, he crossed the Rivanna River, which was swollen by flooding. The account passed down through his family was that William's horse was swept away, but he managed to swim to shore and get to Cloverfields, his wife's family home. Within days of this incident, his health deteriorated; he contracted pneumonia and shortly thereafter passed away. He was buried at Cloverfields, about seventeen miles east of Locust Hill.[14]

According to Arend Flick in a revealing article in *We Proceeded On*, Lucy's husband William was voted into the Virginia regular army as a lieutenant in September 1775 and served in his brother Nicholas's company. Based on his research, Flick presents an alternative hypothetical narrative for the final years of Williams's life, stating that "there is no evidence that William Lewis served in the regular army in any capacity after the summer of 1776" and therefore could not have been returning to the army following a leave at the time of his death.[15]

Based on documentation in the daybook of William Lewis's physician, George Walker Gilmer, Walker made over forty visits to see William in the four years between 1771 and 1775. Flick proposes that Meriwether Lewis's father may have suffered from a respiratory ailment, depression, and possibly a venereal disease, the latter based on Gilmer's entry of "Neopol" as a medical diagnosis of William Lewis. This might refer to the so-called Neopolitan disease of syphilis, which is how some in Europe referred to this sexually transmitted ailment. Such a diagnosis in that era would have been presumptive—not confirmed by any lab test or any other medically reliable study (see chapter 6). Such a diagnosis is medically intriguing and certainly has some support within the historical record, as Flick argues. If Flick's research is accurate, those who believe that William was returning to military service after a leave at the time of his death are not correct as William would not have been a part of the military in the years 1779–81. Some physicians of that era espoused cold water treatment for various illnesses. Flick writes:

William Lewis may have gone to the Rivanna on that cold November day for what he hoped would be its medicinal, or at least palliative value, whether counseled to do so by Gilmer or by the folk medical practices of his time and place. If so, it would not be surprising that a man who was apparently unhealthy with a pulmonary-related disease caught pneumonia and died as a result.[16]

Flick's discovery of Dr. Gilmer's forty medical treatments of William Lewis lends significant credibility to Thomas Jefferson's written comment after Meriwether Lewis's death that William Lewis suffered from "hypochondriac affections"— fear, anxiety, or unreasonable concern about disease and the depression this sometimes produced—that was passed on to his son Meriwether and affected him in his final days. The diseases that Gilmer diagnosed in his daybook regarding William may have been real. Regardless, the repeated treatments by an eighteenth-century physician were likely not effective in curing any real disease, and without question they produced significant and unpleasant side effects. In fact, such illnesses and their often dangerous and unpleasant treatments, as documented by Gilmer regarding William's condition, might have produced "hypochondriac affections" in nearly anyone. We will cover this issue in more detail in the chapter on malaria (chapter 8). Other authors have incorrectly interpreted this term and its meaning and relevance to the death of Meriwether Lewis.

It is highly probable that after Meriwether Lewis's father died when he was five years old, Meriwether would have observed his family members grieving the loss of a person whom they described as possessing very positive attributes of character, such as strength and bravery—a man who was a military hero and whose life was cut short by the intervention of unfortunate circumstances. It seems likely that, on some level, Meriwether internalized this image or representation of his father. His own life and that of his father had quite parallel courses, in the larger scheme of things. Both served in the military and both of their lives ended tragically—William at age forty-four and Meriwether at age thirty-five.

As already noted, it was not uncommon in this era for a woman to remarry relatively quickly following the death of her spouse, and such was the case with Meriwether's mother. Family narratives passed down through the generations report that Lucy remarried, within six months of Meriwether's father's death in May 1780, to another military officer, Captain John Marks (1740–91).[17] Family members have passed down the report that on his deathbed William told his wife to remarry this particular gentleman and that she had his blessing to do so.[18] Lucy bore two children by her second husband: John (Jack) Hastings Marks (1785–1822) and Mary (Polly) Garland Marks (1788–1864). Meriwether was eleven years old at the time of his half brother's birth and fourteen at the time of his half sister's birth. Although Meriwether had a stronger blood bond with his full siblings Jane and Reuben, letters he wrote during his life indicate that he cared deeply about the health and welfare of his half-siblings as well. Such brotherly concern on the part of Meriwether is reflected in a letter he wrote to his mother on March 31, 1805, when he was thirty-one and was co-leading the Corps of Discovery, which was camped at Fort Mandan in present-day North Dakota. Lewis wrote,

> I must request of you before I conclude this letter, to send John Markes to the College at Williamsburgh, as soon as it shall be thought that his education has been sufficiently advanced to fit him for that ceminary; for you may rest assured that as you regard his future prosperity you had better make any sacrifice of his property than suffer his education to be neglected or remain incomplete.[19]

An incident occurred in the Charlottesville area when Lewis was almost seven years old that had to have had a strong impact on him in terms of forming a very negative view of the British, who were trying to defeat Continental troops at that time in the American Revolution. In June 1781, a colonel in British General Charles Cornwallis's army named Banastre Tarleton, who had earned a reputation as a particularly vicious and cruel man based on his history of inflicting mass destruction on buildings and people during the war, descended upon the Piedmont region of Virginia and Lewis's neighborhood in Charlottesville. Tarleton, the "Hunting Leopard," had been commanded to capture all of the members of the Virginia legislature and was in the process of hunting them down when Virginia militia captain John Jouett spotted the more than two hundred cavalrymen and infantrymen under Tarleton en route to Charlottesville. Jouett sped on ahead and warned the legislators of the approaching soldiers; the legislators were then able to flee to safety and avoid capture.

Even though they did not find Jefferson at his home at Monticello and did not damage it (he fled first to Carter's Mountain, a property he owned that was about three miles from his estate house, and then to Poplar Forest, another family plantation farther south), Tarleton and his men wreaked havoc on a nearby property owned by Jefferson, Elk Hill, where they burned crops and barns, slaughtered animals, killed some individuals, and carried off about thirty slaves.[20] It seems likely that Lewis would have heard about and been personally affected by the destructive rampage of Tarleton during what must have been a terrifying few days in Albemarle County. There is no record of how Lucy and John Marks protected themselves and their children during this time, but young Meriwether and his siblings most likely would have felt their lives were in real danger until word came that the enemy had moved on to pursue other victims.

In fact, Tarleton's Green Dragoons are known to have stopped at two estates on Meriwether family lands. Tarleton's men stopped at the Castle Hill property (owned by Thomas Walker and his wife, a Meriwether), where they ordered the Walkers to prepare breakfast for them and then rode to the Belvoir plantation of Meriwether Lewis's paternal grandparents, who had passed the estate down to their son Nicholas Lewis. At the time of Tarleton's visit to Belvoir, the estate was owned by John Walker, a colonel and aide to General George Washington in 1777. Tartleton captured two guests there. Since Belvoir is located only about eighteen miles from Locust Hill, there can be little doubt that young Lewis was aware of the presence of a menacing British army officer in the area and on land owned by his relatives.[21]

Previous biographers of Meriwether Lewis have recorded that he soon moved from Virginia to Georgia with his mother, stepfather, brother Reuben, and half brother John Hastings Marks, probably living there for about four years (i.e., between the ages of eight to twelve). These same authors reported that Meriwether remained in Georgia until he returned to Virginia to receive tutoring by three different mentors during most of his adolescence.

In-depth documentary research on events during this period of Lewis's childhood presented by Guy Meriwether Benson of the Meriwether Society indicates that it is more likely that Lewis lived mostly in Virginia between the ages of eight and twelve. Existing records indicate that his stepfather, Captain John Marks, was appointed sheriff of Albemarle County in 1785 when Lewis was eleven and that his half brother John Hastings Marks was born and baptized in Virginia in 1786 when Meriwether was twelve. It appears unlikely that Meriwether moved with his mother, stepfather, and two half-siblings when they relocated from Virginia to Georgia, which occurred probably no sooner than 1786 when Meriwether was twelve because, on September 14, 1786, William D. Meriwether (the nephew of Lewis's mother) was appointed Meriwether's guardian by the Albemarle County, Virginia, court along with Meriwether Lewis's paternal uncle Robert Lewis, who posted a $3,000 guardian bond. The reason for the guardianship was probably to ensure that the young Meriwether remained in Virginia in order to receive a formal education. He likely visited his mother and family in Georgia during summer vacations but did not spend the majority of his time there, as biographies of Lewis published between 1948 and 2012 have reported.[22]

The activities Lewis most likely engaged in during these formative years between the ages of eight and twelve included the development of his hunting and fishing skills in the mountains and forests surrounding Locust Hill. His proficiency with these early frontier abilities would become essential to his survival during his subsequent years in the U.S. Army and during the expedition he led between 1803 and 1806. This is also undoubtedly when he learned from his mother Lucy how to identify and use medicinal plants—also instrumental skills during the expedition, during which he was responsible for gathering and identifying flora and fauna on the Corps of Discovery's epic journey to the Pacific Ocean. Lucy was widely known in Albemarle County as a "yarb" (herb) doctor; she was known to travel throughout the county to treat sick people with her "simples" (i.e., simple home-grown herbal remedies believed at the time to possess medicinal value), riding on horseback to tend to their ailments.[23]

Adolescence, 1787–92
(Ages Thirteen to Eighteen)

The majority of Meriwether's teenage years were spent under the formal tutelage of three individuals contracted by his legal guardian, William D. Meriwether, to teach him subjects that included Latin, Greek, natural sciences, classical literature, mathematics, and—apparently his favorite—geography. Since there was no formal public school system in place in Virginia in the late 1700s, it was the usual practice for members of the Virginia gentry to apply for and be accepted for tutelage by the most educated and learned figures in the communities where they lived. Lewis's first teacher was Parson Matthew Maury, who mentored him between March 1788 and fall 1789, when Lewis would have been between about thirteen and a half and fifteen years old. After waiting for his application to be accepted, Lewis attended to his studies in a small log cabin used by Parson Maury and resided in the home of his uncle Peachy Gilmer, with his room and board paid for by his mother's nephew and his guardian. His studies there included mathematics, which he referred to as "figures" in a letter to his mother, then living in Georgia.[24]

In the fall of 1789, Lewis transferred to his second formal tutor, Dr. Charles Everitt, a physician who was generally unliked by his students due to his strictness and harsh discipline. Lewis's schoolmate and cousin (five years his junior), Peachy Gilmer Jr., wrote that Everitt had an "atrabilious [ill-tempered] and melancholy temperament: peevish, capricious, and every way disagreeable." His method of teaching, according to Cousin Peachy, was "as bad as anything could be."[25] This description of the doctor leaves us to imagine the discussions that might have been held between the cousins about their course of study and their cheerless tutor. It was also Cousin Peachy who wrote one of the most insightful perceptions of Lewis that we possess today, as follows:

> always remarkable for perseverance, which in the early period of his life seemed nothing more than obstinacy in pursuing the trifles that employ that age; a martial temper; great steadiness of purpose, self-possession, and undaunted courage. His person was stiff and without grace, bow-legged, awkward, formal, and

almost without flexibility. His face was comely and by many considered handsome.[26]

In 1790, at the age of sixteen, Lewis transferred to his third formal mentor, a Presbyterian minister named Rev. James Waddell, who held an honorary doctor of divinity degree from Dickinson College and was highly regarded by Virginians for his strengths as a moralist and orator. Lewis described him as a "polite scholar" and no doubt thought of him as a much more respected teacher than his previous one.[27] He wrote to his mother in August 1790 that he hoped to stay on and study with Rev. Waddell for another eighteen months to two years.

This hope was not to materialize, for in the early summer of 1791, within a month or two of Meriwether's seventeenth birthday, his mother's second husband died in Georgia, leaving her a widow at the age of forty with three young children to raise—Reuben (fifteen), John or "Jack" (six), and Mary or "Polly" (three). Lucy wrote to her daughter Jane, then married and living with her husband Edmund Anderson in Richmond, of the news of the passing of Captain John Marks and communicated her desire to have her oldest son Meriwether come to Georgia to help her and the children move back to Locust Hill. Based on his understanding that his mother was anxious to return to Virginia by the spring of 1792 and his sister Jane's (presumed) encouragement that he suspend his studies to accomplish this, Lewis no doubt felt torn between his desire to continue the formal education he was pursuing (he possibly wished to attend college at a respected nearby institution, such as the College of William and Mary) and his felt need to fulfill his obligations as his mother's oldest son and heir to his father William's plantation. Lewis chose the route of the dutiful son. He dropped out of school and wrote to his mother in April 1792 that he had ordered a carriage to be built by an artisan at Thomas Jefferson's estate of Monticello for the journey south. One can surmise that Lewis's neighbor and friend Thomas Jefferson was probably aware of the situation and felt compassion for the family—he knew Lucy Meriwether Marks and reportedly always ordered her cured hams, considered the best in the region, for his table. Lewis informed his mother that spring that he expected the carriage would be ready by May 1 and that he would depart the Charlottesville area by May 15, 1792.[28]

In the fall of 1792, just after turning eighteen, Lewis completed what was essentially an administrative dress rehearsal for his future journey across North America, although he could not have known this at the time. In this mini-expedition, he formulated his plan, prepared for the necessities of the trip, traveled from Virginia to Georgia, and transported his mother and siblings with all of their belongings back to Virginia to reside again at Locust Hill.

During this period, Jefferson was serving as the country's first secretary of state under President George Washington. It is highly likely that during Meriwether's boyhood, since Jefferson was a relative (by marriage), friend of the family, and source of useful knowledge, Lewis visited Jefferson and they conversed about common interests including agriculture, history, and the natural sciences. The young Lewis's strong mental and physical constitution, his characteristics of conscientiousness and integrity, and his values of hard work and a strong degree of responsibility would have made a positive impression on the future third president of the United States. There can be little doubt that Jefferson's high regard for Lewis led to his determination to ask Lewis to serve as his personal secretary during his administration; he viewed him as a reliable, loyal, intelligent, and industrious person who would assist Jefferson in his presidential duties.

Plantation Owner, 1792–94 (Ages Eighteen to Twenty)

Lewis had barely turned eighteen when the death of his stepfather resulted in his life taking a path he didn't expect. It is impressive, and speaks to Lewis's strong and steady character and constitution, that he rose to the occasion and met his responsibilities conscientiously and wisely. Upon the death of Col. Marks, his wife Lucy, Lewis's mother, inherited his entire estate and would, upon her death or remarriage, leave his estate to Marks's biological children, John and Mary.

As the eldest son, Lewis had inherited most of his father William's estate at the age of five (his mother inherited a smaller percentage through dower rights), which was managed by overseers until he turned eighteen. After relocating his mother and his siblings back to Virginia, within a matter of months Lewis assumed the position of the principal owner and manager of a plantation consisting of two thousand acres and at least two dozen slaves. There is documentary evidence that during the two years preceding his twentieth birthday Lewis conducted all of his business in a highly responsible manner, even adding acreage to the amount of land he already owned and operated. As a Virginia planter/farmer, Lewis's primary crop was probably tobacco.

Army Officer, 1794–1800 (Ages Twenty to Twenty-Six)

Lewis was running his plantation effectively, but when volunteers were sought to join the Virginia militia to help suppress the armed rebellion in western Pennsylvania known as the Whiskey Rebellion, it should be no surprise that he followed in the military footsteps of so many of the men of his family before him, including his father and stepfather. Lewis was surrounded by many male relatives who had served as officers, so the possibility of becoming an officer was very natural for him to consider. Lewis's inherent strengths, talents, and interests suited him to be a relatively more effective military leader than plantation owner, even though he was competent in both positions. From his writings that have survived, including letters he wrote to his mother, it is clear that Lewis found the army to be the place where he could fulfill his true potential—he loved the lifestyle of the army, its challenge, adventure, and the opportunity it gave him to grow and learn.[29]

The Whiskey Rebellion (1791–94) arose as a protest over the first tax imposed (on rum and whiskey) by the newly formed federal government of the United States. Since the American Revolution arose out of the outrage of the early colonists over the British government's taxation of their tea and other trade goods to help pay off Britain's debt incurred during the French and Indian War (1754–63), America's earliest citizens in western Pennsylvania felt as if history was repeating itself. The motivation for imposing the whiskey tax was to help the new federal government, which had replaced British rule, pay off the debt the newly formed country had incurred during the American Revolution.

Washington feared that this revolt by farmers on the Western frontier, if not suppressed, could lead to a sort of second Revolutionary War and the secession of this region from the newly formed United States.

He was so determined to stop this insurrection that, even though he was serving as president, he personally led U.S. Army troops during the conflict. Lewis was determined to aid his country's commander in chief in this endeavor. What is evident here is another strong characteristic manifested in Meriwether's personality—he was an extremely loyal and patriotic individual. He demonstrated these traits in other circumstances (see later sections in this chapter).

Close to his twentieth birthday in August 1794, Lewis answered Washington's call for volunteers to military service to put down the Whiskey Rebellion by enlisting as a private in the Virginia militia for a period of six months. In the fall of 1794, Lewis received his commission as an officer (ensign), and in letters he wrote home to his mother during this same time from his posts in places like Cumberland, Maryland, and in the environs of Pittsburgh he expressed only positive sentiments about his experience of serving in the military and pride about the opportunity to be of service to his country. So pleased was he with the military lifestyle he had chosen that when the time of his discharge approached in May 1795, Lewis enlisted in the federal army and was stationed at Fort Greenville (present-day Greenville, Ohio) under the command of General Anthony Wayne. Wayne was in charge of dealing with conflicts between the Indian tribes in the area and the American citizens encroaching on Indians lands as they pressed to move ever further westward.

Lewis's career in the U.S. Army progressed successfully during the spring and summer of 1795 until September 24, 1795. Within a few weeks following his twenty-first birthday, Lewis's entire military career, indeed his future prospects for success, came under very serious threat at the hands of one of his superiors, Lieutenant Joseph Elliott, a native of South Carolina, who was about twenty years Lewis's senior. Elliott had served in the U.S. Army for eighteen years at the time of his interaction with Lewis. He had been wounded and taken prisoner during the Revolutionary War at the siege of Charleston, South Carolina.[30]

Elliott was hosting a dinner party for four fellow officers, and Lewis arrived uninvited and engaged in a somewhat heated discussion in an adjacent room with one of the officers present at Elliott's party. Apparently, the volume and tone of their discussion disrupted the dinner party, and Elliott intervened in an attempt to quiet the two officers. Lewis then became agitated and argumentative with Elliott. As Arend Flick noted in an excellent article in *We Proceeded On*, "For his [Elliott's] pains, he got a duel challenge from the much younger Lewis."[31] Elliott ultimately accused Lewis of entering his headquarters during a dinner party with his guests and of challenging him to a duel while intoxicated. Lewis was arrested and confined until his general court-martial convened, a trial that lasted from November 6–12, 1795. During these proceedings, Lewis pleaded not guilty to the two charges of conduct unbecoming an officer and of challenging his superior to a duel. After witnesses were called for both the defense and prosecution, Lewis, who served as his own defense counsel, was acquitted "with honor" of all charges. We can only imagine how relieved Lewis must have felt about this outcome as he was no doubt aware of how close he had come to shattering his dream of a career in the army.

Following Lewis's acquittal, it was clear that Lewis and Elliott would no longer be able to serve in the same unit, so Lewis was reassigned to William Clark's Chosen Rifle Company of elite sharpshooters, where he served under Clark's command for approximately eight months between November 1795 and July 1796. Arend Flick notes that Clark was on leave in Louisville for six of those eight months. Danisi's research seems to support the idea that Lewis may have initially met William Clark before the court-martial trial, as records indicate that they were both serving in the same unit at Fort Greenville, Ohio, in September 1795.[32]

Whenever Lewis came into prolonged contact with Clark, it is apparent that he gained respect for his company commander and his leadership abilities. When the time came for Lewis to select someone he could trust and rely on to collaborate with him on a momentous endeavor, he chose Clark to co-lead the Corps of Discovery with him. In a good illustration of every dark cloud having a silver lining, Lewis's transfer into Clark's unit turned out to be a blessing in disguise. Although Lewis served for only a few months under Clark, the upside of his distasteful court-martial experience was that if it had never occurred, Lewis would not have become so well acquainted with his expedition co-captain as well as his most trusted and loyal friend.

Much more could easily be written about the history of Lewis's military career between 1794 and 1800, but, to summarize, these six years when he was between the ages of twenty and twenty-six were marked by several promotions in rank and duties, from private to ensign to lieutenant (March 3, 1799) and then to captain (December 5, 1800).[33] Evidence of recognition by his superiors of his excellent service to his country and his promise as an officer included his assignment to tasks that he had no way of knowing at the time would prove to be excellent training exercises in preparation for the westward expedition. These included extensive travel throughout the Ohio River frontier during which he rode both horseback and on watercraft resembling those he would use during the expedition up the Missouri River, delivering dispatches for General Anthony Wayne and having frequent contact with Indian tribes.

Another pursuit that Lewis managed to attend to while he was on active duty was his application for admission, on December 31, 1796, to the Masonic Lodge in Albemarle, Virginia. On January 28, 1797, he was accepted into membership there. On April 3, 1797, he advanced to the degree of past master mason, and in October 1799 he achieved the status of royal arch mason.[34] Lewis was a very active and dedicated member of this organization throughout the course of his life; in fact, one of the items found in his possession following his death and returned to his mother was his Masonic apron.

Records indicate that Lewis took an approximately six-month leave of absence between May and November 1797 to return to Charlottesville, where he engaged in buying and selling property within his own plantation (Locust Hill) and his mother's estate in Georgia.[35] Toward the end of 1797, Lewis resumed his military duties as commander of an infantry company under Captain Isaac Guion's command at Fort Pickering on the Mississippi River, which had been constructed near today's Memphis, Tennessee.[36] This indicates that during the last days of his life, when Lewis stopped and stayed there en route to Washington, D.C., to clear his name and try to address his financial difficulties with the War Department, he was in a place that was familiar to him. One cannot help but wonder whether, when he returned there in 1809, he thought back to his first visit to that place as a younger officer. It is not hard to imagine that it was with very mixed feelings that he returned, in September 1809, to a place that would remind him of how far up he had climbed the ladder of success by the age of twenty-three and how far he had then fallen by the age of thirty-five.

Early in 1798, Lewis was reassigned to Charlottesville as commander of recruitment, where he stayed for the next year and a half, undoubtedly glad to be close to home, family, and friends. This experience was also helpful when he later was recruiting members for the expedition. John Bakeless, in his biography of Lewis, notes that "[s]ometime in 1800, he went north again and was assigned to Captain Ferdinand L. Claiborne's Company of the First Infantry, when it was organized at Detroit in September."[37] This leg of Lewis's military service gave him the opportunity for additional travel in the Western wilderness, mostly between Detroit and Pittsburgh, as regimental paymaster, a position requiring not only travel but also the skill of keeping account records and logs of his daily activities—yet another area of competence useful for the future expedition.

President Thomas Jefferson's Personal Secretary, 1801–02 (Ages Twenty-Six to Twenty-Eight)

On February 23, 1801, shortly after his election as the third president of the United States, Jefferson penned a letter to Lewis that dramatically changed the course of Lewis's life. The letter invited him to come to Washington as soon as reasonably possible to serve as the new president's private secretary. Lewis replied promptly and enthusiastically accepted what he no doubt felt was a high honor and privilege. He was granted immediate leave by his company commander and traveled on horseback to the nation's capital, arriving on April 1 to take up his $500/year salaried position, which Jefferson described as "more in the nature of that of an Aid de camp, than a mere Secretary."[38] When Lewis moved into the mansion, his living quarters were located in what is known today as the Green Room, adjacent to the East Room (which was confirmed for us by White House Police when we toured the White House in 2017, contrary to Stephen Ambrose's report in *Undaunted Courage* that Lewis's residence was in the East Room[39]). For the next two years, Lewis fulfilled with dedication, diligence, and responsibility the duties that his commander in chief requested of him. These included reviewing a War Department roster of all commissioned officers and ranking them according to his judgment of their worthiness to hold commissions. (Lewis's nemesis Elliott escaped the cut of Lewis's administrative knife; he had left the army in December of 1800).[40] Jefferson also gave Lewis the responsibility of copying and then delivering his first State of the Union Address to the U.S. Congress.

Lewis, Jefferson, and the servants Jefferson had brought from his Monticello estate in Virginia were the only residents of the White House, save for a few weeks in May 1801 when James and Dolley Madison stayed there. Dolley reportedly acted as a hostess for regular dinner parties. Guests were regularly served the finest of French wines that Jefferson had imported along with food prepared by Jefferson's personal chef. At these dinner parties, Lewis had the opportunity to meet with a long list of interesting and distinguished personalities—other politicians, cabinet members, writers, and scientists. Jefferson was a Renaissance man; he had diverse interests that included philosophy, religion, geography, and the natural sciences. Lewis's presence at these events enhanced his interest in many of the topics Jefferson was exploring.

It was at one of these dinners that Lewis first met Mahlon Dickerson, a Philadelphia lawyer and politician who became a very good and cherished friend. Dickerson provided Lewis with a friendly contact in Philadelphia when Lewis's duties in preparation for the upcoming expedition took him to the "city of brotherly love" in May of 1802 and then again in the spring of 1803. It is certain that during the two years that Lewis and Jefferson resided together in the "President's House" they dreamed and schemed about their mutual passion—that of sending an expeditionary party into the regions of Western North America not yet settled by Europeans. During a two-month summer vacation in August 1802, with Lewis staying temporarily in a clapboard house about three miles from Monticello, the two men undoubtedly pored over maps together and talked about their mutual interests, with Jefferson opening up his library to Lewis and sharing valuable information about botany, geography, and weather patterns.[41] In March, Lewis left Washington and stopped in Harper's Ferry, Virginia, to consult with and order weapons from the National Armory. Lewis's creative imagination cost him several weeks of preparation as he worked with the army to construct an iron-framed, portable boat that would prove to be a bust in the coming trip. He was then off to Philadelphia.[42]

In February 1803, a month after receiving approval from Congress for the funding of the westward expedition, Jefferson wrote letters to five individuals in Philadelphia who were his colleagues and members of the American Philosophical Society, asking them to meet with Lewis and train him in the areas he would need to ensure the success of his upcoming epic journey.[43]

For about seven weeks between April 19 and June 10, 1803, Lewis met with the leading scientific experts in their fields at that time for what amounted to a crash course in land surveying, astronomy, botany, geology, and medicine. His tutelage began with mathematician/astronomer Andrew Ellicott, whom Lewis described as "extreemly friendly and attentive" while Lewis visited at his home in Lancaster, Pennsylvania, for two weeks.[44] Lewis received instruction there in how to make celestial observations, survey land, and use the instruments required for these endeavors. Ellicott then provided Lewis with a letter of introduction to his colleague, mathematician Robert Patterson, who furthered the instruction of Lewis in the science of taking celestial observations and their application to geographical exploration. Records indicate that on May 17 Lewis met with Benjamin Rush, professor of medicine at the University of Pennsylvania, and received medical recommendations, research questions regarding Native American health, and advice about how to treat various maladies encountered en route to the Pacific Ocean. At this time, Dr. Rush also provided Lewis with medical instruments, including penile syringes for use with anticipated venereal disease, forceps, and lancets as well as fifty dozen pills that Rush had concocted himself to treat all manner of diseases. Rush's pills contained ingredients guaranteed to purge the intestines of any illness-producing contents in a very intense way[45] (see chapter 5 on common medications used by physicians of this era).

Lewis then visited with Benjamin Smith Barton, professor of botany at the University of Pennsylvania and author of the first botany textbook published in the United States. Barton taught Lewis how to preserve both plant and bird specimens as well as animal skins. Lewis also received instruction from the winsome Caspar Wistar, who was at the time an adjunct professor of anatomy, midwifery, and surgery at the University of Pennsylvania. Wistar eventually became chair of the anatomy department and author of the first anatomy textbook published in America. He was also the foremost American authority of his time on fossils. Wistar instructed Lewis about bones that he (and Jefferson) thought might be discovered along the route covered by the expedition.[46]

Following his preparatory studies in the Philadelphia area, Lewis took charge of the practical side of moving all his purchased goods, some 3,500 pounds, from Philadelphia to Pittsburgh. Lewis turned over the job and its cost to the U.S. Army and left for Washington. Once in Washington, political considerations involving the expedition into a foreign land took center stage. Madison, Jefferson's secretary of state, brought up the issue of taking an expedition into French-owned and Spanish-administered territory. Attorney General Levi Lincoln warned of the virulent attacks that would be made by the Federalists against Jefferson's plans, in addition to its costs. Lincoln also suggested that the expedition be, at least in part, an attempt to learn more about native religious beliefs so that this knowledge could be used in the future to "civilize & instruct them" in Christianity. This proposal garnered support from New England clergy, and Jefferson agreed to Lincoln's suggestion.[47]

On June 19, 1803, Lewis wrote a letter to his friend William Clark, inviting him to co-command the pending expedition and enlisting his trusted fellow army officer to select physically tough men to become members of the Corps of Discovery. Then, on July 4, Secretary Madison's concern about entering into foreign territory became a moot point. American newspapers announced that the United States had purchased the Louisiana Territory from France for a mere fifteen million dollars, one of history's greatest real estate deals. Any pretense of purely scientific progress could be ignored as Americans would now be exploring their new backyard. Some Federalists who opposed the purchase criticized the deal as spending money "of which we have too little, for land of which we already have too much."[48]

Lewis left Washington on July 5, on his way to Pittsburgh. He stopped at Harper's Ferry and picked up the weapons and the iron boat frame he had ordered the previous March. On July 29, Lewis received Clark's letter expressing his enthusiasm at being invited to join the expedition, and on August 31, 1803, Lewis was set to sail out of Pittsburgh, heading westward down the Ohio River. He navigated over the Falls of the Ohio River near Louisville, Kentucky, on October 15 and joined Clark at his home in present-day Clarksville, Indiana Territory. This moment marked the start of the greatest wilderness adventure in American history.

Expedition Co-Leader, 1803–1806 (Ages Twenty-Eight to Thirty-Two)

It could be easily argued that the three-plus years (1803–06) that Lewis spent co-leading the famed expedition of the Corps of Discovery represented the high-water mark of both his personal happiness as well as his life's accomplishments. It is not our desire to rehash the history of the entire expedition, which many authors have accomplished in great detail. Since numerous works have covered the epic journey and this period in Lewis's life, we simply summarize here what we consider to be some of the highlights. To do so, we have roughly followed the time segments suggested by Gary Moulton in his 2018 summary of the expedition's journals titled *Day by Day*. As a result, we elaborate on about a dozen of the events that occurred between May 14, 1804 (the day Lewis left St. Louis to ascend the Missouri River) and September 23, 1806 (the day the entire party returned to St. Louis). These are key events during the expedition that we believe illustrate Lewis's personality characteristics we address in more detail later in this book.

Lewis and Clark and the Corps of Discovery spent the winter of 1803–04 across the Mississippi River from St. Louis at Wood River, Illinois Territory. During these months, Lewis spent a good deal of time gathering much-needed information and hiring additional boatmen to aid in the upriver rowing as well as the last-minute purchasing of supplies in St. Louis.

On the afternoon of May 14, 1804, with Clark in command, the Corps of Discovery left their winter camp, crossed the Mississippi, and started up the Missouri River. Meriwether Lewis was in St. Louis making final arrangements and joined the expedition a few miles upriver at St. Charles. This event marked the end of months of meticulous preparation by Lewis as the expedition's commander, including decisions about the recruitment of additional members for the expedition, purchasing of needed supplies, and procurement of goods destined for gifts to various

Indian tribes they would encounter along their route. This period of preparation illustrates Lewis's strong organizational ability and innate intelligence.

The key goals of the expedition, as ordered by Jefferson, were to
- find, if possible, an all-water route to the Pacific Ocean;
- explore the Missouri River, noting tributaries and other geographic parameters;
- establish American authority over the Louisiana Purchase;
- map the area through which they traveled, taking measurements of the latitude and longitude of key geographical areas;
- encourage peace among the Native Americans and tell the tribes of the new "great father" in Washington who was now in control but desired only commerce with the Indians, not their lands; and
- gather new species of flora and fauna and other information for science.[49]

One of the key goals of the expedition was to contact and inform the various Native American tribes of the new authority governing their territories and of their chief living in Washington. Depending upon the tribe, these interactions on occasion were tense. Although no blood was shed in any of these encounters until the expedition reached modern-day North Dakota in 1805, this prime directive from Jefferson was accomplished with varying degrees of success. In May and July, during their interactions with the lower Missouri tribes of the Otos and Missouris, Lewis and Clark's school of American diplomacy opened for business.[50]

Any effective commander of such an expedition would need to possess the ability to improvise when faced with unexpected situations. Such an occasion arose during the expedition's interactions with the chief of the Otos when he made a request/demand for some whiskey from the captains, with the veiled threat that if they did not receive any whiskey the young warriors of those tribes would attack the Pawnee and Omaha tribes.[51] This was the first such surprise that Lewis experienced, and it challenged his resourcefulness in dealing with Native American culture and politics and would be but the first of many diplomatic difficulties encountered by Lewis and the expedition. James Ronda, noted Lewis and Clark scholar and author of the highly respected book *Lewis and Clark among the Indians* (1984), states that the captains had neither "the time nor the talent to understand and control" the intricacies of centuries of established Native American culture.[52]

On August 27, the expedition made contact with part of the greater Sioux nation, the Yankton tribe. Jefferson had told Lewis, "On this nation, we wish most particularly to make a favorable impression due to their immense power."[53] The Yanktons were peaceful, friendly, and cooperative with the expedition, but once the tribe was informed by a White interpreter, Mr. Dorion, of the desire of the American government for peace among all of the tribes along the river, the expedition members were informed that the Teton Sioux, a bit farther up the river, was probably not going to listen to such talk. Chief Half Man of the Yanktons warned, "I fear those nations above will not open their ears and you cannot I fear open them."[54]

The Teton Sioux tribe, made up of several bands of Lakota Sioux (Miniconjou, Brulé, Oglala), controlled the middle Missouri River and thereby controlled and benefited from any tribe or trader who desired to pass through their lands. John Truteau, a knowledgeable trader, stated that "all voyageurs who undertake to gain access to the nations of the Upper Missouri ought to avoid meeting this tribe, as much for the safety of their goods as for their lives."[55] With the obvious disadvantage of not having a Sioux interpreter, the expedition's limited ability to communicate through George Drouillard's sign language and Pierre Cruzatte's knowledge of a few words of Sioux made any attempt at an effective discussion nearly an impossibility. This visit with the Tetons led to a contentious and occasionally dangerous three-day layover, and finally, through a bizarre set of interactions that included drawn bows and cocked rifles, the expedition was able to proceed upriver. The captains displayed remarkable courage in the face of this strong military threat to their success, but they had nevertheless suffered another setback for American-Indian diplomacy.[56]

By October 24, the expedition had rowed, poled, and sailed their way 1,600 miles up the Missouri River (against the current) and arrived at their winter headquarters among the relatively friendly Mandan and Hidatsa tribes, who lived in separate villages along the Missouri and nearby Knife Rivers. These tribes were active traders with British merchants and along with many other tribes were at war with the Teton Sioux and their sometime ally, the Arikara. The Mandan tribe had been severely weakened by smallpox in 1781 and had moved north to ally themselves with the Hidatsa tribe in hope of mutual protection. Lewis spent the winter gaining intelligence on the geography they would encounter in the next year and attempting to consolidate peace with the surrounding tribes, trying to pry the Arikara away from the influence of the Teton Sioux. The captains maintained security for the Corps by directing the construction of Fort Mandan, a log structure that served as a house, American consulate, and military fort during the sometimes −40°F temperatures of the harsh winter. One of the significant events of this winter occurred on February 11, 1805, when Lewis assisted in the birth of Sacagawea's baby boy, Jean Baptiste Charbonneau.[57] This little boy would travel with the Corps across the entire remaining course to the Pacific Ocean and back and probably not remember anything about his epic journey.

By April 7, 1805, the Corps had spent over five months in their winter quarters, and when the spring thaw came they were eager to proceed on their journey westward. On this date, Lewis wrote of his joy upon leaving Fort Mandan:

> Our vessels consisted of six small canoes, and two large perogues. This little fleet altho' not quite so rispectable as those of Columbus or Capt. Cook were still viewed by us with as much pleasure as those deservedly famed adventurers ever beheld theirs; and I dare say with quite as much anxiety for their safety and preservation. we were now about to penetrate a country at least two thousand miles in width, on which the foot of civilized man had never trodden; the good or evil it had in store for us was for experiment yet to determine and these little vessels contained every article by which we were to expect to subsist or defend ourselves. . . . I could but esteem this moment of my departure as among the most happy of my life.[58]

We believe that Lewis was sincere in this emotionally revealing journey entry and that this may have been the happiest day of his life up until that point in time and perhaps even of his entire life (see chapter 13). This was what he was made to do. This was the day he had been preparing for over the previous months and years.

Between the day the group departed Fort Mandan until the end of May 1805, the Corps had no hostile contacts with Native American tribes. They did, however, have some rather terrifying encounters with grizzly bears, who sometimes chased the men after being wounded. Some bears required six or more shots from the men's flintlock rifles before they died (see chapter 9), and while initially Lewis discounted the toughness and ferocity of "these gentlemen," he eventually came to respect the real danger they represented to the expedition members. His courage under fire was never so apparent as when he had a very personal encounter with one of these furry monsters far upriver, near the Great Falls in present-day Montana. This episode displayed his cool character under threatening circumstances perhaps better than any other in the entire twenty-eight months of the expedition. The men of the Corps had nearly three dozen close encounters with grizzlies between May and July of 1805.

During this leg of the journey, the Corps passed the confluence of the Yellowstone and Missouri Rivers, viewing wildlife and plants they had never seen before. On May 31, 1805, the expeditionary party arrived at an area in present-day north-central Montana known today as the White Cliffs. We believe that Lewis's journal entry describing this forty-three-mile-long area along the Missouri River area illustrates not only his accomplished ability to observe his environment but also his eloquence in describing what he observed. The following is a quote from his journal on this date:

> The hills and river Clifts which we passed today exhibit a most romantic appearance. . . . The water in the course of time in descending from those hills and plains on either side of the river has trickled down the soft sand cliffs and worn it into a thousand grotesque figures, which with the help of a little imagination and an oblique view at a distance, are made to represent ranges of lofty freestone buildings, having their parapets well stocked with statuary. . . . As we passed on it seemed as if those Seens of visionary enchantment would never have an end; for here it is too that nature presents to the view of the traveler vast ranges of walls of tolerable workmanship, so perfect indeed are those walls that I should have thought that nature had attempted here

to rival the human art of masonry had I not recollected that she had first began her work.[59]

At the beginning of June 1805, the captains faced a dilemma—they had come to a major fork in the river and were not certain which branch was the true Missouri. To ensure that they would make the right decision, they spent several days camped near the fork and sent reconnaissance parties up both branches, conducting an assessment of the rivers. Based on a review of all of their observations, Lewis and Clark decided the south fork was the correct path. They named the alternative branch the Marias after Lewis's cousin Maria Wood. This series of events illustrates not only Lewis's critical thinking skills but also his ability to collaborate well with his co-captain.

On June 7, 1805, an incident occurred that offers a great example of Lewis's ability to keep a cool head in a crisis. While walking along the slippery edge of the Marias River, with a ninety-foot drop to the river below, Lewis heard a voice cry out behind him, "[G]od, god, captain, what shall I do?" He turned around to see Private Windsor dangling over the edge of a cliff, holding on precariously with his left leg. Lewis calmly instructed Windsor to take out his knife, dig a hole with it for his right foot, and raise himself to his knees. He then instructed Windsor to remove his moccasins, use his knife and rifle to gain a foothold on the slope, and crawl forward on his hands and knees until he reached the top of the bluff.[60]

One week later, Lewis became the first Euro-American to see the Great Falls of the Missouri—another spectacular natural wonder that he witnessed during the journey westward. He was so overcome by the beauty of the falls that, try as he might to describe "this sublimely grand specticle," he felt that he could not do literary justice to the falls. He was so profoundly moved by this scenery that he called it "the grandest sight I ever beheld."[61] Lewis witnessed many novelties, including flora and fauna, during the three years he and the Corps traveled to the Pacific Coast and back to St. Louis; his rating this event as the pinnacle of all the landscapes he had encountered gives a clear sense of how impressed he was by the Great Falls.

One of the characteristics exemplified by Lewis was his seeming contentment to be by himself a fair amount of the time, in addition to spending time in the company of the other members of the group. Before he came upon the Great Falls, he had sent several members of the party in other directions to hunt for meat for their meals while he proceeded upriver alone. His solitary ventures also included the not infrequent times he set off by himself, with his Newfoundland dog Seaman, to collect flora and fauna specimens during the twenty-eight-month expedition.

Lewis's talent for keeping his presence of mind under what we would consider terrifying circumstances was evident on June 14, 1805, when Lewis set out on his own and hiked over the grassy and sagebrush-covered hills surrounding the Missouri River near the Great Falls. Lewis found himself among a large herd of over a thousand buffaloes. Lewis selected an appropriate bull from the group, cocked his single-shot rifle, and shot the animal. With his attention directed toward the dying animal, he failed to see a grizzly bear approaching him to within a distance of about twenty paces. Thinking very quickly and assessing that there was no time (or point) to reload, he sprinted into the nearby Missouri as the grizzly bear gained ground with every step. Once in the river, Lewis pivoted toward the onrushing bear, raised his espontoon, and stood his ground against the charging bear, which likely weighed more than three hundred pounds. The charging grizzly was apparently surprised by Lewis's courage; the bear pivoted and retreated and, in fact, ran away for quite a distance. Such quick and appropriate reactions resulted from Lewis's years of outdoor experience facing a myriad of challenging and dangerous situations. In the face of danger, Lewis seemed to be at his very best. This bear incident was a very close call and an amazing story he could tell for the rest of his life.[62]

The most arduous activity of the expeditionary force during the summer of 1805 was the portaging of all of the Corps's supplies in canoes for a distance of approximately sixteen miles over the hot, prickly pear-infested plains around the series of five falls in the Missouri River near present-day Great Falls, Montana. As if the spectacularly physical work was not sufficient discouragement, the plains were inhabited by numerous rattlesnakes that required "great caution to prevent being bitten."[63]

At the end of July 1805, the Corps reached the convergence of three separate rivers now known as the Three Forks of the Missouri River. At this juncture were a southeast fork (which they named after Gallatin, the secretary of the treasury), a middle fork (which they named after Madison, the secretary of state), and a southwest fork (which they named after Jefferson, the president of the United States). The party was eager to push up the southwest branch (the Jefferson River) to the area where they anticipated meeting with members of the Shoshone Indian tribe, who they were hoping would sell them horses to help them travel over the mountain range they knew lay between them and the distant Pacific Ocean. It was here in the foothills of western Montana that Sacagawea had been kidnapped several years earlier by the Hidatsa, and as the group came closer to this area, she began to recognize familiar landmarks.

A prominent tendency in Lewis's personality was to quickly erupt into anger when he perceived his honor was being questioned or betrayed or when in general he was not getting what he wanted. This is a theme that we visit frequently in this work as it is vitally important in Lewis's personality analysis. All historians seem to agree about Lewis's quick temper. One of the occasions when this disposition appeared was in early August 1805, when the party had entered into Shoshone territory. It was vitally important for them to make peaceful contact with this tribe.

On August 11, Lewis was the first to see an Indian, who was on horseback and descending the gentle hill while moving slowly toward the group. Lewis proceeded slowly toward the man with words and gestures (e.g., laying down his rifle and his blanket, rather than waving them, to indicate his desire for a friendly meeting). The Indian, having discovered Lewis, was understandably very wary, as he could also see Drouillard and Shields approaching on his flanks. When Lewis realized this, he turned and signaled to them to halt. Drouillard saw the command, but Shields did not and continued on his course. The Indian at that point turned and rode away, leaving Lewis frustrated; he later wrote in his journal that "with him vanished all my hopes of obtaining horses for the present."[64] Gary Moulton wrote in *The Lewis and Clark Expedition Day by Day* about this incident: "He was also upset at the men, particularly Shields, whom he blamed for bungling the encounter, and reprimanded them for their inattention."[65]

The happy ending to the August 11 disappointment occurred the very next day. On August 12, Lewis, Hugh McNeal, George Drouillard, and John Shields were following an Indian road and creek that was ascending the gradual uphill plain that would ultimately be known as Horse Prairie Creek, one of the feeder creeks to "the mighty & heretofore deemed endless Missouri."[66] When the path disappeared, Lewis sent Drouillard to his right, with orders to stay near the creek, and Shields to his left, both in search of the Indian road. Lewis instructed the men that if any of the three were to find such a path, they were to signal each other by waving their hats on their uplifted rifles. Lewis, Drouillard, Shields, and McNeal located the headwaters of the Missouri near the Continental Divide at Lemhi Pass, the present-day border between Montana and Idaho.

Their good fortune continued, for within days they made contact with the Shoshone tribe and began negotiations for the horses they needed. One of the many amazing stories in the history of the expedition was that, to everyone's surprise, when Sacagawea was called forth to speak to the chief of her tribe and participate in the English-French-Hidatsa-Shoshone translation chain, she recognized the chief as her brother, Cameahwait.

After obtaining the horses they needed to cross the "tremendous" Bitterroot mountain range, the expedition members began their long and sometimes treacherous journey, guided by a Shoshone man they named "Old Toby." The passage in mid-September was arduous. They were often cold, waking up to shake off a layer of snow on the blankets they slept under during the frigid nights, and they even had to resort to eating fat-based candles when they ran short on food.[67]

In mid-October 1805, the Corps reached the junction of the Columbia River, and on November 7 Clark triumphantly wrote, "Great joy in camp we are in View of the Ocian."[68] In actuality, Clark's view that day was of the estuary of the Columbia River, not the open Pacific Ocean. Once they reached the coast and had endured some of the most uncomfortably cold and wet weeks of the expedition, the group voted to construct their winter quarters on the southern side of the Columbia, which they named Fort Clatsop after the neighboring Indian tribe. The months of December 1805 to March 1806 proved to be wet, cold, and mostly miserable for the group.

Having grown thoroughly weary of the Pacific coastline in winter, on yet another rainy morning of March 23, 1806, the men of the Corps of Discovery with their loaded canoes bid a welcome farewell to their rainy and cold home of the past several months. By 1 p.m., the last remaining man stepped off the shore, pushed away from the riverbank, and once again headed upriver, this time on the Columbia, with their ultimate goal being to return to civilization, which by Clark's estimation was 4,134 miles away. Their return up the Columbia was both physically and emotionally demanding as the level of river flow in the spring was significantly more forceful and dangerous than it had been the previous fall. Some very negative interactions with various native tribes took place in April, the result of a clash between the stark difference in the values and personality of Lewis and those of some of the Pacific tribes.

By April 16, already noting the drier air, the Corps arrived at the beginning of the open prairie of today's eastern Oregon and Washington, which they successfully crossed. A demanding portage of the canoes on the falls at the Dalles began on April 18. As the Corps moved farther inland, nearly depleted of their trade goods, the Lewis and Clark medical clinic opened for business with surrounding tribes. The captains treated a variety of problems, from orthopedic issues to eye problems, with good common sense and a desire to do no harm. Captain Clark became the Indians' favorite doctor, likely due to his gregarious nature. Their treatments varied from "eye water," a mixture that may have helped irritated and infected eyes, to the application of soft flannel. In payment, they received food—chiefly in the form of horses and dogs.[69]

By May 3, the Corps had arrived in the territory of the Nez Perce tribe in modern-day Idaho. This tribe, which had rendered great help to them the previous fall, had kept their horses for the winter. Anxious to recross the Bitterroots, the Corps set out on June 15, a date that would prove to be too early. Even with the amazing outdoor skills of Drouillard, the high banks of snow that obliterated any sign of a trail on their first attempted ascent of the western slope of the Bitterroots forced the Corps to return to the Nez Perce villages and wait until some of the snowpack melted.

A new attempt to recross the mountains that Gass had called "the most terrible mountains I ever beheld"[70] started on June 24, 1806, this time with the help of three young Nez Perce braves who guided them expertly and more quickly over the rugged and often invisible trail that was covered with feet of snow. By June 29, they reached today's

Lolo Hot Springs, about thirty-four miles up the eastern slope from the Bitterroot valley floor and Traveler's Rest. After a several-day rest, the group divided into two. Lewis and his nine men would ascend the modern-day Blackfoot River valley and take a shortcut across the mountains suggested to them by their young Nez Perce guides. Clark and his group, heading toward the Three Forks area, would divide yet again. One small group, commanded by Sergeant Ordway, split off to regather supplies and canoes hidden along the Jefferson River and proceed down the Missouri to the Great Falls area with the intent of reconnecting with the Lewis-led group. Clark's main group traversed on foot from the area of Traveler's Rest to the southeast, across modern-day Bozeman Pass, to the confluence of the Yellowstone and Missouri Rivers, where the groups planned to meet sometime in early to mid-August.

Lewis's prime mission was to reconnoiter the Marias River and find its headwaters, or at least the general area from which they flowed. The fear of dividing the Corps was apparent in the voices and faces of their Nez Perce guides as they parted ways. Lewis noted that "these affectionate people our guides betrayed every emmotion of unfeigned regret at seperating from us; they said that they were confidint that the Pahkees [Blackfeet] would cut us off."[71] In light of what ultimately happened between Lewis and the "Pahkees," one must wonder how worried Lewis was about this unwelcome response. It would seem that Lewis's very high self-confidence eclipsed any fear he might have felt about this tribe. Given the reality of his numerous encounters with other either friendly or militarily weak tribes, his judgment at the time seemed to confirm his confidence in his ability to deal with any potential threat from any tribe. His confidence would nearly cost him and his men their lives.

During March–July 1806, several interactions illustrate Lewis's quick and significant temper. First, on April 11, 1806, Lewis's questionable judgment and anger were evident when some members of the Wah-clel-lar tribe stole his dog Seaman. Lewis "sent three men in pursuit of the thieves with orders if they made the least resistance or difficulty in surrendering the dog to fire on them." In addition, after discovering the theft of an axe from camp, Lewis ordered that all Indians be kept out of camp and that "if they made any further attempts to steal our property or insulted our men we should put them to instant death."[72]

Eight days later, Lewis, after ordering the expedition's horses to be hobbled and allowed to graze at their campsite in present-day Klickitat County, Washington, wrote that "one of the men Willard was negligent in his attention to his horse and suffered it to ramble off . . . this in addition to the other difficulties under which I labored was truly provoking. I reprimanded him more severely for this piece of negligence than had been usual with me."[73]

Two days later, upon discovering that the Indians had stolen "another tomahawk from us this morning," Lewis wrote,

> I surched many of them but could not find it. I ordered all spare poles, paddles and the balance of our canoe put on the fire as the morning was cold and also that not a particle should be left for the benefit of the indians. I detected a fellow in stealing an iron socket of a canoe pole and gave him several severe blows and mad the men kick him out of camp. I now informed the indians that I would shoot the first of them that attempted to steal an article from us . . . [and] that I had it in my power at that moment to kill them all and set fire to their houses but it was not my wish to treat them with severity provided they would let my property alone.[74]

On May 5, 1806, while peacefully seated and enjoying his dinner, Lewis reported that

> an indian fellow very impertinently threw a poor half starved puppy nearly into my plait by way of derision for our eating dogs and laughed very heartily at his own impertinence. I was so provoked at his insolence that I caught the puppy and threw it with great violence at him and struck him in the breast and face, seized my tomahawk and shewed him by signs if he repeated his insolence I would tomahawk him.[75]

In another incident, Lewis, George Drouillard, Joseph Fields, and Reuben Fields, while conducting their reconnaissance of the Marias River drainage, unexpectedly encountered on July 26, 1806, at least eight braves from the Blackfeet tribe at what has come to be known as the Two Medicine Fight Site. After an initially tense interaction in which Lewis utilized his best diplomatic skills, the group descended the grassy hills for a quarter of a mile to a flat meadow along the Two Medicine River, a tributary of the Marias River. They set up a campsite and, after supplying the Blackfeet with some smoking tobacco, Lewis communicated through Drouillard's sign language the surely unwelcome news about the new American control of the area.

Of all the sites we have visited along the Lewis and Clark Trail where one might feel a ghostly presence, this nearly treeless, roughly hilled area is the one that affects us the most. When we were last there in 2016, we felt as if we had been through a time machine. The scene of this violent encounter with the eight Blackfeet men appears today much the same as it would have looked at that time. With the journals in hand and a great thunderstorm brewing overhead, guided by Larry Epstein of Essex, Montana, former district attorney of Glacier County and past president of the Lewis and Clark Trail Heritage Foundation, we walked the surrounding hillsides, looked northward until the horizon vanished, and then descended the same hills that Lewis and the Blackfeet had descended to establish their campsite of July 26. As we walked, we frequently stopped and read Lewis's detailed description of the day from the journals with the slight feeling that we might find ourselves in the middle of the bloody incident of two hundred-plus years ago. It was definitely a bit eerie.

We believe that what transpired on July 27 illustrates not only Lewis's military demeanor but also his hot temper and his occasionally poor judgment. That Lewis would bring a group of only four armed men into a vast territory controlled by a powerful tribe that Lewis himself described as a "vicious lawless and reather an abandoned set of wretches"[76] was at best reckless. He had been warned on repeated occasions by other tribes about the "Pahkees" and knew better, or definitely should have, than to reconnoiter the area with an anemic force of four.

Early on the morning of July 27, Joseph Fields, who was supposed to be awake and standing guard, was instead snoozing and, as Lewis wrote, "had carelessly laid his gun down behind him near where his brother was sleeping, one of the indians the fellow to whom I had given the medal last evening sliped behind him and took his gun and that of his brothers unperceived by him, at the same instant two others advanced and seized the guns of Drewyer and myself."[77] Joseph yelled, awakening his brother Reuben, who chased the brave down and stabbed him in the chest, a wound that was quickly fatal, probably due to direct trauma to the man's heart or major veins and arteries in the area as well as at least one collapsed lung. Lewis, after chasing down two other Blackfeet who were attempting to steal horses, shot one of the young men "through the belly." In the chaos, these circumstances would have been described by both sides as self-defense—i.e., kill or be killed—so anger in these circumstances would be entirely normal, but the hostilities resulted in the loss of two lives and negated Lewis's attempted diplomacy of the previous evening.[78]

What is noteworthy about Lewis's anger during this incident is his prideful decision not to remove the Jefferson peace medal around the neck of one of the deceased Indians "that they might be informed who we were."[79] This arrogant action twisted a knife in the chest of the entire Blackfeet nation, who without question heard about this event within hours. Stephen Ambrose described this as "an act of taunting and boasting that put into serious jeopardy the entire American-empire scheme Lewis was concocting. To turn the most powerful tribe on the Upper Missouri into enemies of the United States was Lewis's biggest mistake."[80] We completely agree.

Within minutes, Lewis and his men were heading rapidly southeast toward their stated goal of the confluence of the Marias and Missouri Rivers. They pushed their horses "as hard as they would bear." They rode without delay except for a few hours' rest and covered nearly one hundred miles through vast herds of buffalo, often on a plain "as level as a bowling green with but little stone and few prickly pears." By late in the morning of July 28, Lewis wrote that "on arriving at the bank of the river [I] had the unspeakable satisfaction to see our canoes coming down."[81] The men in the canoes were the small group led by Sergeant Ordway that had gathered the Corps's cached supplies and portaged their canoes across the plains of the Great Falls while Lewis and his group left for their separate mission.

The final two months of the expedition, except for Lewis's receiving a bullet to his hind end (the result of a hunting accident caused by Pierre Cruzatte, who was blind in one eye, mistaking Lewis for an elk), were relatively smooth. He fully recovered from the wound within about three weeks. The Corps of Discovery returned to St. Louis on

September 23, 1806. This day marked the start of Lewis's meteoric rise in the consciousness of the American public. He became known far and wide for his achievements during the expedition.

Governor of Upper Louisiana Territory, 1806–1809 (Ages Thirty-Two to Thirty-Five)

After arriving in St. Louis on September 23, 1806, one of Lewis's first duties was to send President Jefferson a written report informing him that the expedition party had arrived back safely and that their mission had been successful. The enormity of this event, and its significance at that time in history, cannot be emphasized enough. It is no exaggeration to compare it to the American astronauts' safe return to Earth after they visited the moon in July 1969. Lewis and Clark became national heroes within weeks. Local townspeople a few miles upriver from St. Louis appeared to Clark to be competing for the attention of the newly arrived explorers. Within weeks, as the report of the expedition's arrival in St. Louis traveled throughout the new nation by boat or horseback, news of their safe return was published in newspapers across the country.

Between the time of the ink drying on Lewis's September 24 letter to Jefferson and December 28, 1806, when Jefferson welcomed the returning hero at the President's House, Lewis traveled first to the Charlottesville, Virginia, area to be reunited with his family and friends. All along Lewis's route, parties and celebrations were held in his honor. The exhilaration and incredible sense of accomplishment he felt during these days of public adulation must have been similar to that of the Apollo astronauts after their return to Earth.

Lewis spent the winter months of 1807 with Jefferson in the President's House, working on the accounting for the expedition and negotiating with politicians there to obtain compensation for his men. In March 1807, the Senate approved Jefferson's nomination of Lewis to become governor of the Upper Territory of Louisiana (and unfortunately rejected the nomination of Clark to officially receive a promotion to the rank of captain; this injustice was finally remedied in 2000 during the Clinton administration).[82]

From April to July 1807, Lewis spent time in Philadelphia, where his main goal was to arrange for the publication of the journals he and

Clark had kept throughout the course of the expedition. In this process, he met with the owner of a publishing and bookselling firm. He also met with some of the tutors who had mentored him there four years earlier, including Barton, who agreed to help compile the natural history volume. He visited with the famous portrait artist Charles Wilson Peale, who agreed to work on drawing the animals for Lewis's book and painted the portrait of Lewis that now hangs proudly in Independence Hall next to those of Washington and Jefferson in Independence National Historical Park in Philadelphia.[83] Lewis interspersed these professional engagements with social outings with his good friend Mahlon Dickerson. These outings most certainly included a great deal of personal adulation of Lewis for his heroic journey. After leaving Philadelphia, Lewis proceeded on to Virginia and to his Locust Hill plantation for a visit with family.

From there, in August 1807 Lewis traveled to Richmond, Virginia, where Jefferson had requested that he attend the trial of Aaron Burr. Burr at that time had finished serving as vice president during Jefferson's first term as president and had been accused by Jefferson and other government officials of conspiring to take control of New Orleans and then Mexico. In September 1807, Lewis returned to the Charlottesville area to inform Jefferson of the unwelcome news that Burr had been acquitted of all charges.[84] Between then and early November, Lewis is reported to have attended to matters related to his family's estate, including efforts to extend its size through the purchase of more land in the area of present-day Ohio.[85]

Lewis departed for St. Louis from his Locust Hill home in Ivy, Virginia, in early November 1807 with his younger brother Reuben, where Reuben would begin a career in the lucrative fur trading industry. Along the over 750-mile route, they stopped first at the end of November in Fincastle, Virginia, to visit George Hancock, the father of Julia, Clark's fiancée. They traveled on to Lexington, Kentucky, arriving there in mid-January 1808, and then reached Louisville by mid-February.[86] At the beginning of March, they arrived in St. Louis, where Lewis took over the reins of power from Frederick Bates, the territorial secretary, who had assumed the role of acting governor before Lewis's arrival.

The matters that most preoccupied Lewis for approximately the next year and a half, until he left St. Louis to travel to Washington, D.C., to settle financial disputes he had with the War Department, were related to Indian affairs. He was involved in resolving conflicts between the citizens and settlers of the Upper Louisiana Territory, whose aim was to push farther westward and claim more land, and the Indian tribes, who were determined not to move off their tribal lands. Lewis served as a mediator, striving to settle these disputes with reasonable negotiation strategies rather than through violence. Given his characteristic integrity and strong sense of responsibility, he aimed to try all nonviolent means of confrontation before having to resort to military intervention to try to balance the needs of the settlers to advance and the needs of the Indians (including the Osage, Shawnee, Delaware, Kickapoo, and Iowa) to resist encroachment onto their land.[87]

The thirty-seven-year-old Clark joined Lewis in St. Louis in the spring of 1808 with his new wife, sixteen-year-old Julia. Clark was there to take up his post as a territorial Indian agent. Without a doubt, Lewis would have been glad to partner up again with his expeditionary co-leader to tackle the challenges facing them.

But this period of time between March 1808 and August 1809 would prove to be the beginning of the end for Meriwether Lewis. Unlike many of Lewis's contemporaries, his life would not be cut short by an infectious disease nor as a result of Indian-White conflict. Stressors Lewis had not encountered previously when dealing with native tribes, near-death experiences on the expedition, or the difficulties of a military command were soon bombarding him during his governorship. Some of the key events that occurred in the year and a half of his governorship, which were the punches that had such destructive effects on him, were related to Frederick Bates and to the election of James Madison as the new president of the United States.

Although Frederick Bates was his "Masonic-brother," Bates's and Lewis's views of governing were almost constantly in conflict. In addition to policy differences, it appears that their personalities were like oil and water. Bates, the secretary of Upper Louisiana Territory, was undoubtedly more than a little insulted by having to step down from his role of acting governor when Lewis arrived to take over that position. Bates showed every indication of being a petty bureaucrat; he backstabbed Lewis repeatedly simply because he had the power to do so. The undermining effects of Bates's actions and words on Lewis's authority were immensely frustrating and personally insulting to Lewis. He undoubtedly viewed Bates as his subordinate in government and thus felt he had encountered the equivalent of a disrespectful and disobedient sergeant in the Corps of Discovery (and it is perfectly clear how such an interaction would have played out). The friction between Lewis and Bates became so intense that Clark had to intervene in June of 1809 at a Masonic Lodge ball. We only have Bates's version of the incident, but Lewis reportedly felt so insulted by Bates's apparent snubbing of him that he called on Clark for assistance. In a letter written to his brother Richard, Bates stated that

> the dances were now commencing—He [Lewis] also rose—evidently in passion, retired into an adjoining room and sent a servant for General Clark, who refused to ask me out as he foresaw that a Battle must have been the consequence of our meeting. He complained to the general that I had treated him with contempt and insult in the Ball-Room and that he could not suffer it to pass.[88]

The need for Clark to intervene in this situation and prevent a possible duel indicates that the inescapable and tormenting association with his assistant Bates represented a profound stressor in Lewis's life.

Until the end of Jefferson's second presidential term, Lewis enjoyed the support and understanding of Jefferson in substantial ways in all of his endeavors. Bills for expenditures— submitted by Lewis to the Jefferson led War Department to cover the costs of Lewis's territorial government—were reimbursed without question. All this changed after the 1808 election of James Madison as U.S. president and his appointment of William Eustis as the new secretary of war. In the spring of 1809, Eustis began to deny payment of drafts submitted by Lewis. Eustis, through his subordinate accountant, William Simmons, wrote Lewis a highly insulting letter, dated July 15, 1809, refusing payment for a substantial amount of requested funds.[89] Referring repeatedly to Lewis in the letter as "your Excellency," which was likely an insult, Eustis gave notice that the unquestioned support of the previous War Department was at an end. Lewis received this letter on August 18, 1809, his thirty-fifth birthday. Likely enraged and offended by this correspondence,

Lewis replied that same day. With undertones of restrained righteous indignation, he responded that the message he had received compelled him to do nothing short of departing for Washington, D.C., to represent himself and clear his name. Lewis wrote that he intended to leave "with all dispatch. . . . Be assured, Sir, that my Country can never make a Burr of me—She may reduce me to Poverty, but she can never sever my Attachment from her."[90]

In this same letter, Lewis wrote that the outstanding bills "from the Departments of War and Treasury have effectively sunk my Credit: brought in all my private debts amounting to about $4000, which has compelled me, in order to do justice to my Creditor, to deposit with them, the landed property which I had purchased in this Country, as Security."[91] Lewis undoubtedly could see the writing on the wall—his financial situation was dire and would only become worse if he did not go directly and immediately to the sources who were squeezing him more and more tightly.

Meriwether Lewis's Final Journey, September 4–October 11, 1809 (Age Thirty-Five)

The most important events during the last five weeks of Lewis's life are as follows. Lewis left St. Louis on September 4, 1809, on a boat filled with supplies he had purchased for his journey. A ledger that belonged to his physician, Dr. Antoine Saugrain, documents the purchase of medications by Lewis at the end of August 1809 (this included a total of forty-seven "purgative pills"). Dr. Saugrain is known to have prescribed medications for Lewis throughout the year and a half that Lewis resided in St. Louis.[92]

A critical entry by Lewis in his personal account book of private debts due, dated August 22, 1809, mentions an IOU to Isaac Miller for $202.87 1/2 cents. Lewis recorded other debts, but the entry of the debt to Mr. Miller is of particular interest. Several other authors have reproduced Lewis's account book of these same debts, but they have not identified the specific item Lewis purchased from Miller. We address this vitally important issue in chapter 4. Lewis is believed to have also packed several trunks containing clothes and weapons as well as the expedition journals with the apparent intent of taking the journal on to Philadelphia following his meetings with War Department officials in Washington, D.C.[93]

On August 25, 1809, Lewis's friend William Carr of St. Louis wrote a letter to his brother stating, "Our Governor left us a few days since with his private affairs altogether deranged. He is a good man, but a very imprudent one—I apprehend he will not return."[94] On September 11, after leaving St. Louis by boat, Lewis made out a will at Cape Girardeau. Between September 5 and 15, as crewmen on the boat reported to the commanding officer of Fort Pickering when they arrived there on September 16, Lewis was reported to have attempted suicide twice and had to be restrained by members of the crew.

Captain Gilbert Russell, the commanding officer at Fort Pickering, wrote several reports of Lewis's illness while at the fort. Upon his arrival at Fort Pickering, Russell reported, Lewis was observed to be in ill health, so Russell insisted that Lewis remain there for several days to recover. His first letter to Jefferson, written three months after the death of Lewis and dated January 4, 1810, was not specific regarding Lewis's illness. The second letter from Russell, dated January 31, 1810, explained in much greater detail that Lewis's illness was the result of "the free use of liquor," a fact that Lewis "acknowledged very candidly to me after his recovery."[95] Russell, according to his report to Jefferson, weaned him off of the effects of the liquor with a diet that included "claret & a little white wine"[96] (we cover Lewis's abuse of alcohol extensively in chapters 4 and 13). Russell noted that "on the sixth or seventh day all symptoms of derangement disappeared and he was completely in his senses—considerably reduced and debilitated."[97] Lewis wrote a letter to President Madison stating that he was "very much exhausted from the heat of the climate, but having [taken] medicine feel much better this morning. My apprehension from the heat of the lower country and my fear of the original papers relative to my voyage to the Pacific ocean falling into the hands of the British has induced me to change my rout and proceed by land through the state of Tennisee to the City of washington."[98]

On September 18, Major James Neelly, agent for the Chickasaw Nation, arrived at the fort and claimed that he had business in Nashville, and he reportedly offered to accompany Lewis along the Natchez Trace. On September 30, Lewis departed Fort Pickering with his servant John Pernier along with Neelly and his servant.

Tony Turnbow, an attorney in Franklin, Tennessee, has done excellent research on the personal character of Major Neelly. Neelly was the one who wrote the initial letter to Jefferson reporting the suicide of Lewis and is thus an important figure in this story. Turnbow established that Neelly, consistent with reports by both his son and Captain Russell, was a man who enjoyed the fiddle, dancing, and strong drink. Neelly was ultimately relieved of his duties in 1812 for drunkenness, indecent exposure to the Chickasaws, becoming intimate with a woman other than his wife, and self-dealing in land transactions.[99] His finances seemed to be in a constant state of chaos, which resulted in multiple lawsuits being filed against him. Russell, in a letter penned at the end of January 1810, noted that Neelly, "being extremely fond of liquor, instead of preventing the Govr from drinking or putting him under any restraint, advised him to it & from everything I can learn gave the man every chance to seek an opportunity to destroy himself."[100]

For three days, this group traveled about one hundred miles, and Russell later noted that Lewis's "resolution [never to drink again] left him."[101] Neelly later reported to Jefferson that upon their arrival at the Chickasaw Agency, Lewis "appeared at times deranged in mind."[102] They rested there for two days, into October 5. They then left on October 6 and traveled to the vicinity of the village of Collinwood, Tennessee, arriving on October 9.[103]

Lewis, Pernier, and Neelly's servant traveled alone from that site, according to Neelly, "with a promise to wait for me at the first house he Came to that was inhabited by white people."[104] In the afternoon of October 10, Lewis arrived at Grinder's Stand (a small inn). He reportedly checked in and asked for some whiskey but did not drink much of it. According to Mrs. Pricilla Grinder's report, Lewis's behavior was strange. Lewis would "would seem as if he were walking up to her, and would suddenly wheel round, and walk back as fast as he could." While seated at the dinner table, Grinder noted that Lewis was "speaking to himself in a violent manner."[105]

Early in the morning on October 11, Lewis reportedly shot himself twice. The first shot was reported as an apparent grazing scalp wound, and the second was a wound to either the chest or abdomen that exited in the lower back beside the spine. Grinder heard Lewis exclaim "O Lord!" after Lewis fell to the floor. After the second shot, Grinder noted that Lewis opened his door and called out to her, "O madam! Give me some water, and heal my wounds." Lewis reportedly survived until after daylight. The *Franklin Argus* reported that Lewis had used a knife to cut his own throat, and the *Nashville Clarion* referenced Lewis's cutting himself, but Grinder did not report that Lewis had cut himself (according to Alexander Wilson in a letter to Alexander Lawson dated May 18, 1810, recounting his interview with Pricilla Grinder).[106] After Lewis called out to her, Grinder sent her children to get the servants, who were sleeping in quarters nearby. Pernier arrived at the scene, and Lewis reportedly asked him for some water, saying, "I have done the business my good Servant. . . . I am no coward; but I am so strong, [it is] so hard to die."[107]

Sometime after daybreak, within a few hours of the gunshots, Lewis died.

Those who do not believe that Lewis committed suicide have cited multiple arguments against his suicide. Points of attack on the suicide theory include the unreliability of Neelly's and Grinder's reports; Neelly's poor character; the reported wounds suffered by Lewis, both in terms of being self-inflicted and the length of time he survived; and the report that Lewis was drinking and was mentally deranged. Some supporters of the murder theory suggest that Neelly was involved in the murder of Lewis because of his questionable character. Gilbert Russell stated that Lewis landed at Fort Pickering on September 15 in a state of mental derangement that "appeared to have been produced as much by indisposition as other causes."[108] This is of interest. Why was Lewis so sick? Was his poor state of health caused by malaria? Syphilis? Mercury poisoning? Was Lewis depressed, as has been alleged by many? What did Lewis have to be depressed about? Did Lewis suffer from bipolar disorder? Wasn't Lewis, as one author has asserted, an "anti-suicide type"? Many have used various angles of attack to deny that Lewis had a problem with alcohol. Did Lewis become emotionally unhinged, the result of posttraumatic stress disorder acquired during the expedition, a theory put forward by David Nicandri in *River of Promise*, or did he return to St. Louis in 1806 emotionally intact (as Stephen Ambrose argues)? Some Lewis and Clark enthusiasts believe that the Natchez Trace was a dangerous place and that Lewis was murdered and that Pricilla Grinder was involved in the coverup. Some believe that General Wilkinson, the commander of the U.S. Army at the time of Lewis's death, was involved in a plot to murder Lewis because Lewis knew damaging information about him and was going to Washington to "spill the beans" to the federal government—a theory for which there is no reliable evidence, so we will spend little time on it.

Each of these factors has been addressed from multiple angles. We note that other authors have done outstanding work in their analyses of these issues. But, these points of contention have never been analyzed by a physician and a clinical psychologist. We thus have something new to contribute to this argument. The remainder of this book will document in detail our appraisal of all these issues, and you can decide for yourself how you believe Meriwether Lewis died in October 1809.

Chapter 3
Philosophical Influences on Meriwether Lewis: Thomas Jefferson and the Enlightenment

> *No conclusions can be more agreeable to scepticism than such as make discoveries concerning the weakness and narrow limits of human reason and capacity.*
> —David Hume, Enlightenment philosopher

In our effort to appreciate the entire life and personality of Meriwether Lewis, it is necessary to briefly examine some of the important cultural influences operating within his life and times. The philosophical thinking of Aristotle and other ancient Greeks and the development of philosophical thinking that had laid dormant for many centuries were resurrected during the humanistic awakening of European academics in the fifteenth and sixteenth centuries. Since the disintegration of the Roman Empire in the fifth century, European scholars had lacked exposure to and knowledge of ancient Greek texts on medicine, science, and philosophy. After the defeat of the Islamic forces at the Battle of Tours in 732, European knowledge of ancient Greek learning started to reemerge in the late eleventh and twelfth centuries and fully blossomed into a great resurgence during the Italian Renaissance. This movement ultimately spread across Europe during the fourteenth through sixteenth centuries. Translations from Greek of the Hermetic Corpus fueled the development of alchemy in Europe, and other ancient writings were translated into Latin, chiefly by Roman Catholic scholars. This was also the era of the Scientific Revolution, generally accepted by historians of science as occurring between 1500 and 1700.[1]

Due to this new infusion of ancient Greek learning into European culture, Greek philosophical thinking about the use of human reason was reapplied to Christian thinking by the great Catholic theologian Thomas Aquinas (1274–1323). Aristotelian and Platonic influences increased the dependence on human reason in biblical interpretation, but Aquinas still gave biblical revelation and church-formulated doctrines priority over reason in arriving at an accepted theological conclusion.

Some historians equate the onset of the European Enlightenment with the beginning of the Scientific Revolution. They reference the natural philosophical work of Bacon, Copernicus, Galileo, Descartes, Leibniz, and Newton, along with the Protestant Reformation and the invention of the printing press, as the inciting events that caused an intellectual reevaluation of the reality of both the physical and philosophical worlds. The Enlightenment, which was highly influential in the lives of Lewis and his contemporaries, was full of optimism about the future of the human race. It was a heady time of tremendous scientific discoveries that seemingly promised great human progress and happiness.

René Descartes was a remarkable figure due to his vast talents in philosophy, mathematics, and other scientific fields. He believed that only through applied scientific progress would the human race be able to achieve "freedom, autonomy, and self-realization," which was Descartes's idea of human happiness.[2] Toward the end of his life, Descartes, exhibiting some of his optimistic self-confidence, believed that "given sufficient research funding, he would be able to solve all the outstanding problems of physiology [the study of the function of the human body] and learn thereby the cures of all diseases."[3] Even though humans have traveled nearly four hundred years further along the path of scientific discovery, we are still nowhere near Descartes's predicted scientific outcome.

Due to this proliferation of human scientific knowledge, the Enlightenment was also the age when scientific societies appeared throughout Europe, and their members shared their discoveries with other natural philosophers and physicians. Although much scientific progress was seen, particularly in the fields of math and physics, medicine languished in a seemingly hopeless quagmire. The British medical profession aggressively treated their patients with often harmful medications and procedures, while the French medical system was busily making observations of the sick in an effort to discover the causes of various diseases. With the English stressing treatment over theoretical knowledge and the French medical establishment emphasizing theory and clinical observation of patients, the English often killed their patients with unneeded and dangerous interventions and the French simply observed their patients until they died.

Topics considered by Enlightenment philosophers extended beyond the bounds of natural philosophy (the physical and biological sciences) to philosophical topics such as how humans think, reason, arrive at truth, and consider the substance and meaning of their lives. Truths that had been accepted for centuries came under the scrutiny of human reason, often with contrasting results; the Enlightenment thinkers did not represent a monolithic point of view. The new tidal wave of human philosophical analysis washed over nonscientific fields as well. Great philosophers of the Enlightenment, such as the German Immanuel Kant (1724–1804), who wrote the influential book *Critique of Pure Reason* (1781), did not agree with the dire skepticism expressed by the Scottish philosopher David Hume (1711–76) in his work *A Treatise of Human Nature* (1739). The medical mechanists, whose theories viewed the body as simply a sophisticated machine, fought over treatment and philosophy with the vitalists and their view of a spiritual component to life.

In the end, the Enlightenment thinkers believed that their input into human thinking and knowledge would profoundly change the world for the better. They believed that human reason would result in liberty, progress, religious toleration, and fraternity and would vastly improve the human situation.

The youthful Thomas Jefferson's introduction to Enlightenment thinking came by way of a much respected and loved professor at the College of William and Mary, Dr. William Small of Scotland.

Sixteen-year-old Jefferson entered this college in Williamsburg, Virginia, in March of 1760, where he met this professor who had a dramatic effect on the course of his life. Dr. Small taught math and natural and moral philosophy and was heavily influenced by European thinkers such as Kant, Bacon, Locke, Newton, and philosophers of the Scottish Enlightenment. Jefferson's biographer Jon Meacham notes that Small "introduced Jefferson to the key insight of the new intellectual age; that reason, not revelation or unquestioned tradition or superstition, deserved pride of place in human affairs." Small's profound influence on Jefferson is reflected in Jefferson's comments that his beloved professor was "to me . . . a father."[4]

In the early America of Jefferson and Lewis, orthodox Christianity was involved in philosophical battles with Deists, who believed that God had wound up the universe and stepped away from the creation and its control. Deists favored the belief in one God but rejected the Bible as a book given by divine revelation, demoting its teachings from authoritative and God-given to the category of mythology. Controversies swirled among other groups as well. Roman Catholics were at theological odds with Protestants and vice versa. Monarchists attacked Republicans.

Thomas Paine, whose pamphlet *Common Sense* (1776) had galvanized colonial American attitudes against Britain during the Revolutionary War, likely under the influence of British Deists, wrote a scathing review of orthodox Christianity in his 1794–95 work entitled *The Age of Reason*. Although originally written for the French during their revolution, Paine's work became popular reading in America when Meriwether Lewis was a young adult. Paine and Jefferson established a longtime friendship in 1786 during Jefferson's diplomatic stay in Paris. However, America's culture in the late 1790s was not the same as it had been in 1776. Paine's diatribe against Christianity was so vitriolic that even Jefferson, once he was elected president in 1801, gave him the brush-off. In a critical letter, Ben Franklin rebuked Paine with his own scathing comments, writing, "He who spits in the wind spits in his own face. . . . If men are wicked with religion, what would they be without it?"[5] It has been reported that every American founding father ultimately renounced Paine and that only six people showed up for his funeral in 1809.[6]

Jefferson, during his years in France (1784–89), enjoyed nearly constant interaction with French society in salon conversations and his developing friendships with leading French thinkers. This all served to further his hoped-for benefits of the Enlightenment, which were ultimate human freedom, religious toleration, republicanism, and scientific progress to improve the human condition.

Considering the large amount of time that Meriwether Lewis spent with Jefferson at both Monticello and in Washington, Jefferson without a doubt would have recommended various Enlightenment texts for Meriwether to read. These would have included the writings of the Enlightenment figures mentioned in this chapter. Given Lewis's association with various of Jefferson's contemporaries in Washington and with his Philadelphia-based scientific tutors (Madison, Ellicott, Patterson, Barton, and Rush; see chapter 2), the Enlightenment emphasis on observation of nature and reliance on the scientific method and human reason would have been integral to his thinking.

One of Jefferson's French contacts, the Marquis de Condorcet, "believed the destinies of America and of France were bound up with each other"; he added, "Everything tells us that we are bordering the period of one of the greatest revolutions of the human race. The present state of enlightenment guarantees that it will be happy."[7] Judging from what happened in the French Revolution during the reign of terror in 1793–94 and the world's sad history since that date, it is impossible to argue that his statement is accurate.

The personality of Thomas Jefferson is connected in various ways to the story of Meriwether Lewis. Jefferson was in many ways the proverbial enigma wrapped in a mystery. He was a devoted idealist, but when it suited his purposes he became an arch pragmatist. It is probably the most generous conclusion to note that his acts often did not align with his stated principles. Jefferson accomplished some great advances for humanity when he wrote the Declaration of Independence and penned the words "all men are created equal." Yet, the same Jefferson who reportedly disagreed with the institution of slavery nevertheless owned slaves, and although he freed two during his lifetime and five in his will, most of the African Americans he owned continued in slavery after his death.[8] Many historians have generously argued that these issues in Jefferson's life show that he was "complicated" and sometimes "contradictory." We believe his life effectively illustrates the inability of human reason to achieve its stated purposes.

Jefferson's life, attitudes, behavior, and inconsistencies are significant because he likely had a profound effect on the thinking and worldview of Meriwether Lewis and Lewis's apparent rejection of his mother's Christian faith (this topic is covered in detail in chapter 7). There can be little doubt that Lewis heard numerous lectures from Jefferson regarding these issues and adopted a great deal of Jefferson's philosophy for his own personal mantra during his stay with the president in 1801–02. What we wouldn't give for the opportunity to attend dinner parties at Monticello or the President's House in Washington, sip a glass of Jefferson's imported French wine, and participate in the discussions among Jefferson, Lewis, and Madison.

Due to his enormous infatuation with the Enlightenment as well as the work of scientists, during the final year of his stay in Paris (1789) Jefferson made contacts with art dealers with the goal of obtaining either paintings or plaster busts of the men who were in his opinion the greatest to have ever lived. Once he returned to Virginia, these works of art would allow him to bring the images of these savants home with him to Monticello.

Who were these members of Jefferson's elite, his intellectual Hall of Fame, his philosophical mentors and heroes? They were Francis Bacon, John Locke, Isaac Newton, and Voltaire.

Francis Bacon (1561–1626)

Bacon is perhaps most remembered as the politician/philosopher who described and encouraged the use of the scientific method to investigate natural phenomena. This investigative process is based on the assumption that the answer to any natural philosophical question can be arrived at through the process of forming an initial explanation of the problem to be explored (a hypothesis), then designing a process (experiment) by which data is gathered, and finally interpreting the data to form a conclusion. The conclusion either supports the original hypothesis or provides evidence against it. Bacon's method put into question the validity of some of Aristotle's method of argument based on pre-accepted facts, which was accepted by some academics as a legitimate tool for arriving at the truth. For Bacon, Aristotle and his scholastic methods were out. The scientific method became all the rage.

Bacon, as was true for many other European natural philosophers before and after him, was not quite in line with some of the Enlightenment's anti-religious dogma. Bacon believed it was necessary to learn about the natural world as a contribution to the magnifying of God's glory. With this goal in mind, his plea for the growth of scientific knowledge is understandable.[9]

Bacon's method of inductive reasoning is illustrated by the following; "Five thousand crows were examined from various parts of the world and all were found to be black . . . therefore all crows are black." This statement progresses from a particular statement to a general statement of truth. Deductive reasoning, on the other hand, proceeds from a general statement and ends with a particular statement, such as, "All men are mortal. Francis Bacon is a man. Therefore, Francis Bacon is mortal." Bacon's scientific method relied on the former design, on experimentally obtained data (particular data), and he used that information to reach a general conclusion.

As mentioned, this method directly threatened the age-old scholastic method in which disputation was carried out to satisfy an already accepted conclusion. This type of reasoning was viewed by Enlightenment figures as an example of superstition. For example, Aristotle believed and taught that heavier objects, when dropped from a height, would fall faster than lighter ones. This was an accepted truth. Aristotelians would argue the case using various philosophical reasonings, without any reliance on actual experimental data. No experiment needed be done, from this point of view, and thus Aristotle did not do any. So, higher education prior to the introduction of the scientific inductive method simply accepted Aristotle's philosophical conclusions as fact. When Galileo dropped two objects of different weights and noted that they hit the earth simultaneously, Aristotle's scholastic method was doomed. This was in part why the science of Galileo ran into trouble; his experiments and mathematics disproved the accepted Aristotelian view of reality.

John Locke (1632–1704)

An English philosopher and medical researcher, John Locke is the author of *An Essay Concerning Human Understanding* (1689), which is considered one of the great defenses of modern empiricism. The book addressed the limits of human understanding concerning a variety of topics. In addition to scientific works, Locke also published *The Second Treatise of Government*, in which he argued that "sovereignty resides in the people and explains the nature of legitimate government in terms of natural rights and the social contract."[10] From his work sprang the ideas of human cultural equality and the novel idea that kings and nobles were no better than the commoners. Locke believed that government should be the institution to manage the happiness of humankind. Kings should be the servants of the people they rule. It is no accident that Locke's ideas were pointing more and more toward Jefferson's thinking as well as the content of Jefferson's Declaration of Independence.

Isaac Newton (1642-1727)

Newton's pioneering work in physics not only set the standard for that basic science but also encouraged philosophical applications to medicine through the establishment of the medical mechanists, another example of humanity's medical misadventures. His influence on scientists' thinking about the natural world and the development of mathematical tools with which to explore it was profound. Newton's reliance on the use of mathematical and reason-based evidence must have attractive to a man of Jefferson's mentality. Newton's genius was manifested in many fields, from his discovery of calculus to his work in optics, gravity, alchemy, and theology (Newton's theology was unorthodox), and his genius no doubt qualified him for induction into Jefferson's group of elite individuals.

Voltaire (1694-1778)

François-Marie d'Arouet was better known by his pen name, Voltaire. His often witty writing attacked the philosophy that this world was the best of all possible worlds as proclaimed by the optimism of his fellow Enlightenment philosopher and mathematician Gottfried Leibniz. Many of Voltaire's political viewpoints were displayed in his book *Lettres Philosophiques* (1733), with its scathing comments on the French government. He was a great supporter of the scientific method and believed science would banish the forces of fanaticism and superstition and all the human ills that proceeded from these perversions of goodness. His religious views were highly critical of orthodox Protestant and Roman Catholic practices. Voltaire, like Jefferson and many other early Americans, was a Deist. Because of his maverick beliefs, he became a philosophical outlaw in eighteenth-century France. Voltaire supported and popularized a synthesis of British and French philosophies in support of Newtonian science.[11]

Voltaire's support of liberty, hedonism, and skepticism (expressed in his hostility to clerical and church authority) was an attitude that Jefferson held throughout his life. Jefferson's "epicurean" life philosophy—that the highest good is "to be not pained in body, nor troubled in mind"—seems to reflect European Enlightenment thinking.[12] Jefferson so respected Voltaire's philosophy that he had Voltaire's bust installed at Monticello next to the paintings of the above three luminaries.

The thinking of each of these four men would have undoubtedly, through a process of philosophical osmosis, had an influence to some degree on the life of Meriwether Lewis. Jefferson was a rationalist, Anglophobe, religious maverick, and believer in the ultimate ability of human reason and the scientific method to find the answers of life, and Lewis, we believe, shared these personality characteristics of his mentor.

Some of the aspects of the European Enlightenment, such as religious skepticism and undying faith in the ability of human reason to understand all realities, were not expressed by every enlightened thinker. Virtually every noteworthy European scientist during the Scientific Revolution was devoutly religious.[13] Some of the luminaries of American science and medicine, such as Dr. Benjamin Rush, were orthodox and devout Christians even though they believed in the importance of observation and scientific investigation in the attainment of scientific knowledge. The common thread in the lives of all leading thinkers of that era, who are also figures in our story of Meriwether Lewis, was their emphasis on using human reason to observe, describe, and formulate scientifically based areas of study of the physical world.

Enlightenment influences on Lewis during his adulthood were saturated with voices that challenged previously accepted thinking about politics, religion, and the natural world and stressed the value and importance of societal improvement along with the importance of individual liberty, scientific (natural philosophical) progress, and democratic values—all achieved through the application of human reason. The most influential voice on these issues that Lewis heard was that of Thomas Jefferson, whose unfettered faith in the goodness of human nature and the reliability of human reason was certainly manifested in Lewis himself. It is not possible to determine whether Jefferson's influence changed Lewis into a kindred spirit or whether Lewis and Jefferson were already of the same mind by the time Lewis arrived in Washington in 1801. In either case, it is difficult to underestimate the influence of Jefferson on Lewis's thinking. Jefferson's influence likely contributed to the formation of Lewis's worldview, which not only colored his view of reality and human nature but influenced his personality and his reactions to his later life circumstances.

A profoundly influential aspect of American culture, one based in substance and not in philosophy, is the next stop along our path of the story of Meriwether Lewis. The next chapter addresses the topic of alcohol in early America and in the life of Meriwether Lewis in particular.

Chapter 4
Intoxication Nation: Meriwether Lewis and Alcohol

Drink does not drown Care, but waters it, and makes it grow faster.
—*Benjamin Franklin*

Many historical events of Lewis's time, when viewed through the lens of a person living today, may be judged inaccurately and without appreciation of the reality of the situation for people living in that era. Perhaps none of the cultural differences between that world and our own is as profound as the difference regarding the drinking of alcoholic beverages. Due to our removal by over two centuries from the world of Lewis and Clark and the changes in how American culture views the use of alcohol, we run the risk of seriously underestimating its use and its effects on the world in which Meriwether Lewis lived his entire life.

The effects of alcohol on the body are of paramount importance in our story about Meriwether Lewis. Many authors (including my own superficial coverage of this topic in *Or Perish in the Attempt*) have written about Lewis's possible problems with alcohol. Some have completely discounted any possibility that Lewis was a heavy drinker. Responding to Captain Gilbert Russell's report that Lewis's death "may be attributed solely to the free use of liquor," James Starrs and Kira Gale wrote in *The Death of Meriwether Lewis* that "Lewis had absolutely no history of alcohol abuse," adding later that any drinking toward the end of his life "had to be quite an exceptional matter for him. His worst enemy, Frederick Bates, never once said that Lewis had any kind of drinking or drug problem."[1] John Guice admitted that Lewis drank alcohol some in his testimony at the coroner's jury concerning Lewis's death in 1996, noting, "We know from letters to his buddies, we know he'd been drinking a little bit."[2] Others propose that Lewis was a heavy drinker but seem to excuse or attempt to minimize his alcohol intake by noting that many men during that time also drank a lot—as if that would make a difference in the outcome of alcohol abuse. How much truth is contained in these authors' opinions about Lewis and his use of alcohol?

Of all the subjects we researched in the writing of this book, we were most surprised by the utterly amazing extent to which alcohol influenced early American culture. This aspect of the cultural history of early America is a huge piece of the jigsaw puzzle of Lewis's life.

This is not to imply that alcohol has little influence on our modern society. During my (David's) career in medicine, I saw hundreds of patients with alcohol-related problems, and Marti has treated the psychological ramifications of alcohol abuse for over thirty years. In 2018, more than eighty-eight thousand people in America and 1.8 million worldwide died from alcohol-related causes. Estimates vary, but public health officials surmised that in 2020 fifteen to twenty million people could be diagnosed with alcohol use disorder in the United States, based on the parameters in the *Diagnostic and Statistical Manual of Mental Disorders* (DSM-5) of the American Psychiatric Society. In 2018, an additional sixty-five million Americans reported binge drinking in the past month, and the majority of those were men.[3] Alcohol abuse results in multisystem organ damage; it affects nervous, gastrointestinal, cardiac, musculoskeletal, hematologic (blood), and metabolic processes, and it plays an important role in a significant number of both chronic illnesses and suicides.

The Making of Ethanol Beverages

In discussing alcohol abuse, it is important to understand how the alcohol within various alcohol-containing drinks is produced. The basic concept of producing alcohol is fairly simple. Alcoholic drinks come in two basic varieties. The weaker of the two types is fermented, including beer, wine, and hard cider. The much stronger "ardent spirits," to use Dr. Rush's phrase, are rum, vodka, gin, tequila, whiskey, brandy, and applejack. Drinks in the former category have an alcohol content that is generally between 8 and 15 percent, and the latter have an absolute alcohol content ranging from as low as 20 percent to theoretically nearly 100 percent (200 proof). Distilled beverages such as rum and whiskey have an alcohol content of approximately 40 percent, but it can be higher if the distiller so desires.

Fermented drinks are produced by the action of living yeast organisms that metabolize (change) simple sugars obtained through the breakdown of starches present in various cereal grains, usually barley for beer or a type of fruit (such as grapes, apples, pears, currants, chokecherries, or elderberries) for wine or hard cider. As the yeast metabolizes the sugars (in the absence of oxygen), one of the resulting products is ethyl alcohol, also known as ethanol. In beer making, a mixture called a mash is made of heated water, grain, hops (for flavor), and any desired additional flavoring and yeast.

In early America, various types of beers were produced at home, usually by the women of the house. They used various fruits for flavoring and did not use hops as hops in rural areas was scarce (hops were difficult to grow, particularly when tobacco, a very labor-intensive crop, was being tended to by the men of the family). As the alcohol content increases in beer and wine during fermentation, or as the sugar content decreases due to fermentation, the yeast either dies as a result of the increased presence of alcohol or runs out of sugar and the alcohol fermentation ends, resulting in a beverage of alcohol content from 4 to 18 percent.

If a distiller decides to distill "ardent spirits," the mash mixture is heated to a temperature at which the ethanol will reach its boiling point (173.1°F for ethanol vs. 212°F for water), and then the liquid ethanol boils off and becomes a gas. This gaseous ethanol rises into the collecting tubules of the still, where it cools and condenses, thus turning once again into liquid ethanol. The concentrated ethanol is ultimately collected and is either distilled again or is aged in charred oak barrels to make whiskey. Whiskey, apparently one of Meriwether Lewis's favorite alcoholic beverages, can be produced from a variety of ingredients, including barley, corn, rye, and wheat.

How Ethanol Affects the Human Body

When an alcoholic beverage is consumed, the ethanol that is present in it passes easily and readily from the stomach and small intestine into the bloodstream and is distributed by the blood into all bodily tissues in proportion to its concentration in the blood. About 10 percent of the alcohol in the body is passed out unchanged in sweat, urine, and breath. The presence of alcohol in the breath provides one way to test the amount of alcohol in the bloodstream. In this test, the person blows through a testing device, such as the type provided by a friendly law enforcement officer by the side of a road. The legal limit for being an intoxicated noncommercial driver in the United States is a blood alcohol level of 0.08 percent. This limit is usually reached, in a 160-pound male, by drinking either two mixed drinks (containing 1.5 ounces of 80-proof liquor), two twelve-ounce bottles of beer, five ounces of 12 percent wine, or three ounces of 80-proof straight "ardent spirits."[4]

Once the ethanol is present in the blood and begins flowing away from the gastrointestinal system (stomach and intestines), it passes first through the liver and then into the general circulation (bloodstream). The blood carries the ethanol throughout the body. Some of the ethanol easily traverses the capillary walls of the blood vessels supplying the brain (the so-called blood-brain barrier), enters the brain, and acts on brain neurons in a similar fashion to general anesthetics.

Chronic alcohol abusers can tolerate higher blood alcohol levels than nondrinkers. In large part, this ability is due to the chronic alcohol abuser metabolizing the alcohol more quickly than the teetotaler.[5] The ability to more rapidly metabolize ethanol is a result of the liver's supply of alcohol-metabolizing enzymes (alcohol dehydrogenases), which metabolize and inactivate the alcohol molecules. These enzymes build up slowly over months in response to high alcohol intake so that frequent heavy drinkers are able to tolerate a blood alcohol level that would kill a teetotaler.

I (David) vividly remember a patient I saw who presented to our clinic after falling and injuring themself. The person's speech was slurred, and they smelled of ethanol. After my exam, and since there was no history or physical evidence of a head injury from the fall, my suspicion of their intoxication was confirmed when their blood alcohol level was measured at over 0.3 percent. This person was a chronic alcohol abuser and was able to function reasonably well with a very high blood alcohol content, one that would have put many nondrinkers into a stupor.

Is there a relatively simple method by which a level of intoxication can be predicted? Yes, there is. It was formulated during Prohibition (ironically) by a talented Hungarian immigrant named Alexander Gettler who loved chemistry and worked himself through college and graduate school to get his Ph.D. from Columbia University. From there, he became a forensic chemist with the New York City Coroner's Office during Prohibition. Gettler noted that "no other poison causes so many deaths or leads to or intensifies so many diseases, both physical and mental, as does alcohol in the many forms in which it is taken."[6] Many of the bodies brought to his morgue were people who had died due to drunkenness—the result of alcohol poisoning or fatal injuries received during a state of intoxication. Gettler and his assistants performed exacting experiments on the brains of those whose deaths were noted in some way to be associated with alcohol and correlated their findings with observed behaviors prior to death as noted by a physician, police officer, or other observers.[7]

Gettler's studies over a period of years yielded the following results, with the number of plus signs signifying levels of drunkenness ranging from the least intoxicated (+) to the most intoxicated (++++). His results provide a quick overview of the effects of intoxication.

- \+ In all cases in which there was an alcoholic content of the brain below 0.1 percent, the patients showed no obvious alcohol impairment.
- ++ From 0.1 to 0.25 percent blood alcoholic content. Subjects showed slight inebriation; they were a little more aggressive than normal, a little less cautious in their behaviors.
- +++ From 0.25 to 0.4 percent blood alcoholic content. In the hours before death, subjects were unsteady on their feet, loud, and judged drunk by everyone who saw them.
- ++++ From 0.4 to 0.6 percent alcoholic content. These subjects had died after becoming falling-down drunk. They had consumed so much liquor that they succumbed to ethyl alcohol poisoning, usually within several hours after reaching a hospital.[8]

Using Gettler's standards to assess my former patient with a lab-documented 0.3 blood alcohol level, the individual in my memory was someone who would be "judged drunk by everyone." If we apply this scale to a member of the U.S. military in early America who was given four ounces of hard liquor as a daily ration, that amount of alcohol would have likely put the soldier into the ++ category, with a 0.10–0.25 blood alcohol content resulting in "slight inebriation, a little more aggressive than normal, a little less cautious in their behaviors." This amount would be sufficient to qualify them as a drunk driver today.

Drinking alcohol was part of American military culture during this era; troops were furnished with sufficient hard liquor every day (when available) to make them observably alcohol impaired. Considering that some U.S. Naval Special Warfare Command troops (SEAL team members) were recently disciplined for drinking while on deployment during off-duty hours, the *routine* supplying of hard liquor furnished by their commanders to early American troops seems rather scandalous today. The desired effect was no doubt appreciated by U.S. Army officers as they lined up their troops to march into fire directed at them from close quarters during Revolutionary War battles. It would certainly help a line of American infantrymen to stand strong against an oncoming line of Redcoats and make them "a little less cautious in their behaviors," as the above scale puts it. This practice continued into the days when Meriwether Lewis joined the Virginia Militia and then became a member of the U.S. Army.

Other effects of alcohol fall outside of Gettler's intoxication formula. Ethanol in low doses acts to decrease social inhibitions, influencing normally quiet and shy people to magically become talk show hosts at cocktail parties. Others react differently and may become hostile and belligerent. Increasing amounts of alcohol result in progressively slowed reaction times and loss of physical coordination, as shown by drivers taking roadside tests who are unable to walk a straight line heel to toe. It is important to note that significant intoxication can lead to an acute psychotic state. The severely intoxicated person can lose touch with reality and suffer from visual hallucinations and paranoia—suspicion and mistrust of others.

With continued drinking, as the blood alcohol level rises, many negative things happen to the body. High blood pressure, heart arrhythmias, dehydration, stupor (at 0.3 percent), and coma may follow. If the victim drinks excessive amounts of alcohol quickly, the blood alcohol content will continue to rise after they lose consciousness. When the level rises to above approximately 0.5 percent, the medulla of the brain—which controls vital life functions like breathing, swallowing, and heart-related functions—fails and death from alcohol poisoning is the sad result. On average, six people die every day in the United States from ethanol poisoning, with most of those being men between the ages of thirty-five and sixty-four.[9] This can be a very sad fate for teenagers who are experimenting with binge drinking and do not realize that they might pay the ultimate price for their ignorance and experimentation.

It is worth noting here that chronic alcohol abusers often suffer from malnutrition, particularly in the B vitamins. The brain is particularly sensitive to vitamin B deficiency, which predisposes to significant mental disorders such as Wernicke-Korsakoff syndrome, which leads to symptoms of psychosis and confusion and visual changes (double vision). Difficulty walking and controlling the eye muscles may occur in about 1 percent of chronic alcoholics and is due to damage to the brain's cerebellum region that controls muscle coordination.

I doubt that Lewis was exhibiting a classic case of Wernicke-Korsakoff in his final days when he exhibited his state of "mental derangement" as his symptoms can be assigned to other more likely causes. However, as a physician, if I wanted to provide the Lewis and Clark world with yet another novel medical theory concerning possible medical issues that Lewis suffered from, this syndrome would be a good candidate to exploit.[10]

A much-feared result of chronic alcohol abuse that results from the sudden cessation of drinking after prolonged abuse is seen in a minority of alcohol abusers. This problem is called delirium tremens (DT) and involves profound changes in the brain and body. Symptoms of DT usually occur within two to four days after the person had their last drink (in chronic alcoholics), as well as in alcoholics who suffer head injuries, illness, or infection. The symptoms include

- a sudden state of confusion
- body tremors
- changes in mental function
- agitation, irritability
- deep sleep that lasts for a day or longer
- excitement or fear

- hallucinations (seeing or hearing things that are not real)
- quick mood changes
- restlessness
- sensitivity to light, sound, and touch
- fatigues, stupor, or sleepiness
- hyperthermia
- irregular heart rhythms
- seizures[11]

The person's restlessness may progress to the point of violence, and they may need to be physically restrained to avoid injury to themself or others. Sedative medication may be necessary to calm the patient, and dehydration may require intravenous fluids. The sedatives that are used today commonly include members of the benzodiazepine family of drugs (e.g., diazepam, lorazepam). This is an important topic in relation to Meriwether Lewis, and we address it in chapter 14.

Disease in multiple organ systems is prominent in cases of chronic alcohol abuse. The pancreas, which controls many aspects of digestion, is often directly poisoned by high levels of alcohol. The pancreas consequently may become inflamed, leading to significant abdominal and back pain, nausea and vomiting, and the release from damaged pancreatic cells of digestive enzymes (amylase and lipase). Patients who present to an emergency room and receive a diagnosis of acute pancreatitis often have gotten the disease from binging on alcohol.

Alcohol is toxic to the heart muscle as well. Severe binge drinking may cause heart failure. Prolonged abuse over time can cause the heart muscle to enlarge and thus become less efficient in pumping blood (cardiomyopathy). Alcoholics also run an increased chance of developing various types of cancers. Chronic alcohol abuse has a negative effect as well on the body's immune system, decreasing its ability to fight off disease.

Alcohol abuse also affects the kidneys. Excessive binge drinking is probably the greatest threat to the health of the kidneys. The kidneys filter the blood, removing metabolic byproducts such as urea (from protein metabolism), and maintain tight control on the pH of the blood by monitoring both acidic hydrogen ions ($H+$) and basic bicarbonate ions ($HCO3-$). The kidneys also monitor and control the blood levels of many important electrolytes (potassium, chloride, sodium, magnesium, calcium) that allow nerves and muscles to function properly. Drinking alcohol temporarily puts to sleep the kidneys' control of the hydration of the body by decreasing the brain's output (from the pituitary gland) of a hormone that influences how much liquid is reabsorbed into the circulation from the kidneys' tubules. For example, a person who becomes dehydrated due to drinking excessively and urinating profusely has excessive thirst the next morning. Alcohol intoxication may result in electrolyte-related problems when the person becomes profoundly dehydrated.

Binge drinking, in particular, may result in death by the poisoning of skeletal muscle cells and the release of muscle proteins into the bloodstream. This process may cause the kidneys to malfunction or even fail, which may lead to a buildup of fluid within the body that can be life-threatening.

Cirrhosis, or scarring of the liver's tissue, is a common disease among chronic alcohol abusers. The liver plays a very important role in the body. The blood, which supplies the intestines and absorbs substances that are eaten and drunk, travels to the intestines and then, without flowing through the rest of the body, goes through the liver. The food nutrients that this blood picks up from the intestines, along with any drugs the person has taken orally or any alcohol they have drunk, begin to be processed during this passage through the liver.

The liver performs some seemingly magical tasks. If a person's diet is low in sugar, various amino acids contained in protein can be changed by the liver into glucose molecules. Since alcohol is changed (metabolized) within the liver's cells, high alcohol levels in the blood act as toxins to these liver cells. If an alcoholic frequently drinks high amounts of ethanol, many liver cells may die, resulting in significant scarring within the liver and a simultaneous loss of liver function. Such problems over a period of years may lead to cirrhosis of the liver, which, if sufficiently severe, leads to death.

Chronic alcohol abuse results in permanent changes in the brain and can damage various systems within the brain that regulate learning, memory, and motivation. The person may experience loss of memory, the inability to form new memories, and emotional instability and depression. In the case of alcohol abuse, some of this dysfunction may be reversible in six to twelve months if an active drinker stops drinking.

It is vital to understand that the abuse of alcohol leads to serious health risks. It should not be minimized with a playful "boys will be boys" attitude, adopted by some authors writing about Meriwether Lewis to minimize the alcohol abuse present in many Americans during his lifetime. When Lewis was an adult, from 1790–1809, America suffered from problems related to alcohol that were nothing less than spectacular.

Ethanol and Early America

From the moment that the first Europeans set foot upon North America, alcoholic beverages have been a part of the story of the continent. Their abuse has led to amendments to the U.S. Constitution, and these beverages have also been an important part of American culture through the centuries.

The consumption of alcohol by early Americans was widespread, and it played a profoundly important role during this period. The alcohol use in 1790–1830 makes alcohol drinkers in the United States today look like teetotalers. As historian W. J. Rorabaugh notes in his masterful book *The Alcoholic Republic: An American Tradition*, "During the first third of the nineteenth century the typical American annually drank more distilled liquor than at any other time in our history."[12] This binge on alcohol during the lifetime of Meriwether Lewis was the result of a combination of cultural factors that encouraged its use. Distilled alcohol was present in nearly every part of American life. As historians Mark Lender and James Martin write in their excellent work *Drinking in America*, "[T]he wisdom of the day held that alcohol was essential to good health," adding that "even children shared the dinner beer."[13]

In the seventeenth century, during the early days of colonization, beer was the colonial drink of choice and rum was the distilled spirit that grew quickly in popularity. Other popular alcoholic drinks included hard cider, a favorite of John Adams, containing about 7 percent alcohol. The Puritan minister Increase Mather, condemning drunkenness in a sermon and 1673 pamphlet entitled *Wo to Drunkards*, wrote, "Drink is in it self a good creature of God, and to be received with thankfulness, but the abuse of drink is from Satan; the wine is from God, but the Drunkard is from the Devil."[14]

In 1708, Puritan minister Cotton Mather taught that spirits had nutritional and medical value and that people could drink moderately to gain strength. Distilled liquor, produced from nutritious wheat, corn, rye, or other carbohydrate-containing plants, was believed by the public as well as the medical establishment to be a healthful and nutritious drink; a small quantity of whiskey (a dram, or about one fluid ounce), taken several times daily and at bedtime, was believed to be an excellent aid to health.

Alcoholic drinks in early America were popular for several reasons. The first and perhaps most obvious reason was the lack of pure drinking water. Early Americans routinely dumped garbage, human excrement, and other waste into rivers and lakes. These bodies of water also contained a vast assortment of naturally occurring bacteria, viruses, and parasites, some of which could cause disease, particularly gastrointestinal problems leading to fever, diarrhea, nausea, vomiting, and, in extreme cases, dehydration and death. Water supplies along the Lower Mississippi River in the eighteenth and nineteenth centuries were so full of mud that even when a glass of river water sat still for days, the mud never settled.[15] Sarah Meacham, in her informative work *Every Home a Distillery*, relates the story of a southern tourist in the United States who recorded in his journal in the early nineteenth century that "we most seriously felt the effects of drinking the water . . . which . . . acts as a cathartic." His culinary review of the taste of this water was that it was "insipid in the extreme."[16]

Even when clean water was available, drinking cold water was considered a dangerous practice. A traveler in the late 1790s related that "several persons die each year from drinking cold pump water when hot."[17] In addition to running the perceived risk of death caused by drinking cold water, drinking water in England marked the user as indigent because water drinkers were assumed to be unable to afford alcoholic drinks.[18] It appears that this attitude sailed along with its believers from the Old World to the colonies in pre-Revolutionary America. An anecdote from the early years of America tells the story of an Italian visitor to Monticello who asked for a glass of water during dinner. The humor of the scene can be imagined; the guest reported that Jefferson leaned over and with a smile asked "if I could not drink something else, because the unexpected request for a glass of water had upset the entire household and they did not know what they were about."[19]

By the early eighteenth century, colonists, in an effort to pump up the potency of their drinks, started distilling the relatively weak hard cider (7 percent alcohol) into its more potent cousin applejack, which could contain four to six times the ethanol of hard cider. Applejack became a particularly popular drink in the colonies where apples were plentiful. Fruits of all types could be fermented and then distilled. A typical Chesapeake Bay small planter in the eighteenth century, whose household contained six people, consumed around ninety gallons of cider and twenty-one gallons of distilled spirits per year, but a large planter's household that might have two dozen slaves could drink 450 gallons of cider and 105 gallons of distilled liquor per year.[20]

Not only did the general public believe that alcohol consumption was beneficial, the medical profession often supported its use as a medication. Dr. John Brown, the infamous Scottish physician whose "Brunonian" medicine taught that disease was the result of either insufficient or excessive nervous excitation, believed that whiskey was a great stimulant. Spirits were believed to have curative powers for a number of diseases. Brown was likely addicted to both alcohol and opium. During his lectures on his system of medicine in London, he often took at least four "doses" from his bottles of whiskey and laudanum (a preparation containing opium). Brown's ridiculous theories had a greatly negative influence on colonial American medicine as well as the public that it professed to serve.

Dr. Benjamin Rush began his anti-liquor stance, at least for nonmedical uses, in the 1770s due to the frequent health complications that he, engaged in the Enlightenment-influenced practice of observation, frequently saw in his patients. When he advised Meriwether Lewis during the spring of 1803, Rush still thought whiskey was a good stimulant, and he suggested that Lewis should use it to massage tired feet.

Alcohol, which flowed so freely through American society in those years, led to social situations that most twenty-first-century people can barely imagine. Many physicians making house calls were invited for a drink of liquor when visiting a sick home; Dr. David Hosack of New York City estimated that forty in one hundred physicians in that city were drunkards. Dr. Joseph Speed of Virginia wrote, "I often hear the people saying, that they scarcely know of a single sober doctor but myself."[21]

Whiskey and wine also served well as solvents into which physicians could dissolve the sixteen different pharmacologically active ingredients in the opium poppy. If whiskey alone were not potent enough, then mixing whiskey and opium produced the liquid medication laudanum, which was included in the Lewis and Clark pharmacy. The captains used laudanum for a variety of illnesses, most notably to treat the severely ill Sacagawea near the Great Falls, the paralyzed Nez Perce chief, and the Nez Perce woman suffering from "histeria" in May 1806. The alcohol as well as the morphine (or codeine or other narcotics) contained in the raw opium did lessen pain, decrease intestinal action, and lead to a euphoria-producing delirium. But opium-prescribing physicians and the public who received opium used it for a variety of other symptoms as well as it was thought by many physicians to be a great tonic for the system. Dr. Rush believed it to be a powerful stimulant and prescribed it for a number of different diseases (see chapter 5).

Before the American Revolution, while British ships were still actively supplying Britain's American colonies with goods from the West Indies, rum grew in popularity during most of the eighteenth century. The raw ingredients of rum were also shipped north, and rum distilleries in colonial America gained an increasingly large base of fans. Americans continued to drink rum until the Revolution. During the war, British merchant shipping came to a stop and rum became much more difficult to obtain.[22]

Given the ample supplies of various grains such as rye, corn, and wheat, colonial farmers and distillers starting producing whiskey to take the place of rum. After the Revolution ended, western farmers produced bumper crops of grains, which in turn yielded a handsome profit for those who started to produce whiskey. Ardent spirit distilling was more common on American farms in our early history than baking bread is in American homes today. The immigration of the Scots-Irish, who brought their knowledge of making Scotch whiskey to America, accelerated the public's preference for whiskey over rum and most other alcoholic beverages.

Drinking was not solely an activity for people who sat around a fireside at night, as we might imagine today. Drinking in Lewis's time was done at all times of the day.²³ According to Rorabaugh, "Virginia gentry gathered at 1 p.m. an hour before dinner for the purpose of taking juleps compounded of peach brandy or whiskey, sugar and ice."²⁴ Mint leaves were crushed and added to sugar and distilled spirits to create a julep. This potent and lively beverage was popular near Lewis's boyhood home near Charlottesville and was used in the cause of colonial independence in June 1781. During the closing days of the Revolution, General Cornwallis's British cavalry officer Banastre Tarleton was terrorizing the county of Albemarle, Virginia (as noted in chapter 2) in his attempt to pursue and capture all of the members of the Virginia legislature, including Thomas Jefferson. Meriwether Lewis's family lore has it that when Tarleton stopped to feed and rest his soldiers at a Castle Hill property outside Charlottesville, the lady of the house and those who were helping cook the breakfast plied Tarleton and his men with mint juleps in an effort to slow down their pursuit of the American officials. The ploy seemed to have worked. Tarleton missed capturing Jefferson by ten minutes.²⁵

In most of America, afternoon dinner (today's lunch) was washed down by hard cider or distilled spirits diluted with water. Another break came in the late afternoon, when supper was washed down with more alcohol, and finally, in the evening with friends and family, one might look forward to a relaxing evening sipping on a glass of whiskey.²⁶

Alcohol was expected to be served at nearly every social occasion. Rorabaugh notes that "[g]uests at urban dances and balls were often intoxicated and so were spectators at frontier horse races. Western newlyweds were customarily presented with a bottle of whiskey to be drunk before bedding down for the night."²⁷ Elections, explained one Kentucky politician, depended upon understanding that "the way to men's hearts, is, down their throats," and during trials, a bottle was often passed to all present, apparently in hopes that the defendant might be acquitted.²⁸ The early American barbeque offered not only a feast on roast beast but the opportunity to indulge in some very serious drinking. The "barbecue law" in the South required every attendee to drink to intoxication, and "the only excuse for refusing a round was passing out."²⁹

Many clergymen also drank freely. Although the leaders of the Methodist Church in America joined with the Quakers in the 1780s in their opposition to the free or recreational drinking of spirits, this abstinence was not practiced by all men of the cloth. One minister of an unknown denomination, most certainly not a Methodist or Quaker, reportedly considered himself temperate because he only drank four glasses of spirits to help him make it through a Sunday.[30] In 1767, Jefferson was involved in a case in which the parishioners of St. Anne's Anglican Church in Albemarle tried to remove a priest, in part on a charge of drunkenness, who had compounded his sin by drinking the sacramental wine.[31]

As we cover more fully in chapter 7, post-Revolutionary America was a much more markedly republican and egalitarian society than it had been prior to the Revolution, and early Americans often went out of their way to prove their egalitarian attitudes. The old habits of cultural leaders (gentry, clergy, physicians, and attorneys), who had been readily accepted as authority figures by colonials—particularly due to unquestioned obedience to the church and political leadership, genetic bloodlines, and the resulting class demarcations—were tossed out in favor of an "every man is equal" attitude that was noted in every area of American life.

The parameters of this high level of alcohol drinking in early America are startling. When Meriwether Lewis was sixteen years of age, an entirely accepted age in Virginia for him to be drinking hard liquor, the average annual consumption of pure alcohol was 5.8 gallons/year.[32] Between the years of 1790 and 1830, Americans drank more pure alcohol per capita than they did any time prior to or after those forty years, peaking at 7.1 gallons/year in 1830.[33] Between 1800 and 1830, annual per capita alcohol consumption actually was higher than it was in 1790, when the rate was nearly double the present rate.[34] It is worth repeating: during the first third of the nineteenth century, the typical American annually drank more distilled liquor than any other American ever has, averaging about half a pint per day![35] Meriwether Lewis lived in the middle of that era in a culture that accepted such hardcore drinking, which is, at the very least, intriguing.

The early American love affair with drinking often shocked foreign visitors. A visiting Englishman retired from the British Royal Navy and perhaps aiming some arrows of hostility toward the former colonies noted that outsiders to the American culture would be "perfectly astonished at the extent of intemperance."[36] When traveling by stage, travelers could buy liquor at the inn while their teams of horses were switched. During one very demanding seventeen-hour trip of sixty-six miles across Virginia, the stage stopped ten times, and two of the passengers had drinks at each way station.[37] The amount of alcohol they consumed during their two-day stage trip could have been equivalent to two to three pints of hard liquor. The supply of whiskey available to a thirsty America was ample to meet the demand. By 1810, fourteen thousand distilleries were operating in the United States.[38]

With American adolescents drinking as a rite of passage with their fathers, uncles, and friends, the routine drinking of hard liquor often began at an age that might shock many modern Americans. Some young males did not wait until they turned fifteen. "It is no uncommon thing," wrote one man, 'to see a boy of 12 or 14 years old . . . walk into a tavern in the forenoon to take a glass of brandy and bitters."[39]

The extraordinary amount of drinking done by the average early American led to numerous societal problems and, in response, to a strong temperance movement that started within the American religious and medical communities when Lewis was a young man, albeit with little results. Per capita annual alcohol consumption continued to increase until 1830. John Adams, hoping to encourage temperance, proposed that the number of taverns be reduced in 1760. In 1764, Ben Franklin's *Pennsylvania Gazette* noted that taverns were "a Pest to Society."[40]

The extensive use of alcohol in America spawned the same social problems in Lewis's time that its abuse does today. Dr. Rush, noting the severe problems caused by drunkenness among the citizens of Philadelphia, wrote a medical treatise titled *Notes on the Use of Ardent Spirits* in 1794 that detailed his observations of chronic illnesses and accompanying problems of those addicted to strong drink. As early as 1743, the general rules of the Methodist church prohibited its members from buying or drink ardent spirits except as needed for medicine.[41] Rush became so alarmed at the state of American intoxication that he warned that unless the country's liquor intake diminished, "Our country, would soon be governed by men chosen by intemperate and corrupted voters" rather than by good Republicans filled with virtue.[42]

Why So Much Booze?

There are multiple probable explanations of why early Americans drank so much alcohol. Humans and their ability (or inability) to reason have undoubtedly not changed very much in this regard since the dawn of time. The reasons people drank too much in early America may have included some that were unique to their day, such as the sometimes difficult task of obtaining sufficient food, physical danger, and sudden untreatable and potentially fatal diseases. But their emotional responses to their unique stressors were essentially the same as our emotional responses to different stressors today. Many people who drink do so to relieve emotional stress.

Rorabaugh argues that although the supply of distilled spirits was plentiful in the early nineteenth century, the *supply* of liquor does not fully explain why the people of that time took to the bottle in such an aggressive manner. He believes that between 1790 and 1830, "[A]lmost every aspect of American life underwent alteration, in many cases startling upheaval."[43] The socioeconomic classes that were most affected by the alcohol binge were also those who experienced the greatest change. He points out that the greatest change in America during those years was the great increase in the population, which grew from four to seven million people. Since the American economy was largely based on farming, the amount of cultivated soil needed to support this population gain required as much new land as had been farmed during the prior two centuries. The resulting push westward also necessitated the settlement of lands that were not directly in contact with rivers, which could be used for transportation of crops and other goods both to and from the east. These situations, as Rorabaugh notes, resulted in "significant numbers of Americans living detached from the effects of traditional society." He concludes that "It should not be surprising that these isolated and lonely western pioneers had a reputation for drinking more alcoholic beverages than residents of other sections of the country."[44]

Much of the early American diet was boiled or roasted meat and vegetables, so alcoholic beverages and their neurologic effects were no doubt a welcome relief from a boring, limited diet. In addition, any mental disorder would be demonstrably affected by both alcohol and opium—suggesting to the naive that these substances might be beneficial in the treatment of mental disorders. During the days of Lewis, there was no psychiatric *Diagnostic and Statistical Manual* to help distinguish the numerous different mental illnesses of our modern era. If alcohol were used to treat mental health issues, it was a one-size-fits-all prescription.

Alcohol use was not confined to the home or to social occasions as it was customary for employers to provide some liquor to their employees during worktime breaks around 11 a.m. and again in the afternoon.[45] Of course, when payday came workers would enjoy a social time at the local watering hole. This alcohol indulgence resulted in a severe labor problem, cited by one employer, as "noxious habits continued to increase in many places with unabated ardor, until the evil had become so great as scarcely to be endured."[46]

Another interesting cultural situation was the difference between the social class hierarchy of pre- and post-Revolutionary America. Prior to the Revolutionary War, as historian Mark Noll notes in his authoritative book *America's God*, colonial Virginia culture was a mirror of the English system, from social class distinctions and their inherent attitudes to theology and church-associated life. As their social counterparts did in England, the aristocratic men in pre-war colonial Virginia wore powdered wigs, rode in fancy carriages, and occupied respected positions within the hierarchy of the Anglican church. Attorneys, physicians, and ministers held exalted places within this upper crust of society.[47]

The rapid and important changes that took place in post-Revolution America changed the cultural landscape in relation to medicine, religion, social hierarchies, political structure, and leadership in profound ways. These cultural changes, in addition to the difficulty of simply living one's life in a safe and healthy manner, would without question create a cultural dust storm. Until the dust settled, these changes created a cultural angst that fostered emotional insecurity in numerous Americans. Cultural angst and emotional insecurity yield personal anxiety, and anxiety is not a pleasant human emotion. Given the ready availability of alcohol, which always works in relieving anxiety, many early Americans resorted to alcoholic drinks, as is still true today.

Thomas Paine, whose pamphlet *Common Sense* galvanized the colonies into a state of revolution, further influenced the behavior of his admirers when he published an attack on orthodox Christianity in

1794. Rorabaugh notes that the great popularity at the time of Paine's "irreligious radicalism" (*The Age of Reason*, 1794) among the younger generation was a contributing social force that led to "unprecedented lusty drinking" in many American colleges.[48] A student at Dartmouth reported to the college's president "that the least quantity he could put up with . . . was from two to three pints daily."[49] This undoubtedly was either cider or beer, as two to three pints of hard liquor is highly dangerous as a daily intake. This type of serious partying led most colleges to ban drinking by 1800. It would be fanciful thinking at best to believe that the social forces that created this degree of alcohol intake and attitudes toward drinking would be present only among the young men in the nation's colleges. This type of behavior would likely be equal or greater in the young men who were enlisted in the U.S. Army, which routinely supplied its troops with a daily ration of ardent spirits sufficient to produce mild intoxication.

These cultural realities make Lewis's comment to his mother in his letter after joining the militia in 1794 much more meaningful than if simply viewed on its own. One may legitimately question Lewis's total truthfulness regarding the extent of his participation in drinking, given his reference to "oceans of whiskey" in his letter to his mother. He did on occasion mildly tease his mother about various issues, such as a letter in which he asked her to remember him to all the girls of his neighborhood. The motive behind such comments to a Methodist woman who was probably a teetotaler who likely did not approve of recreational drinking is a bit of a mystery. If Lewis was teasing his mother, such a scenario suggests a lack of sensitivity on his part, given her probable deeply held, religiously based view against recreational alcohol. Was he being a bit of a naughty child with his mother or was he telling her the truth—that he was enjoying drinking the ample supply of whiskey available with his fellow soldiers? We are not certain, given his culture and the prevailing heavy and frequent drinking, why anyone would believe the former scenario.

The Behavior of Alcohol Addicts

Human addiction to alcohol has been part of the human story for nearly as long as the ethanol molecule was first sipped. No chronic disease has affected more people in a more profound way than alcohol use disorder. Cleary, alcohol abuse has represented a significant problem throughout history.

It is also frequently alleged by authors writing about Lewis and Clark from different academic perspectives that Lewis at times abused alcohol or perhaps suffered from alcohol use disorder. As we already reported earlier in this chapter, other writers have objected to such claims, asking questions such as, "If Jefferson knew Lewis was an alcoholic, why would he have given him command of the expedition?" or "If Lewis was a drinker, wouldn't his hypercritical nemesis Frederick Bates have known about it and blown the whistle on him?" Others, in their attempts to discredit every possible report of Lewis's alcohol use, have asked why the boatmen who witnessed Lewis's reported drunken suicide attempt on his way down the Mississippi in September 1809 did not report it. More than one author simply ignores any report in the historical record of Lewis's alcohol abuse or claims that such reports reflect a different health problem.

It is enlightening to review some of the known factors that make some people more prone to alcohol use disorder than the average person:

- If their family history includes alcohol use disorder, there is a greater risk. We are not aware of any such issues within the Lewis or Meriwether families, but given the history of early America, it must be a consideration.
- Alcohol abusers in close familial relationships are a major factor in a person becoming an alcohol abuser later on in life. This is especially true if the abuser is the person's biological parent.
- While people are growing up, they live in a particular social environment. Individuals from certain demographics have been shown to be more likely to develop alcohol use disorder. Psychologist Kay Redfield Jamison writes, "Substance abuse . . . usually begins early in life, often in adolescence or the early twenties, and, once it has set in, has a stubbornly progressive course."[50] There is solid evidence that this factor was at play in the life of Lewis.
- The emotional health of the person plays a role. If someone is significantly depressed or anxious, they are more likely to turn to alcohol to numb their symptoms. This is a major factor in many people suffering from mood disorders (various types of unipolar

depression and bipolar disease) and often leads to an alcohol habit. Alcohol, as a central nervous system depressant, relieves their anxiety but aggravates their depressive symptoms. There is perhaps no stronger association in this area than that between the abuse of alcohol and depression.
- Many people with social anxiety drink to decrease their anxiety and become more open to conversations with others.

There is strong merit to the argument that an "alcohol use disordered personality" exists in the population. Certain behaviors are commonly noted by psychologists and psychiatrists as well as other medical specialists who work with people with alcohol use disorder on a daily basis. Some of these behaviors are as follows:
- The alcohol abuser finds it difficult to control their alcohol intake and suffers from both a physiologic and psychological addiction to alcohol.
- The alcohol abuser often attempts to hide their abuse and drink in secret.
- The alcohol abuser often treats others with verbal and emotional abuse. At times, they may become physically abusive.
- The alcohol abuser often engages in dangerous sexual or physical risk-taking behaviors.
- The alcohol abuser often suffers from other psychological issues such as anxiety, depression, and various personality disorders.

People with various personality types react differently under the intoxicating influence of ethanol. Some gregarious people may show increased laughter and excitation. Others may become angry and belligerent toward others. People who suffer from depression or other mood disorders frequently use alcohol to numb their emotional pain.

Meriwether Lewis and Alcohol

Meriwether Lewis was born in 1774 just before the onset of the American Revolution, and Rorabaugh's observations on Lewis's generation are fascinating. He states, "Between 1790 and 1830 the United States underwent not only a period of unprecedented heavy drinking but also a period of unprecedented and extremely rapid change."[51]

This is a valuable insight into the culture in which Lewis lived and a very important factor for us to consider. Taking into account that Lewis turned fifteen in 1789, the association between his youth and an American nation that encouraged the liberal drinking of alcoholic beverages is remarkable.

The cultural history provided by Rorabaugh does not automatically make Lewis an alcohol abuser. But these factors place him in a time and place where the opportunity and encouragement to overindulge in alcohol were common and were an accepted part of society. To our knowledge, these factors have never been acknowledged by those who attempt to deny any reports that Lewis had a problem with alcohol. Many books on Lewis's life either minimize or completely ignore the influence of his culture.

Historical evidence brought to light in recent years supports the idea that Lewis never moved with his mother to Georgia in the 1780s, as had been previously accepted by historians. As we covered in chapter 2, according to Guy Meriwether Benson (Meriwether's first cousin five times removed), Lewis was appointed a guardian for the time he lived in Albemarle County, Virginia, when his mother, stepfather, and siblings moved to Georgia. This is the time when Meriwether would have become of drinking age, in terms of cultural expectations, and he would not have suffered any disapproval from the Virginia gentry for drinking alcohol. (In reflecting on what a difference two centuries make, I (David) believe I would not have made it to the age of sixteen had my police captain father caught me drinking hard liquor at fifteen years of age.) It must be noted that Lewis's mother's presumed influence as an abstainer was not directly present in the life of Meriwether during his early teen years. She was hundreds of miles away in Georgia.

Not only was Lewis a member of a culture that overindulged in alcohol, but at the age of twenty he became a member of the U.S. militia, which certainly had an established culture of alcohol abuse. Militia musters often became excuses for drinking. One newly elected militia colonel pledged, "I can't make a speech, but what I lack in brains I will try and make up in rum."[52]

That whiskey was available and was believed to be necessary to the proper functioning of military units is painfully apparent. Even though Dr. Rush did not approve of the daily whiskey ration given to

Revolutionary War soldiers, believing that it caused fevers and fluxes (in its place, Rush proposed giving vinegar), it is a fact that many U.S. Army personnel received a gill (four ounces) of whiskey as a daily ration. As noted earlier, this amount of liquor was sufficient to put Lewis and his fellow militia members into an intoxicated state daily. Men were rewarded extra whiskey on numerous occasions during the first half of the expedition of the Corps of Discovery. Although the Corps's supply of whiskey was largely intended for recreational use and gifts, it was also included in their medicine box upon the orders of Dr. Rush. The expedition's supplies included 120 gallons of whiskey when the Corps of Discovery disembarked on its epic journey in May 1804.

The Lewis and Clark Expedition's supply of whiskey was well guarded during the first winter that the Corps spent across the Mississippi River from St. Louis at Camp Wood, Illinois. One guard, Private Collins, unable to resist the temptation, broke into a barrel and drank himself numb. Private Collins was once again charged with "getting drunk on his post this morning out of whiskey put under his Charge as a Sentinal and for Suffering Hugh Hall to draw whiskey out of the Said Barrel intended for the party" on June 29, 1804, in present-day Missouri.[53] The jury hearing the charges against Collins consisted of Sergeant Nathaniel Pryor and Privates John Colter, John Newman, Patrick Gass, and J. B. Thompson, with John Potts acting as "Judge Advocate." The whiskey drunk by Collins and Hall was "intended for the party." So, these men not only got drunk but did so with the *other* men's whiskey. Collins pleaded "not guilty," and Hall pleaded "guilty." Collins paid a dear price for his bad judgment; he was given one hundred lashes to his bare back. Hall, admitting his error, received only fifty.[54] One of the main points in this story is that the jurors considered stealing from *their* share of whiskey a serious offense.

Whiskey use was mentioned during the expedition in various circumstances. One of these occasions was when Lewis, ever the resourceful leader, used some large hailstones to chill his whiskey mixture on the plains near the Great Falls on June 28, 1805, and made himself a batch of "punch." Punch was an alcoholic beverage in those days, not a mixture of fruit juices.

If the men of the Corps did not have any alcohol for a prolonged period of time, as was the case on July 4, 1805, near the Great Falls of the Missouri, their body's ability to metabolize ethanol would revert to normal, the physiologic result of their livers not being constantly challenged by ethanol. Such a prolonged lack of alcohol would stop their body's increased stimulation of the enzyme needed to inactivate it—alcohol dehydrogenase. The drinking of their 4th of July whiskey treat from the captains would have produced obvious signs of intoxication, as was confirmed in the journals by Lewis's comment on their celebration: "our work being at an end this evening, we gave the men a drink of spirits, it being the last of our stock, and some of them appeared a little sensible of its effects."[55]

From July 5, 1805, until September 1806, the men were on a dry expedition. In their last miles of paddling along the "Musquetors"-infested Missouri River, on September 6, 1806, the expedition encountered a trading riverboat owned by Auguste Chouteau. He was headed upstream with a good supply of whiskey. The captains purchased a gallon from him and "gave to each man of the party a dram which is the first Spiritious licquor which had been tasted by any of them Since the 4 of July 1805."[56] The gallon of whiskey would have been of a sufficient quantity to supply around two ounces to each man, somewhat more than the dram that was reported, but not enough to supply a gill (four ounces). Then, on September 14, the Corps encountered a boat captain who "pressed on us Some whisky for our men." The men "received a dram and Sung Songs untill 11 oClock at night in the greatest harmony," according to Clark.[57] Surely, this whiskey that was pressed on them amounted to more than a dram per person—a dram would not cause anyone to break into song. The men received another supply of whiskey on September 17, this time from Captain McClellin of the U.S. Army, "for which our party were in want." On September 20, they bought two gallons of whiskey from a private citizen "for our party."[58]

But the greatest wingding came on the night of Wednesday, September 25, 1806, after the Corps's return to civilization, when Lewis's old friend Major William Christy, owner of a St. Louis tavern, hosted a party for the returning heroes. Eighteen toasts were presented, with the opening one going to President Jefferson, "[t]he friend of science, the polar star of discovery, the philosopher and the patriot."[59] After seventeen drinks of what was most likely straight whiskey from a bar that was undoubtedly well stocked, the final toast was proposed in what was probably an extremely slurred tongue. The toaster finally got around to acknowledging the accomplishments of Captains Lewis and Clark with a shout of, "Captains Lewis and Clark—Their perilous services endear them to every American heart."[60] The report of this party, when viewed within the context of the American love of liquor in that period, seems something more than a very special celebration to honor the expedition's return to civilization served up with carrot cake, balloons, and fruit punch. Without a doubt, that party was a drunken spectacle that would not have represented anything out of the ordinary *for that era*.

It should be remembered that Lewis was reported to have attempted suicide in September 1809 while on a boat descending the Mississippi River from St. Louis to New Orleans due to a derangement of his mind and/or excessive alcohol intake. John Guice has questioned the veracity of the report, asking why such a report was not circulated by the workers on the boat once it arrived in New Orleans. He argues that the men who worked on the boat would have shared the news of this incident and Lewis's drunkenness because such an event related to excessive alcohol intake would have been sufficiently novel in the eyes of the boat workers for them to report it.[61] But, Rorabaugh notes that "[a]mong the lustiest consumers of alcohol were stage drivers, lumberjacks, river boatmen, and canal builders," adding that "[t]he typical boatman combined mobility with frontier exuberance, cockiness, restlessness, and daring," resulting in a group of independent men who "literally floated outside society."[62] He sums up the typical boatman as a person who "drank heartily, lustily, frequently, excessively. In whiskey was solace for the uncertainty of his condition, confirmation of his independence, and fellowship that reassured his empty soul."[63] Being intoxicated was a way of life for many boatmen, and the presence of another drinking man, even Governor Lewis, would not have been much of a surprise. Workers on keelboats and rafts were responsible for tending to virtually all of the interstate commerce of goods being shipped down the river systems of western America. There were obviously no interstate freeways carrying trucks and no trains for the transportation of goods; it all went on slow-moving boats on river systems until the advent of steam-powered boats in 1812. So, it is entirely probable that such a mode of transportation for Lewis's departure from St. Louis in 1809 provided him with not only the alcohol but also a group of people who would gladly join him in their alcohol-fueled party.

To give an idea of alcohol consumption closer to Lewis's home in Charlottesville, Virginia, an English traveler coming through the area after the American Revolution described a typical Albemarle gentleman:

> He rises about eight o'clock, drinks what he calls a julep, which is a large glass of rum sweetened with sugar, then walks, or more generally rides, round his plantation, views his stock, inspects his crops, and returns about ten o'clock to breakfast on cold meat or ham, fried hominy, roast, and cider ... About twelve or one he drinks a toddy to create him an appetite for dinner, which he sits down to at two o'clock. [He] commonly drinks toddy till bedtime; during all this time he is neither drunk nor sober, but in a state of stupefaction. ... [When] he attends the Court House or some horse race or cock fight he gets so egregiously drunk that his wife sends a couple of negroes to conduct him safe home."[64]

An interesting and important observation here is that the Englishman writing this report apparently did not consider "a state of stupefaction" as either drunk or sober. What in the world did he think "stupefaction" was? One must wonder what that planter was like when his slaves came to bring him home—and pity his wife.

This comment also leads to questions surrounding the denial of Lewis's drunkenness during his court-martial hearing in 1795. During the trial's testimony, the witness was asked, "Was Mr. Lewis at the time of his coming into Mr. Elliott's house as mentioned intoxicated?" The witness, Mr. Sterrit, responded, "My acquaintance with him will not enable me to say whether he was or was not." Another witness was asked the same question and answered, "I am not sufficiently acquainted with him to determine—he appeared agitated but I did not then know the cause—previous to his leaving the room the first time, he appeared to have some difficulty in expressing himself and shed tears." Yet another witness was asked about Lewis's possible intoxication and answered, "I can't say that he was—he might have been drinking a little." Another witness stated, "I did not think he was intoxicated with liquor," and then another testified "I did not conceive him to be in the least."[65]

One witness did believe that Lewis might have been drinking some, but three others denied that he was intoxicated. We believe it is very possible that he drank some alcohol that day, fueling his interaction with Lieutenant Elliott, given Lewis's tearful response. Unless alcohol, with its emotionally enhancing qualities, had been present, why would a grown man respond with tears to a perceived offense by Elliott? Alcohol can make any mood more prominent, which is exactly why it is such a harmful companion to those who may suffer from mood disorders.

At every stop along his route to and from Virginia, Washington, and Philadelphia in 1806–08, Lewis was repeatedly wined and dined and told how wonderful his accomplishments were. Poems were written about his feats in the wilderness. It is not credible that during this time none of the informal parties, formal balls, and get-togethers of a few men and women had substantial amounts of alcohol available. Given the alcohol abuse culture present in America during that time, Lewis was likely drinking a significant amount of alcohol. To believe otherwise stretches credulity. An appropriate analogy one might provide for the near certainty of such a scenario is this: if it looks like a horse, runs on all fours, lives in Africa, and has stripes, it is probably a zebra.

With this evidence, what are we to make of the theory that Lewis was not a heavy drinker? This theory, raised by James Starrs and Kira Gale, seems highly unlikely.[66]

At this point, it is interesting to note that both Thomas Danisi, in his book *Uncovering the Truth About Meriwether Lewis*, and Vardis Fisher, in his work *Suicide or Murder?*, published a copy of the personal account book prepared by Lewis during his final days in St. Louis in 1809. Both authors listed a text from Lewis's account book that reads, "To Isaac Miller for which a note is left with Genl. Clark, $202.87 1/2."[67]

The copies of Lewis's account book, as printed in Danisi's and Fisher's books, do not specify what Governor Lewis purchased from Mr. Miller.[68] It is not clear to us why these authors failed to identify the item purchased, but this detail is both relevant and very significant. What was this mysterious item? We need not wonder any longer. Lewis spent his own funds on a personal purchase of eight barrels of whiskey. The original IOU, signed by Meriwether Lewis, is held in the Special

Collections of the University of Virginia Library in Charlottesville, Virginia. It reads:

> St. Louis August 22nd, 1809
> I so acknowledge myself justly indebted to Isaac Miller the sum of two hundred and two dollars and eighty seven 1/2 cents for eight barrels of whiskey. −($202.87 1/2)
> Meriwether Lewis

This IOU signed by Lewis, two weeks prior to his departure from St. Louis, raises the possibility that Lewis both indulged himself with some of this whiskey while living in St. Louis in the months before he left for Washington as well as brought along a personal supply on his trip to Washington. It is entirely within reason to assume that he did not plan to and did not take all eight barrels with him but was stocking up for his anticipated return to St. Louis. Perhaps some of the purchase was furnished to Clark, as references to Lewis furnishing Clark with some whiskey occur in Lewis's writings of that era. Whiskey barrels in 1809 reportedly contained forty gallons—which would mean Lewis purchased 320 gallons.[69] This amount represents three times the amount of whiskey taken along on the expedition. This IOU signed by Lewis is inconsistent with a man who was not a heavy drinker.

The date on the IOU of August 22, 1809, does not necessarily indicate that Lewis purchased and took possession of this whiskey on that date, only that Lewis had purchased on his credit this amount of whiskey on a prior date. Before his departure for Washington in September 1809, he acknowledged in this IOU that he owed Isaac Miller $202 for whiskey he had taken possession of in the recent past. It makes little difference when Lewis took possession of the whiskey, just that he did at some point buy and take possession of a very large amount of whiskey that he did not have the money to pay for when it was delivered. The further in the past Lewis took possession, the more likely it was that he was using it during the spring and early summer of 1809. If he was drinking it, how much and how often did he drink? With a purchase of over three hundred gallons, he must have had some plans about the quantity he would need for his future use. Lewis apparently decided that he needed quite a bit. When read in the context of the multiple reports in the coming weeks of his alcohol abuse, it seems to be only wishful thinking to argue that Lewis did not have an alcohol problem in these last months of his life.

If we wanted to deny that Lewis abused alcohol, what would be *plausible* explanations for why Lewis, with money that he did not have, bought a personal supply of such an impressive quantity of whiskey? Some might claim that he needed whiskey to provide entertainment to guests in his role as governor. If that were the case, why would he buy the whiskey on credit—with money that he did not have—and assume personal responsibility for it on August 22, 1809? In addition, if it was necessary to supply governmental social events with vast amounts of whiskey purchased on his own account, then such an explanation actually confirms the high level of alcohol consumption occurring in every level of American society in 1809.

Others might say, in their attempts to explain this purchase, that Lewis was the governor and needed to provide gifts to the Indian tribes, his friends, and the Masonic Temple in St. Louis, of which he was the "Worshipful Master." Gifts to tribes and to friends would again represent government purchases, and if the Masonic Temple meetings required such a large amount of whiskey, that would just serve to confirm that many males in St. Louis in late August 1809 were heavy drinkers. Why would Lewis purchase whiskey for the Masonic Temple for men who could probably better afford such a purchase than he? Perhaps the chief Mason was responsible for providing whiskey to every member. Even if this was one of Lewis's responsibilities as the leader of the lodge, are we to believe that he was not drinking some of the whiskey that he bought? Truly, this line of thinking strays out of the lane of believability.

This scenario is similar to the many times we have taken a medical/social history of a patient and asked about their use of alcohol. Patients who drank excessive amounts of alcohol would often say, "Oh, I drink about a six-pack a day" or "I have a few glasses of wine every night with dinner." For medical and mental health professionals, such statements are a red flag for possible alcohol abuse. We would follow up with the question, "Do you think you have a problem with alcohol?" They would invariably deny any problem whatsoever.

In these drinkers' defense, their denial of having a problem with their use of alcohol does not make them into liars and people with an alcohol use disorder. But, when drinking to excess, it is extremely common to be in denial about any problems that the drinking is causing, and such denial is a hallmark of alcohol use disorder behavior.

Could Lewis have just been binge drinking several times a week or month and not be considered to have an alcohol use disorder? No; such a scenario would be evidence of alcohol abuse. We have often heard from those abusing alcohol, in their attempt to minimize their destructive habits, comments such as "Hey, Doc, I'm just partying pretty often" (binge drinking) rather than the more accurate statement "I'm an alcoholic" (chronic addiction).

With the very real possibility of Lewis showing the typical behavior of an alcohol abuser of hiding his drinking, it is no surprise that Frederick Bates, Lewis's nemesis, did not report it. If Lewis went home from work at night while in St. Louis and drank on a fairly regular schedule, it would be easy for him to hide that from others, especially in a culture where so many were doing the same thing. And it should not be assumed that Bates himself behaved any differently regarding alcohol. Bates was sufficiently popular with his male friends to be named the worshipful master of the Masonic Temple in St. Louis within months of Lewis's death. Are we to believe that he did not himself drink? At the risk of beating a dead horse, frequent intoxication from alcohol was standard in society in those days, so *if there was no deviation from that standard, there was no recognized problem.*

In a parallel matter of cultural differences, did the marriage of men in their thirties to fifteen-year-old girls merit a report of suspected child sexual abuse to the authorities? No. It was normal for that generation and culture. Marrying one's cousin, which in our culture is considered incest and is the subject of jokes about rednecks, was also entirely acceptable to the people of Lewis's world.

How would Lewis's drinking have affected Jefferson's choice of Lewis to head the expedition? Why would Jefferson pick an alcohol abuser for such an important task? We believe that Lewis did not have a significant alcohol problem during his time with Jefferson, which is why Jefferson felt no hesitation in assigning the job to Lewis. Lewis's time with Jefferson in the exciting world of 1801–02 Washington was no doubt a happy, challenging, and stimulating time for Lewis. These great times for Lewis occurred long before the unhappy years after his return from the expedition when the "demons" during his governorship in St. Louis materialized.[70] If those demons were not causing him great emotional pain, he would have had no incentive to self-medicate with hard liquor in his attempts to suppress those emotions.

The profound health-related effects of alcohol use, in conjunction with the IOU written by Lewis for his whiskey supply in 1809, effectively nullify any attempt to minimize or dismiss Lewis's alcohol-related problems and his resulting mental derangement. The reports from Russell, Neelly, Grinder, and others, including Jefferson's reference to the "habit" into which Lewis had fallen, are entirely consistent. The jigsaw puzzle is nearly complete, and no puzzle pieces need to be pushed into places where they do not fit. No historical evidence needs to be ignored, and no distortion of the historical record requires a novel interpretation to fit a predetermined conclusion.

Alcoholic beverages were but one part of the cultural and medical scene in Lewis's world. Other substances used by the medical profession have been blamed by some authors for Lewis's reported illnesses during his final weeks. In the next chapter, we describe some of the medications that Lewis may have used that we can all be thankful are no longer prescribed by physicians.

Chapter 5

Pleasures and Poisons: Medicine in the World of Meriwether Lewis

We think our fathers fools, so wise we grow. Our wiser sons, I hope, will think us so.
—Dr. Benjamin Rush

In today's world, television viewers are subjected to a substantial number of advertisements for pharmaceuticals, everything from anti-clotting medications to treatments for diabetes, rheumatoid arthritis, depression, high blood pressure, dermatologic problems, etc. Although these commercials immediately get the mute button in our household, I (David) admit that I have listened to a number of them, and they often feature a rapid-fire voice listing the numerous potential side effects of these new miracles of the pharmaceutical industry. The unwanted side effects range from fatal problems such as blood-related malignancies (lymphoma) to nausea and vomiting. Perhaps today's new pharmaceutical medication will in several years provide malpractice attorneys with opportunities to file lawsuits against the pharmaceutical companies that are advertising their state-of-the-art medications as near miracles. This is in no way meant as a blanket condemnation of the pharmaceutical industry as many of these medications will provide benefits in alleviating the symptoms and complications of significant diseases. New medications are constantly in the pipeline, and older medications that were state-of-the-art a few years back are now laughed at by physicians in their discussions around the lunch table. Many medications that I used early in my career sometimes come up in conversations with former colleagues. "Hey, remember when we used _____ for a first-line medication?" The prescription of certain medications that were used routinely in the 1970s and 1980s would now be considered malpractice. This is the nature of medicine and the process of discovery of ways to improve the collective life of the human race.

When considering the medications suggested for use by Dr. Benjamin Rush and included in the medicine box of "Drs." Lewis and Clark in 1803–06, we have an even stronger negative reaction. Given the two hundred-plus years of medical progress since that time, these "ghosts of medications past" present a very easy target for criticism. Most of these substances were toxic and grossly ineffective treatments. The medical practice's shortcomings of that day resulted from the inadequate knowledge base of the physicians of that era. There was no modern general chemistry, organic chemistry, biochemistry, microbiology, or other basic medical sciences to provide a basis for understanding the disease process or the medicines that the physicians of that period prescribed in their often vain attempts to treat these diseases. I addressed this subject in detail in my book *Or Perish in the Attempt*, so I will not repeat that material here. What I will do is focus on the medications that Lewis may have taken during the final months of his life and explore their possible indications for use as understood by the physicians of that era, how the medicines affected the human body (its mechanism of action), their effectiveness (and efficacy), and potential side effects that may have either benefited or harmed Lewis's health. Medications of that era were heavily weighted on the side of negative side effects and lightly weighted on their actual benefits. My chief hope is that this discussion will be interesting and offer new insights into Lewis's life and death. Stick with me in this discussion, and you will likely know more about this issue than you did before—and will be very happy that you are living in today's world.

Mercury

Mercury is found in nature and is one of the currently known 118 fundamental building blocks of nature (the chemical symbol Hg represents mercury in the list of elements (called the periodic table). These building blocks are called elements. Some of these elements are key to our very life. Our bodily structures are made from elements such as carbon, hydrogen, oxygen, nitrogen, and many others. You may already be familiar with the names of many other elements, such as sodium, potassium, iron, magnesium, and calcium. All of these elements were produced when God flipped the switch for the "Big Bang" some fourteen billion years ago. All the elements were produced within the intense heat of an uncountable number of stars somewhere within the forming universe. Thus, we are all made of this "stardust," and the fact that we can breathe, think, and love is amazing. Knowing this may deepen our understanding of the biblical saying, "For you were made from dust, and to dust you will return."[1]

But, as important as many elements are to life, mercury is not on the list of wonderful life-supporting elements. We do not need it within our bodies, and it is significantly toxic to us. It is found in nature in its elemental liquid form in the earth's crust, bonding with other elements to produce a rocky cinnabar, a crystalline combination of mercury and sulfur. This ore can be crushed, allowing the silvery liquid form of mercury to be separated from the other substances in the ore. If you played with this element as a kid, as I did, you may remember that if you touched liquid mercury, it would break into many little silver balls (but let me caution you not to let your kids play with liquid mercury). Alchemists of years gone by called mercury "quicksilver" because of this characteristic. Mercury exists in three different forms: (1) elemental—the silver liquid just discussed, (2) inorganic—mixed in its ionized form with other non-carbon-containing elements, as found in calomel, and (3) organic—mixed with a carbon-containing subgroup such as a methyl (CH_3) or ethyl (C_2H_5) group. This is important in our discussion of Meriwether Lewis.

In case you have forgotten your high school chemistry, chemical elements and compounds are different. Elemental atoms may only be broken down into their component particles (neutron, proton, and surrounding electrons). The most simple element is hydrogen, which in its elemental form has one positively charged proton in the nucleus and one negatively charged electron zooming very rapidly around the nucleus. Thus, an elemental hydrogen atom is neutrally charged because the positive nucleus and the negative electron result in an overall neutral charge of the atom. Any elemental atom is neutrally charged because, as an element, the number of its negatively charged electrons equals the number of its positively charged protons (this is an important detail).

Any element, including hydrogen, may become charged by losing (or gaining) one or more of the electrons that are whirling around the nucleus, resulting in an imbalance of positive and negative charges. When this happens to elemental hydrogen, it becomes a hydrogen ion (an ion is an element that is charged). The hydrogen ion and the hydrogen element behave differently, particularly in the body, just because one is charged and the other is not. Ions of various elements (including potassium, calcium, sodium, and chloride) are common in our bodies and are important in maintaining our health.

The element mercury, also known as one of the heavy metals, is significantly larger than the little hydrogen atom, and it has eighty protons in its nucleus and eighty electrons orbiting the nucleus. If the elemental form of mercury loses one or more electrons, it becomes a mercury ion. This information is necessary for understanding the effects of medications on Lewis's body as ions inside the body behave differently than elemental forms of elements.

Chemical compounds are combinations or mixtures of various elements. A simple compound is table salt, which is a combination of sodium ($Na+$), and chloride ($Cl-$) ions. In table salt (NaCl), the sodium atom has lost one electron and thus is a positively charged ion and the chlorine element has gained one electron and thus is a negatively charged ion. As a result, these two elements have opposite charges and are held together in the compound by a force called an ionic bond. These elements become broken when you eat salt as the water in your digestive tract breaks the weak bond and the compound NaCl (sodium chloride) is broken into individual sodium and chloride ions and absorbed into your blood in their ionic components. These ions are necessary to your life, especially to the healthy functioning of your nervous system.

NaCl (the compound we call table salt) + water = Na+ and Cl– (ions)

Before the time in the United States when the Federal Drug Administration administered the control of all medications and tested them for effectiveness and safety, American physicians all too often prescribed poisonous substances to their patients. One of the most common and nasty were mercury-containing medicines. These were sold both by prescription and over the counter as recently as the early twentieth century for the treatment of tonsillitis.

The mercury-containing medicines that Lewis had in his box of medications (poisons), which he erroneously believed to be beneficial, were calomel (mercurous chloride) as well as an elemental form of mercury found in mercury ointment. Calomel was one of Dr. Rush's favorite medicines; he included it in his Bilious Pills of Dr. Rush (the Corps of Discovery carried fifty dozen of these pills with them). This mercury-containing compound was created by combining ionized mercury (missing two electrons) with chloride ions. Calomel is Hg_2Cl_2—a compound containing two mercury ions and two chloride ions.

As I previously mentioned, mercury is a heavy metal. Heavy metal elements are very toxic to humans. In certain forms, mercury is an extremely toxic substance. The most toxic form of mercury occurs when the element is bonded to an organic compound (a carbon-containing compound) and thus becomes an organic mercury. Once mercury becomes attached to a carbon-containing compound, it becomes soluble in body fats (lipids), which are present throughout the human body. Thus, organic mercury can then be dispersed throughout the human body, which is harmful to the body. Organic mercury was considered medicinal in the Lewis and Clark era. Inorganic mercury, like calomel, although it is not lipid soluble, is nevertheless toxic to humans. A number of other heavy metal elements are also poisonous, but they are not relevant to our discussion (these are lead, arsenic, cadmium, chromium, and thallium).

Sometime in the distant past, people decided that drinking liquid elemental mercury (the silver liquid) might resolve their constipation. The element went through their intestinal tracts without much apparent harm.[2] Elemental mercury is poorly absorbed by the intestines. If the cells of the intestines do not absorb it, it will not enter the circulation and will not be systemically toxic. The toxicity of mercury is based on its ability to attack important molecules within our bodies that are themselves held together by chemical bonds. Many biomolecules, particularly proteins, that we need to live and be healthy can be destroyed by the action of mercury.

Proteins are long chains of many amino acids (links in the protein chain) held together by chemical bonds. Some proteins are assembled in bodily structures (found in the gums, muscles, organs, and elsewhere) that may be attacked and destroyed by mercury. The kidneys are largely made of highly organized and specialized proteins. Enzymes are very special types of proteins that catalyze thousands of chemical reactions within our bodies that keep us healthy and alive. Without properly functioning enzymes, which come in a dizzying array of thousands of different kinds, we either become sick or die. Mercury attacks all these proteins by destroying a very important bond within the proteins' structure, resulting in those proteins becoming broken and thus inactive. It is identical to removing a link in a chain; if you remove a link, the chain is broken. Broken chains do not work, and neither do broken structural proteins and their special protein cousins, enzymes. As the mercury attacks structural proteins in the mouth and gums, the gums become softened and sore and teeth may loosen or fall out.

Mercury can also attack the kidneys, damaging their ability to produce normal urine. If mercury in a non-elemental form (organic mercury) enters the nervous system, neurologic damage and other very nasty side effects result.

Lewis and Clark's medicinal mercury ointment may have contained either (1) elemental mercury (dispensed in a lard/fat medium as elemental mercury dissolves well in lipids) or (2) ionized mercury (calomel). This medicinal mercury was used to treat syphilis and a variety of other medical problems. Intestinal worms, a common problem during that era, were treated by Dr. Rush with what he called "large doses" of calomel (as well as an extensive list of other anti-worm medications ranging from rum to gunpowder). Treating various skin diseases as well as syphilis with mercury had been popular since the time of Paracelsus, the Swiss Austrian physician who popularized its use for syphilis in the sixteenth century.[3] The mercury ointment was applied to the patient for several days until the mercury started to poison the salivary glands as well as the kidneys. At this point, the patient started to salivate and urinate excessively as a result of being poisoned. Of course, modern medicine now realizes these signs to be evidence of mercury poisoning, but in Lewis's day it was believed to be a sign that the body was ridding itself of the cause of the syphilis.

Could the mercury-containing medicine have been beneficial to these patients? That would depend on one's definition of the word "beneficial." Clearly, mercury is toxic to all life forms. If a patient had parasites living within their intestines, the mercury could attack and kill them by disrupting their proteins in the same way it did the patient's body. It would also be potentially toxic to the bacterium that causes syphilis, but the administration, dosage, and terms of treatment of the medicinal mercury were so variable and unmonitored (and not understood) that using mercury as a medication was somewhat like hunting for ducks with an anti-aircraft gun on the tarmac of an airport. If some ducks flew through the airport and you opened fire, you might hit a few ducks, but the collateral damage to the surrounding aircraft would be a spectacularly negative result of this approach.

Ionized mercury in the form of calomel behaves in a slightly different manner than the mercury that is either nonionized or organic. Calomel, which was a component of Rush's bilious pills, is only slightly soluble in water and thus is not well absorbed in the intestines after being ingested. Only 7–15 percent of calomel enters into the blood circulation after being absorbed from the intestines. But that does not mean it was harmless. Its localized toxicity to the intestinal wall and the proteins that were present made it a potent irritant to the intestines and therefore the potent laxative that Rush meant it to be. Rush would have prescribed perhaps one or two of these pills per day for almost any medical complaint. The five of these pills that William Clark took on July 27, 1805, near the Three Forks of the Missouri River in present-day Montana, would have had a strong effect. As he reported in his journal, they "operated" on him very well the day after he took them.[4] The calomel that was absorbed into Clark's bloodstream was chiefly toxic to his kidneys, resulting in a condition called polyuria, which is the state of increased urination. This symptom may sound benign, as if the victim is just urinating a little more than usual. But it is definitely not harmless; it is the result of poisoning of the kidneys, reducing their ability to filter blood and reabsorb water. So, the signs that Clark reported of Dr. Rush's pills "operating" on him were, in fact, signs of the mercury poisoning his kidneys and his intestines. Without repeated poisoning, his kidneys and intestinal lining would recover at least most of their normal function. If only 15 percent of that mercury was absorbed by Clark's body, then 85 percent of it went out of the body through his very irritated intestines. Any amount of calomel taken orally will produce diarrhea due to intestinal poisoning. Five of Rush's pills would have caused severe diarrhea.

This same process of mercurial intestinal poisoning happened en masse at Traveler's Rest, at the western base of the Lolo Trail in the Bitterroot Mountains near present-day Missoula, Montana. In September 1805 and again in late June and early July 1806, the Corps dug a latrine at the campsite. When the members of the Corps urinated there, the mercury was deposited in the earth in its ionized form (the same form as in Rush's pills), and there it stayed for two hundred-plus years until archeologist Dan Hall and his research team discovered the site and found high deposits of organic mercury and mercury vapor within a localized underground area in 2002. This discovery established the actual location of the Traveler's Rest latrine. The campsite turned out to be located in a different place from the site officially designated by the National Park Service. Some have challenged the significance of this finding, claiming that the mercury that Hall found was organic and not the ionized form found in Rush's pills. However, inorganic mercury is converted by microorganisms to organic mercury by the addition of an organic (methyl-CH_3) group. Thus, all the inorganic mercury that was deposited in 1805 and again in 1806 by the Corps of Discovery was converted over the intervening two centuries into organic mercury (methyl mercury) courtesy of microorganisms in the dirt at Traveler's Rest.

Ionized mercury, such as that in calomel, does not readily pass from the blood into the brain due to the blood-brain barrier created by the structure of the walls of capillaries in the brain, which prevents mercury ions from passing through. Ionized mercury is not soluble in fat (lipid). If there is no mercury passing into the brain, then its toxic effects are not directly produced in that organ. However, the brain is not completely independent from the rest of the body, and damage to other structures and organs may ultimately affect the brain. Calomel (ionized mercury) is chiefly toxic to the kidneys.[5] So, the calomel that was used for a variety of medical reasons in Meriwether Lewis's time would not have produced symptoms due to central nervous system damage. Even during the 1950s and '60s, when I scraped my knees I was treated with applications of mercurochrome from my mother's medicine chest. This over-the-counter first aid treatment is now a thing of the past due to its mercury content. It worked because the mercury in the liquid killed the bacteria on the skin. Some skin-lightening creams, still available today and produced chiefly in Asia, contain mercury as the lightening agent. These are modern-day potential sources of mercury poisoning.

People in the past who drank elemental mercury for medical reasons did not suffer from neurological symptoms as a result, due to mercury's poor intestinal absorption. As an authoritative text on medical toxicology states, "Because of its poor oral absorption, elemental mercury can be ingested without toxicity."[6] Only about 0.01 percent of the mercury they ingested was absorbed into their bloodstream. Nonionized, elemental mercury easily crosses the blood-brain barrier and thus enters the brain, where it wreaks havoc. Elemental mercury could have been present in the fat-based mercury ointment used by the Corps. The ointment allowed the contents of elemental mercury to be more efficiently delivered through the patient's skin and into their bloodstream.

If you are unlucky enough to be exposed to mercury that passes into your brain, you may experience predictable and serious side effects in various parts of your body. Toxic effects of mercury on the brain may result in tremors (shaking hands), loss of sleep, memory loss, headaches, cognitive difficulties, and muscle-brain dysfunction. These types of side effects are usually the result of long-term exposure to low doses of mercury.[7] Industrial mercury poisoning used to occur among hat makers who used mercuric nitrate (a very toxic form of ionized mercury) to treat the fur and felt used to make expensive hats. These hat makers suffered from a neurologic poisoning known as erethism due to the frequent and high doses of mercury they received, which led to the term "mad as a hatter." Miners may breathe in elemental mercury vapors while working underground in poorly ventilated tunnels. Mercury forms a stable complex underground with both gold and silver, but its toxic fumes are liberated when these precious metals are processed and purified using heat.

The disease of erethism is a neurological disease that is characterized by several different personality symptoms, including, irritability, low self-confidence, depression, apathy, shyness, timidity, and, in extreme cases, delirium. Patients also have difficulty with social interactions. Did Lewis suffer from erethism, or mad hatter's disease, in his final days? In some respects, this seems likely. But the argument against this diagnosis is that any mercury that Lewis used medicinally was likely an ionic form (for example, Dr. Rush's pills), which would not readily pass into the brain from the blood and thus would not cause erethism.

Mercury ointment may have been produced for the Corps either by combining elemental mercury or calomel with lard, and these early-nineteenth-century pharmaceuticals were toxic in different ways. Although dermal absorption is limited with elemental mercury, its chief toxic effects occur when its vapors are inhaled or it is absorbed through the skin. The injection route was not available during Lewis's time. A small amount of elemental mercury passage through the skin was facilitated by its dispersion within the lard medium. (This is the same principle that occurs when you use alcohol-containing hand sanitizer after handling a gas pump handle. If you get some gasoline on your hands and then apply a hand sanitizer that contains ethyl alcohol, an organic solvent, this helps transport some of the gasoline molecules through the skin and into your system. In other words, wear gloves at the gas pump.) Alcohol is used in modern-day medications to help facilitate the transdermal (through the skin) medication delivery of various medications such as testosterone supplements.

Ionized mercury (calomel) was also a source of poisoning of the members of the Corps. Mercury ointment that contained calomel was toxic because calomel is passed through the skin's hair follicles, sebaceous glands, and sweat glands when it is mixed with lard.[8] In fact, calomel, which the Corps used extensively, was not very beneficial to their health, regardless of its route of administration.

Elemental mercury, as found in the mercury ointment in the medicine box of the Corps, once on board in the human body, has the ability to pass into the brain because it is lipid soluble. Once it is in the brain, it will remain there for a very long time. Elemental mercury's half-life in the kidneys is estimated to be thirty to sixty days. But once mercury passes into the brain, the half-life is estimated to be as long as twenty years. This does not mean that it all will be gone from one's brain within twenty years. It means that if one gets a toxic dose of twenty units, in twenty years the brain will still have ten units of mercury, and then another twenty years will pass before that is reduced to five, and so on. This very long presence of mercury in the brain is due to the fact that elemental mercury is strongly bonded to substances (selenium or sulfhydral groups) found in brain proteins. In addition to the toxic effects of mercury described above, chronic mercury poisoning also negatively affects the immune system. This complication results in decreased infection resistance.

So, the question arises, Was Lewis suffering from significant mercury poisoning, given some of his apparent difficulties in social interactions, irritability, depression, handwriting problems, excessive excitability, and decreased immunity to various infectious diseases? If Lewis had contracted syphilis during August of 1805 when he was visiting the Shoshones, is it possible that treatment with mercury for syphilis resulted in the symptoms he reportedly had prior to his death? If syphilis was present, then why not mercury poisoning?

My answer is that I seriously doubt that Lewis was suffering from the neurological symptoms of mercury poisoning. If you do a simple online word search for "signs of mercury poisoning," you will be presented with a list of signs that fairly well match the set of signs observed in Lewis. This exercise (a very poor method of diagnosis) would lead to a diagnosis of mercury poisoning.

There are several reasons I do not believe Lewis was suffering from mercury poisoning.

- The extreme symptoms of erethism are present as a result of long-term and significant mercury poisoning of the brain, chiefly obtained through exposure to very dangerous forms of mercury, usually mercury vapors that, when inhaled, go to the brain and stay there for a very long time. Lewis's exposure to mercury was chiefly through calomel and perhaps some elemental mercury (if he ever underwent treatment with mercury ointment). But such treatments would probably have ended long before the time required to produce erethism. In addition, calomel, as an ionized form of mercury, does not readily or extensively cross over from the blood into the brain.

- If Lewis was suffering from erethism and its resulting mental side effects, he would not have recovered in the few days it took for him to recover his senses while resting and on a diet of wine at Fort Pickering during his final weeks. This alone is enough to reject a diagnosis of erethism.
- Other explanations for Lewis's symptoms are much more likely and would account for any reported personality difficulties he was having during his last days.
- The primary symptom of mercury poisoning that Lewis would have suffered from would likely have been decreased kidney functioning, which would probably have been undetectable and clinically insignificant during his life. Any kidney damage that might have been permanent in members of the Corps would have resulted in decreased kidney functioning, which would have had a progressive effect on their overall health. This kidney malfunction would have occurred in later life in all of the members of the Corps of Discovery, chiefly due to the use of Dr. Rush's bilious pills and, possibly, of mercury ointment. They all probably had some degree of kidney disease as a result of this medication.

Of all the medications that Dr. Rush and other physicians of his day included in their pharmacopeia, mercury in its various forms was perhaps the most harmful. Rush used mercury for a vast array of problems, even swelling of the brain. The best that can be said in defense of Dr. Rush and his contemporaries is that they did not understand what they were doing. They were doing what physicians of that era accepted as proper treatment. Today, we know that these physicians knew almost nothing about chemistry and its applications to medicine. As Dr. Rush honestly commented toward the end of his life regarding his practice of medicine, "Of the poor services I have rendered to any of my fellow creatures I shall say nothing. They were full of imperfections and have no merit in the sight of God. I pray to have the sin that was mixed with them, forgiven."[9] Amen.

Peruvian Bark (Cinchona)

Peruvian bark has a colorful history as a medication and was considered a wonder drug for a variety of problems during the travels of the

Corps of Discovery. In the vast majority of cases, it did absolutely nothing of benefit for its patients.

The medical uses of cinchona bark were discovered by native people in South America at some time in the distant past. These people suffered from malaria, as much of the world still does today, and they experimented with various substances in their surrounding area with which to treat their illnesses. At some point they ground up the bark of the cinchona tree and noted its success in treating an illness that was characterized by fever, shaking chills, headache, nausea, and vomiting. The chills came and went every few days if untreated, but the bark often was successful in treating this unwelcome human malady.

In the early seventeenth century, Spain sent expeditionary ships to the New World, along with Roman Catholic priests who engaged in missionary work with the native population. One of the Jesuit priests working with the natives was informed of the miracle bark and its treatment for the disease previously described. It was a great day for Europe when the priest returned to Spain, bringing with him botanical samples of the tree, its seeds, and the bark. Thus, the bark was introduced into European medicine and the Western medicinal formulary. Ultimately, this knowledge made its way across the Atlantic and into early American medical practice.

What the natives, the priest, and all the rest of the doctors until the middle of the nineteenth century did not know was that the bark of the cinchona contains quinine, an organic (carbon-containing) substance produced by various tree species in the genus *Cinchona*. Quinine was first extracted from the bark in 1820 by French scientists. In the early twentieth century, scientists discovered that malaria was caused by a parasitic organism now called *Plasmodium* contained in the salivary glands of mosquitoes (see more on this in chapter 8).

The Peruvian bark was used in medicine either by brewing a tea or mixing it with wine, if taken internally. It had a very bitter taste that was often disguised with cloves, wine, or other spices. At times, it was also used as some sort of magical poultice, as when the captains applied it to the foot and ankle of Private Joseph Fields when he was bitten by a prairie rattlesnake on July 4, 1804, while walking in present-day Kansas. In some medical writings of that era, the bark is referred to in a general manner as an excellent restorative.

Cinchona bark was used for nearly any illness that was manifested by a fever. Since no oral thermometers existed during that era, a fever could likely mean anything from feeling hot and sweating to an increased heart rate, as monitored by taking a patient's pulse. Sacagawea received a dose of the bark when she suffered from her very severe and potentially fatal disease near the Great Falls of the Missouri River in June 1805. Cinchona appears frequently as a medical treatment, both in the expedition's records and in medical records of that day, for numerous different diseases.

What might have been the possible effects of the bark on Lewis during his final days? The medical records of Dr. Antoine Saugrain, the personal physician of Lewis, show that Lewis was prescribed some "quina quina," a form of Peruvian bark.[10] Although the bark did contain quinine, that plants are little factories that produce various pharmaceutically active substances. The cinchona tree, in fact, produces quinidine in addition to quinine. These two are not the same medication.

Possible side effects of quinine include headache, chest pain, blurred vision, sweating or flushing, unusual bleeding, red spots under the skin, dizziness, ringing in the ears, lowered blood sugar, and heart rhythm problems. The heart-related side effects come chiefly from quinidine, which is used in modern pharmaceuticals to treat some types of heart rhythm abnormalities. These side effects are potentially very dangerous. Due to the couple of centuries of use by the medical profession by 1804, such potential side effects were probably known and physicians (we hope) took these potential side effects into consideration. Topical application of the bark (as used for Field's rattler bite) probably did no good at all because absorption through the skin was likely very little and clinically insignificant.

Some of the side effects of the Peruvian bark are undeniably related to mental status. Dizziness, headache, and blurred vision are all potentially very troubling symptoms. If Lewis had been taking this medication and mixing it with others, which is likely, he had a very real risk of suffering from polypharmacy, a recognized problem of patients suffering from multiple unwanted interactions among their various medications. Mixing quinine with a neurologically active substance such as alcohol or opium could have resulted in the additive effect of a troubling mental status change—a "mental derangement." Any drug interactions Lewis may have suffered as the result of the bark would not have been beneficial.

It is very important to realize that many of the medications that Lewis may have been taking during his final weeks were not used exclusively for one disease. Some authors have pointed out that Lewis was taking "quina quina" as proof that he either had, or had been diagnosed with, malaria. There is no merit to this argument.

Laudanum and Opium

Laudanum and its big brother opium have been around for thousands of years. The opium poppy is the source of raw opium, which contains approximately fifteen different pharmaceutically active substances. Some of these components of opium are drugs that are familiar today. Codeine is the modern cough- and pain-relieving agent present in some cough syrups and codeine-containing pain pills. There is also morphine, a potent intravenous pain reliever and drug used to treat cardiovascular-related problems that not only relieves pain but relaxes vascular musculature, thereby decreasing blood pressure and thus making it easier for the heart to contract. Several others are less well known today: narcotine, thebaine, papaverine, and narceine.

All of these substances are harvested by cutting slits in the opium poppy and collecting the white sap that bleeds out of these slits. Some countries produce opium by bleeding their poppies only once, resulting in the highest morphine content, but others bleed the poppies repeatedly, yielding ever-decreasing amounts of morphine. The biochemical activity within this little plant is phenomenal.

Morphine is the main pharmaceutically active component of opium. Whenever Lewis and Clark used either their raw opium pills or their opium tincture, laudanum, they were administering some morphine as well as the other active molecules found in raw opium.

Synthetic opiates have been made in modern times based on our knowledge of organic chemistry and pharmacology and the necessary chemical reactions required to synthesize various types of opiates. Some of these synthetics, such as heroin, were used in various medications as recently as the early twentieth century. I (David) possess an old prescription for "heroin and turpin hydrate" written in the early twentieth century by a physician in Missoula, Montana—for a cough! This would have been effective in treating a variety of symptom, from pain and cough to diarrhea. Another synthetic opiate, fentanyl, which possesses about fifty to one hundred times the potency of morphine, was synthesized for use in cases of extreme pain. Sadly, these synthetic opioids have become toxic killers of people who buy them on the street in order to get high. Hundreds of Americans are dying every month as a result of these medications that are manufactured in China and Mexico and brought illegally into the United States to sell on the street.

In a recent Lewis biography, *Bitterroot: The Life and Death of Meriwether Lewis*, Patricia Stroud attempts to minimize or eliminate any possible use of opium by Lewis and the other reports of his drug and alcohol abuse by stating that all the reports of such use "have no basis in fact." She does admit, however, that "[h]is drinking, apparently, was heavy."[11] One of the issues is whether Lewis used opium at night, as is implied by his writing down the ingredients of an opium-containing medication in his personal notes.

Lewis's personal account book, written in 1808–09, includes his handwritten prescription for a "[m]ethod of treating bilious fever when unattended by Typhus or nervous symptoms." Lewis transcribed instructions for making "pills of Opium & tartar." He noted the mixture of "9 grains of tartar emetic, 12 grs. of opium made into 18 pills—one every night at bed time."[12] It is not possible to pinpoint when Lewis wrote this prescription, nor to know if he himself took such pills. It is completely possible, given the fact that he bothered to write it down, that he did at some point use it. Stroud states that there is no proof that Lewis was either making or taking this opium-based medication. She notes that he may have simply been writing it down for future reference. Stroud writes that "this statement is a misinterpretation and a fanciful extrapolation from papers in Lewis's possession of medicinal formulas that he planned to take with him in case of illness," further stating that they were likely left over from the expedition and had been furnished by Dr. Rush. Her justification for such a claim is that "there were then no pharmacies in St. Louis to prepare these treatments, one had to make up one's own medication when needed, and for a journey it was especially necessary to take along the ingredients."[13]

Although I agree with Stroud's position that Lewis's papers do not constitute proof that Lewis was actively taking opium during his last days, I do not believe her statement to be entirely accurate. I agree with her that Lewis may have retained some unused medicines from the expedition. But, Lewis was treated by Dr. Saugrain in St. Louis, who gave him medications. It was common practice for American physicians of that time to both prescribe and dispense the medications that they were giving to their patients. If there were no pharmaceuticals available in St. Louis, as claimed by Stroud, why would Lewis have visited Saugrain? If such medications were not available in St. Louis, why would Saugrain have prescribed them? If Lewis lacked access to these ingredients in St. Louis, why would he bother to write down the formulation? If Lewis had no intention of taking such a medication, why would he bother to write it down? If there were no pharmacies available in St. Louis at that time, where did sick patients obtain their prescribed medications?

Two lines of evidence point to the possibility or even probability that Lewis used some form of opium during his years as the territorial governor. The first is the ubiquitous presence of opium and laudanum in the pharmacopeia of physicians of that time. Physicians prescribed opium for multiple misdiagnosed diseases. Dr. Rush believed opium was a great stimulant to the system. As already noted, he used opium for a variety of unrelated diseases. For the most part, his prescriptions did no good for his patients other than to create a temporary feeling of euphoria. Opium certainly was not the great systemic stimulant that Rush believed it to be.

Saugrain, Lewis's point of contact with the pharmaceutical world, like all physicians of that era, lacked a clear understanding of the medicine he prescribed. Some of the medications Saugrain prescribed were, medically speaking, the worst substances he could possibly have given Lewis. If lucky, Saugrain might have accurately diagnosed Lewis, but he would have had no idea of what caused the disease, whatever it was. He was using drugs he did not understand while pushing Lewis toward a profound state of iatrogenic (physician-caused) illness due to the toxic medications he prescribed. This may sound like a harsh judgment, but it is 100 percent true.

The stark reality is that Saugrain was not the only physician who had an ineffective medical practice. Every M.D. at the time was doing exactly what Saugrain was doing. Prescribing cinchona bark for everything from suspected malaria to gout, heart failure, suspected tuberculosis, and edema reflects pharmaceutical confusion. Numerous other poisons, such as calomel and tartar emetic, were used for many other diseases and cured nothing. Using opium tablets for suspected malarial fevers is medical insanity from the perspective of modern pharmacology. But this is all that Lewis had, and this is probably, at least in part, why he was so sick at the end of his life.

In 1996, the Lewis and Clark coroner's jury heard testimony from Dr. Thomas Streed, a criminal psychologist, that applied to Captain Lewis's possible use of opium during his final days. Dr. Streed, summing up his analysis of Lewis's use of opium, stated, "Yes he used opium for malaria, but there is again, no evidence of any kind of an abusive relationship or a dependency."[14]

There are several problems with Streed's statement. We cannot know for certain that Lewis was using the opium for malaria because there is simply no way to establish reliably that he had malaria. His concurrent use of "quina quina," a preparation of Peruvian bark, does not prove Lewis had malaria as Peruvian bark was used at that time for numerous illnesses. Dr. Rush's medical essays regarding his suggested uses of various medications confirms this.[15] Streed's comment that alcohol and opium "may result in some kind of synergistic relation" is inaccurate as the combination of these two medications would *definitely* result in a synergistic action—the depression of the central nervous system.

As already noted, Dr. Rush and the medical community, in general, considered opium to be a stimulant to the body. This is the exact opposite of the actual pharmacologic effect of opiates. These pharmaceuticals are dramatic central nervous system depressants. Opium's pharmacologic benefits of pain relief, slowing of diarrhea, and sedation were used, as was calomel and Peruvian bark, to treat many different diseases. Clark even used opium to treat the "paralyzed" Nez Perce chief in 1806. Opiates have been a dangerous magic bullet for millennia.

Summing It Up

In analyzing the issues included in this book and rendering negative judgments about the medical care available to the people of the early nineteenth century, are we guilty of "historical presentism?" Are we assessing early nineteenth-century physicians based on today's norms? In an online article, Harvard University historian David Armitage wrote that "for most professional historians today, presentism is rather like Augustine's famous definition of time in his autobiographical *Confessions*: if nobody asks them what it is, they know; if you ask them to explain it, they don't."[16] Given that the exact definition of such a term is not even agreed upon by those who most often use it, we plead "not guilty."

We do not judge the physicians who administered poisons to their patients during the time of Lewis. Drs. Rush and Saugrain intended to cure their patients, but they nevertheless administered substances that were poisonous. Their medications were just as toxic to life in 1800 as they are today. The *Plasmodium* that causes human malaria has undoubtedly not significantly changed in its disease course since 1800. The human body's immune response to that disease has not significantly changed either. The physiological effects of alcohol and opium also have not changed since the time of Lewis. They affected humans alive in 1809 in *exactly* the same ways that they do today. So, our judging the effects of these medications (not the intentions of the physicians) two hundred-plus years ago is entirely legitimate.

Human nature has also not changed since 1809. Emotional pain was caused by the same factors then that produce it today, and people still make attempts to mitigate its unpleasant effects in a variety of both beneficial and dangerous ways, just as Meriwether Lewis did in 1809.

We are not passing judgment on cultural issues that were present in Lewis's day. As a physician and a psychologist, our medical and psychological evaluations of the issues involved in Lewis's final days are not evaluations of relativistic social norms such as the age of appropriate marriage partners. We are evaluating unchanging aspects of human nature and of medical issues that have not changed since the death of Lewis.

I (David) have often told audiences through the years that one of the biggest surprises in my study of the Lewis and Clark Expedition is that the captains and the other members of the corps survived relatively unscathed despite the medical treatment that was provided to them. I have covered only a few of the relevant medications in this section and have not discussed such other nineteenth-century therapeutical "wonders" as bloodletting, purging, vomiting, sweating, and blistering.[17] Mercury, Peruvian bark, and opium are all medications that may have played a part in the story of the final months of Meriwether Lewis.

The use of these medications reflects the sad state of medicine and the potentially toxic effects that medicines may have had on Lewis.

It is vitally important to note that it is a *significant error* in evaluating historical medical treatments to equate the prescription of a specific medication with the presence of a specific disease. For instance, we cannot assume that because Lewis was prescribed a form of Peruvian bark that he was being treated for malaria. The bark was indeed a medication used for malaria, but it was not used exclusively for that problem. Opium and other popular medications during that era were used for many different problems. Dr. Rush used Peruvian bark for a variety of problems, including intestinal worms, tetanus, painful legs, consumption (tuberculosis), gout, hydrophobia (rabies), and brain swelling. Opium, mercury, and other medications in the pharmacopeia also were used to treat a wide variety of symptoms and diseases. One might think that opium was used by physicians in 1809 for pain relief or perhaps diarrhea. But an examination of Rush's medical writings shows he used opium to treat a wide array of diseases. Rush even used mercury to treat swelling of the brain.[18] Reading through Rush's medical writings is a fascinating glimpse into his rather complicated thinking process about the often very creative ways and reasons to administer his favorite medications.[19] The inclusion of "quina quina," a form of Peruvian bark, in Lewis's prescription from Dr. Saugrain during his final months in St. Louis is absolutely no proof that Saugrain believed Lewis had malaria.

One of my (David's) favorite words is the German word *schweinerei*, which means "a pig's mess." Our good friend Miriam Krause, M.D., taught me this wonderful German word many years ago when, as a medical student at the University of Heidelberg in Germany, she spent a month with me doing urgent care medicine in San Diego. The word describes well the state of medicine and pharmaceuticals during the life of Meriwether Lewis.

Have you ever wondered what it was like to be a patient during the time of Lewis and Clark? Well, you will not have to strain your imagination to fully appreciate the uneasy feeling of people visiting a physician in the early 1800s. Lest we feel the least bit arrogant about our state of medical sophistication in the twentieth century, as I was typing this chapter on April 2, 2020, our world was in a state of alarm and bewilderment due to the Covid-19 virus. On that date, 1,011,064 cases had been reported worldwide, with 52,885 deaths of Americans, and the peak of the viral epidemic was months away. The number of cases and deaths grew exponentially over the next months. Prior to the administration of an effective vaccine, most healthy people were sheltered in their homes, going out only for groceries and other necessities. Hospitals and ICUs filled up and even overflowed with patients. In some areas of the world, eight to ten family members had to crowd together in a single room with no access to grocery stores or hospitals. A year ago, we had no effective vaccine or medication with which to address this potentially fatal disease. We grabbed at potential cures, just like physicians did in 1793 in Philadelphia when they told people to wear vinegar-soaked cloths at the height of the yellow fever epidemic. In 2020, refrigerated trucks stored the bodies of the dead; in the 1790s, horse-drawn wagons clopped along the cobblestone streets of Philadelphia, taking the dead away to bury. People fled Philadelphia in droves and children walked around smoking cigars in an effort to ward off the yellow fever. We too tried to deal with a modern-day killer that was having its way with humanity, similar to syphilis, smallpox, measles, bubonic plague, influenza, and other infectious diseases in times past. We knew our modern-day tormentor was a virus, a small speck containing some RNA. No one knew of such things during the days of Meriwether Lewis.

Realizing that the physicians in Lewis's day knew absolutely nothing about the chemistry of pharmaceuticals, I am filled with gratitude and humility for the privilege of being alive today. Our modern knowledge of molecular biology and biomedical science has rapidly produced multiple effective vaccines that appear to provide full protection against Covid-19 and even its variants to date. Such progress and pharmaceutical effectiveness could not have even been imagined during the time of Lewis. After a year of feeling a bit helpless and humble, we rejoice at our privileged position in medical history and feel even more empathy and compassion for those who lived long ago.

Chapter 6
Meriwether Lewis: Mental Derangement and Syphilis

The usefulness of an opinion is itself a matter of opinion: as disputable, as open to discussion, and requiring discussion as much, as the opinion itself.
—John Stuart Mill

Several diseases have been proposed as playing a role in the mystery of the death of Meriwether Lewis. The two infectious diseases that have attracted the most attention and discussion are malaria and the sexually transmitted disease syphilis. I (David) covered this in some detail in my book *Or Perish in the Attempt* but will do so again in this work as some physicians have expressed differing opinions in online blogs. As is true of several issues surrounding Lewis's death, the complexities stimulate controversy.

Dr. Reimert Ravenholt, a Seattle-based physician and epidemiologist, proposed in 1994 that the signs of disease that Lewis and others in the Corps of Discovery presented with in September 1805 were "pathognomonic" of syphilis. Ravenholt went on to state that the symptoms of mental derangement reported in Lewis during his final days were the result of the syphilis infection he obtained in August 1805.[1] The word "pathognomonic" refers to a sign or symptom that is distinctively characteristic or diagnostic of a particular disease—say, a particular type of skin rash that, when present, means that a specific disease is present. Given Ravenholt's claim, it is important to have a good understanding of syphilis.

Syphilis is a sexually transmitted disease caused by the bacterium *Treponema pallidum*. Syphilis has four stages whose manifestations may be separated by years. Three of these four stages have clinical signs on the skin, either a typically painless ulcer present at the site of infection (a chancre) or a typically painless, blotchy red rash on the palms of the hands and soles of the feet in later stages.

Regarding syphilis and the Corps of Discovery, we know that
- the Corps of Discovery had in its pharmaceutical box both mercury ointment and pills containing calomel (mercurous chloride), which were common treatments for syphilis in 1804;
- Lewis and Clark noted on repeated occasions that members of the Corps had contracted the "pox" or "Louis Veneri," a creative misspelling by Lewis of the Latin term for syphilis, *lues venerea*; and
- syphilis was present during the expedition; some of the men contracted it through having sex with Native American women, and these men were treated with mercury.[2]

Ravenholt also references the general and severe symptoms of illness displayed by many of the men on the expedition and recorded in the journals several weeks after September 19, 1805, as evidence of his diagnosis of syphilis. Ravenholt quotes these September 24 and 25, 1805, entries by Clark: "Capt Lewis Scercely able to ride on a gentle horse which was furnished by the Chief, several men So unwell that they were Compelled to lie on the Side of the road for Some time other obliced to be put on horses. I gave rushes Pills to the Sick this evening" and "Capt Lewis very Sick. . . . when I arrived at Camp found Capt Lewis verry Sick, Several men also verry Sick, I gave Some Salts & Tarter emetic."[3] Similar entries describing widespread significant signs of illness continue for a number of days.

I agree with Ravenholt that Lewis and many of the Corps "suffered from gastrointestinal illnesses while along the Clearwater River." But I disagree with Ravenholt's claim that, at least in part, these illness symptoms were the result of an epidemic of syphilis due to the concurrent symptom of "skin lesions," which he states are pathognomonic for syphilis.[4] I disagree because skin lesions could be symptomatic of a number of other diseases.

Other physicians have also criticized Ravenholt's diagnosis. Dr. Joseph P. Pollard, a retired Navy captain/physician, noted that if "Lewis contracted syphilis during the time of the expedition as proposed (August 1805), the infection would have progressed for 4 years and 2 months by the time of his death in October, 1809. Syphilis is slowly progressive and in 4 years time should be in its latent state."[5] Pollard theorized that the probable mercury treatment for syphilis was more likely than tertiary (late) syphilis to have produced any mental changes. However, as I have noted in my analysis of mercury poisoning (see chapter 5), that scenario is highly unlikely given that calomel does not pass significantly into the brain and that mercury ointment, although potentially neurotoxic, would likely not have been used for long enough to result in erethism. Pollard makes a good point when he says that perhaps Lewis "misinterpreted the toxic symptoms of his treatment for symptoms of the disease, leading to further overtreatment and, eventually, to suicide."[6] I doubt this was the case, but it is nevertheless a possibility. I doubt this chiefly because it is much more appropriate due to the historical evidence to assign Lewis's end-of-life illness to other causes.

In addition to these two published opinions, I have spoken with a number of physicians over the past twenty years about this situation. One pathologist noted that he had discussed the situation with Ravenholt and was skeptical of his syphilis diagnosis. Another physician, Donald W. MacCorquodale, noted online that Ravenholt stated that expedition members York and William Bratton had syphilis. Ravenholt's medical justification for his diagnosis was that York's feet were so sore that he had to ride a horse in the Bitterroots and that Bratton "had severe pain in the small of his back." The justification for assigning these symptoms to syphilis is greatly weakened when the journals are read in their entirety and these statements are considered in the context in which they were written.

Ravenholt cites a comment in the Lewis and Clark journals about York's feet. On September 1, 1805, Gass wrote: "About the middle of the day, Capt Clarke's black man's feet became so sore that he had to ride on horseback."[7] As stated above, plantar lesions are a common manifestation of secondary syphilis. Dr. MacCorquodale noted that the secondary syphilitic skin lesions found on the soles of the feet are typically not painful. This would certainly be evidence against York's painful feet being the result of syphilis. But, this is not conclusive evidence. Is there another more convincing explanation?

The journal accounts of the preceding days and weeks of the activities of the expedition offer multiple compelling explanations of York's sore feet unrelated to syphilis. These were very hard times for the Corps. They were eating a calorie-poor diet that consisted chiefly of salmon while they engaged in the demanding physical effort of walking and riding over steep mountains with all the accompanying difficulties of moving an expedition through very rough country.

Clark wrote on August 23, 1805: "proceed on with great dificulty as the rocks were So Sharp large and unsettled and the hill sides Steep that the horses could with the greatest risque and dificulty get on." Four days later, he recorded, "[M]y party hourly Complaining of their retched Situation and [contemplating?) doubts of Starveing in a Countrey where no game of any kind except a few fish can be found." The next day, he noted, "Those Sammon which I live on at present are pleasent eateing, not with standing they weaken me verry fast and my flesh I find is declining." Then, on August 31 Clark recorded that "the Countrey which we passed to day is well watered & broken Pore Stoney hilly country" and Joseph Whitehouse wrote, "We proceeded on our way, and crossed over some rough hills, some of them very steep . . . the Stones lay very plenty, & the place full of holes & where we found it almost impossible, for our horses to pass, without breaking their legs. We passed along the Edge of this mountain with great difficulty."[8] I believe that these traveling conditions, described by several journal keepers, were the cause of the sore or red feet.

There are multiple reasons why Ravenholt's diagnosis of William Bratton as having a case of syphilis misses the mark. First, Bratton's back pain lasted through the entire fall and winter of 1805–06. Second, journal entries by members of the Corps frequently mention this problem. A prime example is this entry on May 24, 1806 by Lewis: "William Bratton still continues unwell; he eats heartily digests his food well, and has recovered his flesh almost perfectly yet is so weak in the loins that he is scarcely able to walk (four or five steps), nor can he sit upwright but with the greatest pain."[9]

The pain often prevented Bratton from doing any work during the winter close to the Pacific Ocean. His pain persisted and prohibited him from walking on April 21, 1806, strongly suggesting a musculoskeletal problem. It was not until the return trip, when Bratton was put in a steam or /sweat bath while with the Nez Perce in present-day Idaho, that his condition resolved. This occurred during the third week of June 1806 at the suggestion of Private John Shields, who claimed to have witnessed dramatic cures of this type of ailment through the use of a steam or sweat bath, an icy water bath, and horse nettle tea. Bratton underwent the treatment and the very next day was almost entirely free of pain.[10] This clinical picture in no way supports a diagnosis of syphilis but points strongly toward a diagnosis of a musculoskeletal problem.

Perhaps the strongest and most insightful evidence against the diagnosis of Bratton's syphilis is that William Bratton was singled out by the captains as a man "who had the strictest morals."[11] It would seem virtually impossible for a man who warranted such an observation of his good moral behavior during the expedition, and who achieved a cure by a steam bath, to have obtained his back pain by way of a syphilitic infection contracted by lying with a Shoshone woman. Nothing about the proposed diagnosis of syphilis rings true in light of the historical record regarding either Bratton or York. The evidence against Ravenholt's argument that York and Bratton had syphilis is overwhelming.

My analysis in *Or Perish in the Attempt* of the possibility that Lewis's mental changes at the end of his life were the result of neurosyphilis was criticized in an online blog of the *New England Journal of Medicine* in 2010. The response stated in part:

> I think you're approaching this from a contemporary medical perspective. Obviously, you can't make a definitive diagnosis based on the information available. But we're dealing in the realm of historical speculation. I can't draw a conclusion based on medical training that I don't have but I can look at the evidence the way a juror would and I think from that perspective Ravenholt makes a very good case.

The blogger added that my arguments against Ravenholt's diagnosis seem weak.[12]

In addressing this blogger's critique of my arguments, I have a couple of comments. First, I am the first to agree that we are dealing in the realm of historical speculation and that no concrete diagnosis can be made. This blogger's argument is weakened, however, by his statement that he was looking at Ravenholt's argument as a juror would. A juror's prior knowledge about any subject an attorney is addressing ranges from complete ignorance of the subject to comprehensive knowledge (as an expert). A juror is generally not very knowledgeable about all the facts of a case and is subject to being influenced by the arguments of attorneys depending on their knowledge of the issue being discussed. In arguing for a client, an attorney focuses on facts that support their case. Facts that are not supportive are either ignored or minimized as unimportant or irrelevant. Unfortunately, this is precisely the type of thought process that has been used by many authors, including Ravenholt, who try to analyze the causes of Lewis's death.

We are all speculating, and I would not bet my retirement plan on my diagnosis. However, based on epidemiology and historical statistics regarding untreated syphilis infections (which Lewis may have had, if Ravenholt's theory is correct), it results in insanity (due to the disease's progression to neurosyphilis) in only 10 to 20 percent of patients.[13] I will also cite additional information here that I did not present in *Or Perish in the Attempt*. I believe this collective evidence is strong.

My weak arguments, as noted by the online physician blogger, are as follows:

(1) Lewis could not have known for certain that he was suffering from neurosyphilis because the condition was not even described in the world of medicine until 1882, when Bayle described "dementia paralytica," or paretic neurosyphilis. This was the first psychiatric disease for which a specific pathology and cause were found.[14]

It was suspected during Lewis's time that syphilis, or the pox, was a serious and sometimes fatal illness; some Indian tribes that were questioned by the captains about the presence of venereal diseases stated that members of their tribes had died as a result of what they suspected to be such a disease. Syphilis had already killed many thousands of people throughout the world since its first appearance in the early sixteenth century in Europe. Most medical historians believe that syphilis was brought to Europe by some of Columbus's returning crew and/or by some of the North American natives Columbus brought back with him to Europe in the late fifteenth century.[15]

(2) Although several Indian tribes had offered young women to the captains as bed partners, there is no evidence in the journals that they ever took advantage of these opportunities. In fact, the captains wrote about the various Indian tribes' irritation at their refusals. So, it is presumptive to assume that Lewis contracted syphilis anywhere along the route of the expedition.

Apparently, there were others among the Corps who did not sleep with Indian women. As we have already discussed, the Scots-Irish (and reported Presbyterian) William Bratton was specifically mentioned as "having the strictist morals" during the expedition, which strongly implies that he did not have sex with Indian women. The context of the captains' post-expedition report concerning Bratton makes it intuitively obvious that they were referring to *sexual* morals. There is no other possibility regarding the captains' positive assessment of Bratton's morals. In addition, only some of the men were described as experiencing excessive salivation, one of the nasty side effects of mercury treatments for "Louis Veneri."

(3) Syphilis is sometimes referred to in medicine as "the great imitator" as its symptoms mimic many other diseases. Edmund C. Tramont, in a highly respected textbook on infectious disease, noted that neurosyphilis mimics

> any degenerative neurologic process, or disorder that cause chronic inflammation (e.g. tuberculosis, fungal or sarcoid meningitis, tumors, subdural hematoma, Alzheimer's disease, multiple sclerosis, chronic alcoholism), or any disorder affecting the vasculature of the central nervous system. The axiom that syphilis can mimic any disease is particularly apropos with regard to the central nervous system.[16]

This lengthy list of diseases with which syphilis shares signs and symptoms puts Ravenholt's claims on very thin ice.

(4) As noted earlier, Ravenholt cites the journals' references to "irruptions of the Skin"[17] as evidence of a syphilitic infection. In a very

general sense, this could be true. The great problem in diagnosing the Corps's skin eruptions during this time frame as syphilitic in nature is that the captains, despite their having seen and treated previous skin eruptions as "pox," which was a synonym for syphilis, did not in any way identify these eruptions as such in the journals. Perhaps in not recording them they were just trying to hide their diagnosis. Since they did use the term "pox" as a synonym for syphilis throughout the expedition, though, why would they suddenly refer to a suspected case of syphilis as a "skin eruption?" Did the captains actually believe that many of the men had contracted syphilis from the Shoshones? This possibility must at least be considered, although it seems quite a stretch. There are a number of infectious diseases and localized skin reactions (allergic reactions) that manifest with skin eruptions. We have just explained that York's sore/red feet were undoubtedly the result of prolonged walking on terribly difficult and rocky terrain. On occasion, Lewis mentioned treating syphilis with mercury, as in his journal entry of January 27, 1806: "Goodrich has recovered from the Louis veneri which he contracted from an amorous contact with a Chinnook damsel. I cured him as I did Gibson last winter by the use of murcury."[18] There is no record that Lewis treated any of the skin eruptions mentioned in September 1805 with any mercury product, the accepted treatment for syphilis that he carried in his medicine chest. This is undoubtedly because Lewis did not believe the symptoms to be related to "Louis Veneri" infections.

Let us assume that Lewis *did* contract syphilis during this time frame. If he did not self-treat with one of his mercury medicines, is there any data or scientific information that might predict the outcome of his infection? There have been two major studies on the progression of syphilis in untreated patients. These were performed in Oslo, Norway, and the United States in the twentieth century. These studies were both medically unethical and immoral as effective medication was knowingly withheld from the participants in order to carry out the scientific studies. The data from these studies showed that only about 25 percent of the syphilis victims who were untreated progressed to having complications of late syphilis, which include neurologic involvement.[19] Most people who die of complications of syphilis die from cardiovascular disease; they develop inflammation in the main artery exiting the heart (the aorta) and accompanying complications.

The odds are quite small that Lewis had neurosyphilis that developed from an infection obtained during the Shoshone portion of the trip. First, he did not record that he treated himself with mercury, which he probably would have if he suspected he had "pox," given his tendency toward detail and perfectionism. Given the natural history of the disease as outlined in this chapter, even an untreated Lewis would likely not have progressed to suffering from neurosyphilis. In addition, his mental derangement reported by several people during his final days completely cleared up during his stay and treatment at Fort Pickering (see chapter 4). If this mental derangement had been the result of neurosyphilis, Lewis's symptoms would not have been so transient, nor would the diet of wine prescribed by Captain Gilbert Russell have cured him.

On an entirely different subject, one that actually argues against the point I am making, mercury might have cured syphilis, but its dosage and administration were not standardized, and it certainly was nowhere near as effective against syphilis as penicillin would prove to be in the twentieth century. At best, an appropriate analogy might be that using mercury to treat syphilis was like dropping an atomic bomb on an army of a thousand soldiers. Elemental mercury's horrible side effects make it an extremely poor choice for treating any patient—for any problem. It poisons the kidneys and indiscriminately attacks various proteins throughout the body.

Ravenholt either misinterprets and/or ignores important facts in the known historical record concerning the time period of the Corps of Discovery. He ignores the fact that the symptoms of illness that Lewis and other men had during the weeks after September 19, 1805, were the result of what Lewis diagnosed as a gastrointestinal problem related to several weeks of near starvation while the expedition was in the Bitterroot Mountains. At this time, they were eating their usual portable soup made of a dehydrated, paste-like substance produced from boiling and dehydrating meat products. Following their weeks-long subsistence diet, after contacting the Nez Perce tribe they gorged themselves on salmon and camas bread. Eating these foods produced significant diarrhea accompanied by severe abdominal cramps and gas. The gastrointestinal symptoms were so severe that Lewis was unable to ride on a gentle horse and had to lie down along the side of the path for significant periods, as did many other members of the Corps.

I do think it is entirely possible that Lewis contracted syphilis after his return to civilization in 1806. This could support Ravenholt's general diagnosis that syphilis caused Lewis's mental derangement because neurosyphilis can occur in the primary and secondary stages of syphilis, not only in the tertiary or late stage. Current data shows that this is a somewhat rare situation, however, affecting only 0.3–2.4 percent of patients with primary-stage infections, which usually lasts for only 10–90 days.[20]

The dreaded complication of neurological involvement is not always seen in syphilis patients, even after years of latent infection. In modern days, this is usually the result of a concurrent HIV infection, which affects the immune system. Clearly, Meriwether Lewis did not have HIV. Neurosyphilis that occurs during the primary or secondary phase of syphilis typically manifests as meningitis (inflammation of the covering of the brain and spinal cord), which can affect some of the twelve cranial nerves (so called because they originate in the brain and not as extensions of the spinal cord). Neurosyphilis that affects the cranial nerves usually affects cranial nerve 6, 7, or 8. Cranial nerve (CN) 6 innervates muscles that control eye movement. CN7 controls the sensory and motor functions involving facial expression and taste. CN 8 involves both hearing and balance. Some of the more usual symptoms of these patients include difficulty walking and speaking, headaches, hearing loss, forgetfulness, and personality changes, the result of abnormalities of the involved cranial nerves.

Although I believe that the chance that Lewis was suffering personality changes associated with a case of syphilis is slim to none, what is the likelihood of a mentally deranged Meriwether Lewis in October 1809 suffering from neurosyphilis that he obtained *after* he returned to civilization? Modern medical records documenting personality changes resulting from neurosyphilis are depression, disorientation, uncooperativeness, and self-aggressiveness. One such patient attempted suicide by trying to hang himself. This patient had no previous symptoms of psychiatric illness, prior infections, head trauma, or drug abuse. He was accurately diagnosed with neurosyphilis and was administered appropriate antibiotics (penicillin G). In this fascinating case study, the patient initially improved but then started complaining of visual and auditory hallucinations with persecutory content (he believed that people were out to get him).[21] We need to be very careful not to jump to the conclusion that all the pieces seem to fit and thus that Lewis's mental changes must have been the result of a syphilitic infection that affected his cranial nerves. Again, if we look at the data and the odds, *less than 3 percent* of primary syphilis victims develop such symptoms. It is possible that Lewis was suffering from mental derangement brought on by a case of neurosyphilis that he became infected with after the expedition. But, this is very unlikely. It is even more unlikely given the high probability that other factors were negatively affecting the mental health of Lewis in 1809.

Although early neurologic involvement of syphilis can and does occur, the most common situation in the late stage of infection is an absence of any symptoms. As is true for chronic malaria as well, most late cases of syphilis are asymptomatic, whereas early neurosyphilis usually presents as an inflammation of the meninges (the lining that covers the brain and spinal cord) and, as already noted, possible cranial nerve involvement. The most serious problem with doing a word search of Lewis's symptoms and diagnosing him with neurosyphilis is that all of the many psychiatric changes present in neurosyphilis—cognitive impairment, personality disorders, delirium, hostility, difficulty speaking, confusion, disruption of the sleep-wake cycle, fecal and urinary incontinence, feeling bad about everything, paranoia, hallucinations, and mania—are also present in several psychiatric disorders. This is why neurosyphilis is difficult to diagnose without modern lab work. This is also why syphilis is known as "the great imitator."[22]

Manifestations of late neurosyphilis typically involve changes to the brain and spinal cord (not just its covering or the cranial nerves). This late manifestation of syphilis typically presents with dementia, periodic convulsions, vegetative degeneration, loss of coordination, lack of awareness of the position of the arms and legs—resulting in the inability to walk normally—and bowel and /bladder dysfunction. In addition, it is helpful to note that psychiatric signs and symptoms associated with neurosyphilis (in the current literature) are present in 33–86 percent of patients. Therefore, not all the victims of neurosyphilis will have psychiatric changes. Even if they do develop personality changes, less than half (48 percent) of patients exhibit some component of hallucinations.[23]

Could Lewis have been suffering from simultaneous infections of both malaria and syphilis in his final days? That is certainly a possibility. But if we take into account the probability of both diseases, the incidence of asymptomatic infections (which is high), the incidence of complications even when untreated (which is low to medium), the possible success of the available treatments of cinchona bark and mercury ointment (at best low to medium), it is not probable that Lewis was suffering such severe symptoms as a result of having these two infectious diseases.

How could we verify that Lewis had syphilis? Without examining his body, we cannot. Even exhuming Lewis's remains might not lead to the answer. Neural tissue, which is mainly composed of water, will not likely stand up to more than 230 years of interment in an unembalmed body. When an untrained team of observers last saw Lewis's remains (107 years ago), they noted the presence of skeletal remains. Dr. Glenn Wagner, former chief medical officer of the County of San Diego, has performed over fourteen thousand autopsies in his fifty years of experience as a forensic pathologist. He stated to me that if there was any brain tissue left in the remains of Lewis, even as small as a thimble, which he has witnessed in very old bodies, then it may be possible to detect some *Treponema pallidum*—the organism that causes syphilis—in the DNA in Lewis's brain tissue (see appendix). But without an intact brain to study and the ability to cut it into sections for a microscopic histological exam, any degenerative neurologic disease of the brain that might have been present as the result of a neurosyphilitic infection would be impossible to diagnose.

Ravenholt suggests the interesting possibility that Lewis could have been infected with syphilis during his stay with the Shoshones. Other Native American tribes had offered and encouraged men of the expedition to have sex with women in their tribes. However, the journals record a very different situation in regard to the expedition's stay with the Shoshones. Lewis was greatly concerned that none of the men give any opportunity for Shoshone bad will as a result of sexual relations with their women. On August 19, 1805, Lewis wrote,

> I have requested the men to give them no cause of jealousy by having connection with their women without their knowledge,

which with them strange as it may seem is considered as disgracefull to the husbands as clandestine connections of a similar kind are among civilized nations. to prevent this mutual exchange of good officies altogether I know it impossible to effect, particularly on the part of our young men whom some months abstance have made very polite to those tawney damsels. no evil has yet resulted and I hope will not from these connections.[24]

It seems obvious that Lewis was excluding himself from these encounters in this journal entry. As the commander of the expedition, which required getting horses from the Shoshone, it is nearly incomprehensible that Lewis would jeopardize such an important mission and violate his own stated directive by having sex with a Shoshone woman.

Given this scenario, it seems that Ravenholt's view that Lewis's inquiries about venereal disease among the Shoshone women were motivated by his interest in having sex with them represents a misinterpretation of Lewis's own journal entry. Lewis's questions about this subject were nothing more than the standard questions he asked all the tribes he encountered.

Ravenholt might argue that the captain's refusal of a Shoshone offer of sex was a dangerous negotiation tactic given the Corps's dire need to secure horses and good will from the Shoshones. But the Corps had many other trade items to use in their bargaining, and this tribe was destitute in terms of material goods. They were victims of intertribal bullying by the Blackfeet tribe to the north. They were often famished, as evidenced by their eating of deer hoofs and raw deer intestines after the killing of a deer near Camp Fortunate in present-day southwestern Montana in August 1805. The Shoshones would have traded their horses for almost anything that Lewis and Clark offered them. In addition, the traveling band of White men had a Black man with them who was called by many tribes the "big Medison [Medicine]," a talented dog, and a Shoshone woman who was part of their own band. Lewis would have had nothing to fear from refusing any sexual offers from members of this tribe.

As with many attempted explanations of Lewis's state during his final days, Ravenholt's theory that syphilis was responsible for his mental derangement is somewhat appealing on the surface as a viable explanation for Lewis's behavior in his final months. But when one looks closely at the medical issues involved, other historical documents detailing his life, and the situations Lewis described in the journals, this theory is interesting but very unlikely.

In the next chapter, we look in some detail at the philosophical and religious influences on the life of Meriwether Lewis.

Chapter 7
A Collision of Worldviews: Christianity, the Enlightenment, and Freemasonry

It is the heart which perceives God and not the reason. That is what faith is: God perceived by the heart, not by the reason.
—Blaise Pascal

One of our great joys in life has been studying and attempting to understand various aspects of the human experience. In this chapter, we stray from our career paths and travel another trail of the human experience that is at least as complex and interesting as medicine and psychology. It could be argued that we as a physician and a psychologist (who are not theologians or philosophers) offering our understanding of the matters addressed in this chapter are violating our own critique of those who are not medically trained offering opinions on medical psychological aspects of the Corps of Discovery. We are confident writing about these topics, but doctoral-level theology professors have checked the text of this chapter to ensure its accuracy.

Meriwether Lewis lived in a time characterized by numerous types of change. When he was growing up, the people with whom he had contact and who influenced his thinking differed greatly in their life philosophies. Lewis was, without question, influenced by European Enlightenment thinking, both through his immediate culture and through his close and prolonged contact with Thomas Jefferson. The years of Lewis's adulthood were a tumultuous time that saw quick and dramatic changes in American culture, shifts in the religious influences on his family and friends, and worldwide changes in the fundamental ways humans viewed reality. Synthesizing some of these events and areas of thought and gaining insight into their influence on Lewis is the topic of this chapter.

Religious Influences on Lewis

The entire area of the religious culture of the American nation and its influence on the Lewis family has been scantly reviewed in previous works on the Lewis and Clark Expedition. We firmly believe that gaining an understanding of American religious culture, issues related to Lewis and his spiritual beliefs, and the religious thought he encountered during his early life adds an entirely new dimension to our understanding of who he was, how he thought, and what was important to him in his spirituality. It also explains some important issues surrounding his death. This understanding will in turn provide insight into how he viewed others as well as the factors that led to his ultimate fate. Regardless of your beliefs regarding his death, a look into these important ideas will help round out your understanding of this most interesting American hero.

Many of the societal norms of social class, church, and civic authority that existed in England were transplanted with those who immigrated to the shores of North America in the early seventeenth century. Landholding men in America in the seventeenth and eighteenth centuries became the political leaders who guided much of the course of culture in the colonies. Men who upheld the sovereignty of the English monarchy were appointed as landholders, magistrates, and members of the various colonial houses of government. These early Americans generally ate English-style food, drank English-style beer, and looked on the English king as God's representative on earth who should and must be obeyed. They also looked on the mother country as their protector during the French and Indian War that lasted from 1756 to 1763 and was the American conflict related to Great Britain's Seven Years' War with France in Europe.

As a reflection of religious thought in England, many Americans who were either members of the Anglican church proper or a related version of it held different interpretations of relatively minor points of theology. Such differences of opinion might seem minor, but they were in fact major points of contention within this group. Many of these points of disagreement were significant enough for the Puritans to leave England and set sail for the New World because of the persecution they faced from the established Anglican church.

If you were a church member in colonial America, your minister or priest had likely spent many years obtaining his theological education after completing an undergraduate course of study in college. He had more than likely been appointed by an established bishop who resided in England or by a recognized church envoy in the colonies. Members of the clergy were generally viewed as pillars of respect within the colonies. Unlike present-day America, where aspiring ministers can plant churches without any formal theological training, clergymen in the colonies spent years of training within their respective denominations in preparation for ministering to their flocks, and they enjoyed great societal respect, even reverence, from much of the American colonial population.

Rarely has such profound cultural change occurred in so few years and to such an extent in American society as happened after the American Revolution and the nation's independence. The attitudes that resulted from America's newfound autonomy—republicanism, egalitarianism, and increased dependence on human reason due to the American Enlightenment—made their way into every facet of American life, both secular and ecclesiastical. These viewpoints had a profound influence on American religious thought and thus the culture of Meriwether Lewis.

Many of the pre-Revolutionary War societal norms of civic and clerical hierarchies of the English-based colonial culture not only changed in the years of 1775–83 but were aggressively resisted and detested by many Americans of this period. The results and effects of the American Revolution on the behavior and beliefs of Americans are central to the theme of this section as the egalitarian American spirit influenced many areas of American culture, including its religious beliefs and practices.

Meriwether's education during his adolescence was primarily in the hands of three private tutors, two of whom were clergymen. Starting at age thirteen, he studied for two years under the Anglican minister Matthew Maury (1744–1801) in Albemarle County, Virginia, a tutor well known to Thomas Jefferson. The third tutor was the Irish American Presbyterian minister Dr. James Waddell (1739–1805). Waddell had attended Nottingham Academy in Lancaster County, Pennsylvania, and was taught there by the Reverend Dr. Samuel Finley; interestingly, Finley had also taught Dr. Benjamin Rush, who became Lewis's physician mentor for his future expedition to the Pacific Ocean. Waddell was a talented preacher and a master of several ancient languages. James Madison described Waddell as one of the two greatest orators he had ever heard and reportedly stated, "He has spoiled me for all other preaching."[1] Waddell became blind due to cataracts in 1787, the same year that Lewis became his student. He was characterized as "cheerful, happy and resigned to his physical afflictions."[2] Waddell, who held an honorary doctor of divinity degree from Dickinson College, Pennsylvania, and had established several Presbyterian churches in Virginia, undoubtedly conveyed aspects of his Christian faith and talented oratory in his lessons to young Meriwether Lewis.

It appears, however, that Lewis never became a committed Christian. In the afterword of his excellent book *The Lewis and Clark Expedition: Day by Day*, in which he addresses the end-of-life issues of Meriwether Lewis, Gary Moulton wrote the following sentence that, although brief, reflects deep insight into Lewis's view of life and the world around him. Moulton wrote, "Never deeply religious, Lewis had no reserves of spiritual commitment to fall back on and find solace when problems mounted and demons set in."[3]

Although Meriwether may have rejected the evangelical Christian faith of many early Americans, his mother apparently did not. Considering Moulton's view of Lewis's life and the fact that his mother Lucy was an apparently devout Christian with whom he had a close and loving relationship, what are we to conclude about this apparent disconnect? This provides some stimulating information on the Lewis family and yields some thought-provoking insights into Meriwether's relationship with his mother and how she responded to the reports of his suicide.

If the Lewis family and historians who have reported on Lucy's faith are correct, it is highly likely that Lucy (1752–1836) was originally a member of the Anglican church.[4] Before and during the American Revolution, the Anglican church was the officially recognized church in Virginia, and it was not until 1786, through the efforts of Jefferson, that the Anglicans lost their privileged and state-endorsed position in Virginia.[5] Other Protestant denominations were not allowed to hold services in Virginia prior to the introduction of religious freedom to the state.

It is not known for certain when Meriwether Lewis's mother joined with thousands of other Americans in their increasing disdain and rejection of the English-controlled ecclesiastical organization of the Anglican church, viewed by many early Americans as elitist and nonegalitarian, and became a Methodist, whose clerical hierarchy as well as theological orientation reflected the new American sense of equality. Whether an anti-English attitude served as a deciding factor in Lucy's departure from the Anglican church or whether a true religious conversion occurred that led her to agree with Methodist theology (or some combination of both), we cannot know for certain. The latter is quite likely the case as the Methodism of that era did not encourage members to come to church, sit in a pew for a couple of hours, listen passively, mumble a few hymns, and then go home and live their lives until the following Sunday service. Lucy's gravestone at Locust Hill has the following biblical verse inscribed in it: "Blessed are the dead which die in the Lord" (Revelation 14:13). This inscription reflects a strongly evangelical Christian sentiment.

The Roots of Lucy Meriwether Lewis's Religious Beliefs

As most people understand, Christian denominations reflect a vast spectrum of differing beliefs regarding the essential truths of the faith. For our purpose of understanding Lucy's faith and how it influenced her, we outline here the basic tenets of early American theology.

By the fourth century CE, the Roman Catholic church held the primary position of authority in organized Christianity. Over the centuries, the Roman Catholic church acquired a vast influence over both the spiritual and the political lives of most Europeans. It remained in full control until 1054, when the Eastern Orthodox church split from the Roman Catholic church over issues of papal control of the church and more esoteric doctrinal concerns.

A second major split in the Christian world occurred when the German Roman Catholic priest and doctor of theology Martin Luther (1483–1546) challenged the Roman Catholic church's official dogma on various theological issues. Luther's thinking and disagreements with Rome had been sparked by his reading of the Greek New Testament, which had recently been made available in a critical edition by the Dutch Roman Catholic theologian Erasmus. Rather than accepting the Roman Catholic theology he had been taught during his years of study of the Latin translation of the New Testament, Luther believed it was vital to go to the original language of the New Testament, Koine Greek. His study of the original text, coupled with the great personal disillusionment he suffered when observing some of his fellow priests' corrupt lifestyles, led Luther to some serious soul-searching and internal conflict about his beliefs and the teachings of the Roman Catholic church. As a result, during the years 1517–21 Luther publicly challenged Rome's official doctrine regarding the selling of indulgences, a Roman Catholic practice that involved making a monetary contribution to the church on behalf of a deceased love one who was languishing in purgatory. This is believed to be where faithful Catholics undergo "purification, so as to achieve the holiness necessary to enter the joy of heaven."[6] The purchase of an indulgence, according to Pope Leo X (1475–1521), decreased the time required in purgatory for a departed loved one.

In addition to this disagreement, Luther further split from Rome when he stated that salvation for a Christian believer was the free gift of God, based solely on their faith in Jesus Christ and not as the result of obeying the Roman Catholic church's teaching on the necessity of good works and faithfully performing the Roman Catholic sacraments (baptism, Eucharist, confirmation, reconciliation, anointing of the sick, marriage, and holy orders). Luther's understanding of biblical teaching on these and other theological issues (the sacrament of Communion, the marriage of priests, the priesthood of every believer—which meant that every believer should be able to read and interpret the Bible for themself) differed significantly from Roman Catholic dogma. This resulted in Luther's excommunication by the pope and his condemnation as an outlaw by the Holy Roman emperor.[7]

These theological controversies and the resultant split in the Christian church of Europe ignited religious wars between Roman Catholics and Protestants across Europe for many years to come and fueled the critique of Christianity expressed by some of the European Enlightenment philosophers. Some historians credit Luther's challenge to accepted authority as initiating profound changes within unrelated areas of society such as medicine, science, and political thinking. All of these arenas of human existence had their own accepted authority figures and dogmas, which were soon be opposed by other notable personalities and either changed or completely overthrown. It was as if Luther had let the proverbial genie out of the bottle and enabled other free-thinking adversaries of long-accepted ideas to flourish. Great changes were in store for the panorama of intellectual, theological, political, and scientific thought during the early sixteenth century.

Within just a few years of the revolution in Christian thinking initiated by Luther, an important person came on the scene—John Calvin. Calvin never set foot in North America, but he had a direct and significant influence on early American religious culture. This French church reformer and theologian lived and taught in Geneva, Switzerland, during the 1540s. Calvin's distinct contributions to Christian practices centered around both religious/theological and political thought. He was a talented student as a young man and had learned Koine Greek, necessary for translating and studying the New Testament. As a young man, he underwent a religious conversion and wrote extensively concerning his life of faith. In reference to his conversion, Calvin wrote: "God by a sudden conversion subdued and brought my mind to a teachable frame, which was more hardened in such matters than might have been expected from one at my early period of life."[8] Over his lifetime, Calvin produced his influential theological work entitled *Institutes of the Christian Religion*, which provided the theological underpinnings for numerous Christian denominations. His fundamental theology was a belief in the authority of the Bible alone (without dependence on church tradition or on theology not supported by the Bible) and in predestination, which divides some Protestant denominations even today. In a nutshell, this school of theology teaches that God, based on God's divine authority, elects some humans to salvation and others to damnation. An extension of this idea is that Christ died only for the elect, not for everyone. In addition, Calvin believed in the concept that all humans are born with original sin and thus with the inability to either know or even be interested in the things of God. Calvin held that a believer's salvation has nothing to do with their good works, such as observing the sacraments, or anything else that they might do to contribute to their salvation. Their salvation is accomplished from start to finish by God alone. Calvinists sometimes say that "the only thing I can contribute to my soul's salvation is the sin which required it." Although Calvin believed that the practice of good works is important as evidence of a person's salvation, he firmly believed that God does not keep a balance sheet on individuals in order to weigh their good deeds against their bad deeds. Many of Calvin's theological convictions were included in the faith statements of several early American denominations: Puritan, Congregationalist, Presbyterian, and some Baptist and Methodist congregations.

When the Protestant church became established in England under the rule of Edward VI (1547–53), it took on the form of the Anglican church. Although they maintained some theology similar to that of the Roman Catholic church, as well as much of its liturgical flavor, the Anglicans believed in only two sacraments: baptism and the Eucharist. They granted no spiritual authority to the pope, and the appointment of priests, bishops, and other members of the church hierarchy was controlled by the archbishop of Canterbury. The Protestant Reformation in England had a great influence on its geographical and cultural neighbors, and by 1560 Scotland had followed England and became officially Protestant. Although Anglican theology resonates with some Calvinist doctrines, it is considered by some to hold a separate theological position than that of either Lutheran or Calvinist denominations.[9]

Within the Anglican church, a group of dissenters called Puritans became active in trying to rid the official Anglican church of its Roman Catholic influences. The Puritans fell afoul of both the British Crown and the Anglican hierarchy and were persecuted by the established powers. This led to their emigration from England in the 1620s and '30s to the New World. The Puritans were devotees of Calvinistic theology, and they attempted to create a society whose politics and lifestyle were thoroughly influenced by their faith. Puritan theologians achieved remarkable notoriety within the early colonies. Such personalities as the

Mather family of ministers (Increase, Cotton) and Jonathan Edwards, considered by some to be the greatest American theologian in history, were Puritan "divines" (clergy members or theologians).

Although Puritans entered the New World as a result of the persecution they experienced both politically and theologically, they were not accepting of others' beliefs that conflicted with their own theology. This led to further conflicts and ultimately to divisions within the New World church and to the establishment of other Protestant denominations such as Congregationalists (Puritans who believed that each congregation should remain autonomous) and Unitarians (who were heavily influenced by European Enlightenment thinking and its emphasis on human reason).[10] Unitarians rejected the orthodox belief of most evangelicals in the Trinity as well as biblical miracles such as the resurrection of Jesus. Thomas Jefferson, who adored human reason and rejected divine miracles, believed that Unitarianism would become the most popular sect of Christianity in the United States, but it never experienced the success that Jefferson believed it would.

Many early colonists engaged in institutional religious practices; 75 to 80 percent attended church.[11] In addition to the previously mentioned denominations, colonists also were Lutherans, Quakers, Baptists, Presbyterians (largely immigrants from Scotland and Scots from Northern Ireland), Methodists, Mennonites, Amish, Dutch Reformed, Huguenots (French Protestants), and, in relatively low numbers, Roman Catholics.

Some religious freethinkers adopted the doctrines of Deism, a loose term that describes the views of certain English and Continental thinkers who rejected the orthodox teachings of many of the above-mentioned Christian denominations and adopted their own convictions. This group thought of Jesus as a great teacher of morality (as human, not divine) and subjected all established Christian doctrines to the Enlightenment's cardinal virtue, which was human reason.[12] They believed in a god who wound up the clock of the universe but did not personally intervene in human affairs.

During the pre-Revolutionary era in America, when the chief Christian denominations were both Protestant and heavily Calvinist in their theology, the ecclesiastical governance of the churches was closely controlled by the English. Anglican priests were sent to America from

England and answered to England-based religious authorities. These authorities, such as the archbishop of Canterbury, all believed in the power of the ruling monarchies. The influence of an English king or queen, recognized as the head of the church with the accompanying God-appointed authority over all their subjects, was accepted by these church leaders. In spite of rebels such as Martin Luther, American theology in its early days was largely under the ecclesiastical control of Great Britain. But the cultural landscape and immense cultural changes brought about by the American Revolution, along with the resulting changes in the fundamental thinking of many Americans about authority figures in government, Old World ideas about class distinctions at birth, and ecclesiastical authority, changed many facets of life in the new country. The developing American theological landscape took on a decidedly and distinctively American flavor manifested in the control of and practice of the faith shortly after the end of the American Revolution.

Before the Revolution, young American men who went to college studied one of three main academic courses that led to careers in medicine, law, or theology. A significant number of the men who studied theology in seminaries went on to become leaders in their church denominations.[13] Many young Americans did not find fulfillment within the organized church in post-Revolutionary America, and they started moving away from becoming ministers and choosing secular careers. Many American college students trained for the ministry in the fifty-five years prior to the Revolution, but the percentage of those who ultimately entered the ministry decreased dramatically from the pre-war years to the decade after 1800 from one-third of graduates to only one-sixth.[14] In part, according to historian W. J. Rorabaugh, this reflected the "growing belief that the college's traditional role, that of educating an elite class, was in conflict with the Revolutionary concept of equality."[15] The notion of American egalitarianism was headed downhill and gaining speed.

It is not clear whether, when the Lewis family immigrated to the American colonies in the early seventeenth century from Wales, they were members of an organized religious group, but Meriwether's four-times-great-grand-niece Jane Lewis Henley believes the family was Anglican at the time of their arrival in colonial America. The history of religion in Wales at the time of the emigration of the Lewis family shows a predominantly Anglican influence but also a strong tradition of nonconformist Anglicans. In addition, there were also Methodist influences once that movement came to life in the early eighteenth century under the leadership of John and Charles Wesley.[16]

As noted above, Calvinism was a dominant theological influence in many early American Protestant churches but not all. Some groups of believers, similar to Calvin, accepted biblical authority in faith and practice as well as in the concept of all humans being born with original sin. However, in contrast to Calvinism, they firmly believed in the more egalitarian idea, according to historian Mark Noll, that "God's grace was no respecter of persons—[which] encouraged ordinary men and women to treat their own religious experience with as much respect as the directives of traditional authorities."[17] This egalitarian theological thought held that Christ died for everyone and that each individual not only had the ability but must, by necessity, make a personal decision to follow Christ during their lifetime. These and other tenets of faith—that a believer's ultimate salvation depended on their continuing in the faith, that everyone had to have a personal conversion experience, that people were able to accept or reject God's grace, and that believers were capable of falling from grace and losing their salvation—are not uniquely American. These non-Calvinistic ideas had their roots in the sixteenth-century European theological school of thought called Arminianism, a Protestant theology based on the ideas of Jacobus Arminius, a Dutch Reformed theologian (1560–1609).[18] His beliefs influenced several Christian denominations in America, most notably some Baptists in the seventeenth century and, more importantly for our story of the Lewis family, most Methodists in the eighteenth century.

The Methodist denomination was founded by two brothers, John and Charles Wesley, and it began with John Wesley's profound spiritual experience in 1738. Charles Wesley's influence has lived on in some notable hymn lyrics he composed that are still sung in many churches today ("O for a Thousand Tongues to Sing," "Hark the Herald Angels Sing," "Christ the Lord Is Risen Today").

The Wesley brothers entered Christ Church, Oxford University, in 1720. John and Charles believed, as did other Puritans, that the established Anglican church and many of its priests had become corrupted with ungodly living and practices. John was ordained an Anglican priest in 1728 and began the so-called Holy Club at Oxford University, which at the time was showing rather low enthusiasm for the Christian faith. This Wesley-led group believed in the necessity of daily prayer, Bible reading, fasting twice a week (Wednesdays and Fridays until 3 p.m.), meetings and Bible study with like-thinking believers, partaking in Communion, telling others about their faith, working in prisons, taking food to poor families, and teaching orphans how to read.[19] One may rightly conclude, based on this description of the practices of the Holy Club, that theirs was a very serious form of faith. Many members of the Oxford student body did not react well to the Wesleys or their club, and the name of the group is reportedly a snarky label supplied by Oxford scoffers of the time. The Wesleys would not agree with the characterization of them as founding a separate denomination from the Anglicans as they always believed that their method of Christian living was located well within the established Anglican church.

The Wesleys brought their brand of Protestant Christianity to Georgia in 1736. During the years of the mid- to late eighteenth century and into the early nineteenth century, Methodists as well as other evangelicals such as Baptists and some Presbyterian groups became known for their camp meetings. Many areas of the American frontier lacked established and formal churches, and these events became particularly popular in these areas. Numerous attendees would camp for days, singing hymns and listening to multiple itinerant ministers from various denominations giving emotional messages. One such meeting in Tennessee produced reports that "hundreds, of all ages and colors, were stretched on the ground in the agonies of conviction."[20] Perhaps the most noteworthy meeting was held in 1801 at Cane Ridge, Kentucky; it drew thousands.

In addition to preaching in colonial Georgia, the Wesley brothers established an orphanage, initiated missions to Native Americans, and began establishing the Anglican church in Savannah. John reportedly fell in love with a local girl, and when she disappointed him, it led to a dispute within the church that ultimately influenced John and Charles to leave Georgia and return to England. But the religious thought they brought and the movement it spawned lived on in America.

American Christian thought underwent a remarkable change during the decade of 1730–40, a period referred to as the First Great Awakening.

One of the greatest and most effective ministers of this era was George Whitefield (1714–70), a man referred to by some newspapers of that era as a "marvel of the age."[21] Whitefield would prove to be far more influential in America's religious thinking than the Wesley brothers. In the estimation of some historians, Whitefield was the most famous religious figure in America in the eighteenth century. He reportedly preached at least 18,000 sermons to perhaps ten million people.[22] Whitefield, although a contemporary of the Wesleys and a member of the Wesleys' Holy Club, disagreed with the Wesleys in some areas of doctrine and was a Calvinist in his theological orientation. Regardless, Whitefield practiced the evangelical ideology of the Wesleys, which involved preaching to crowds out-of-doors, traveling to various cities to preach, and following their guidelines for living a Christian life that produced Christian perfection, or a state of being free from any sin in this lifetime.

The Wesleys and Whitefield went against the grain of the Anglican establishment by appointing itinerant preachers who had been converted but did not always have a proper English theological education. Early Methodists encouraged women to become church leaders and to tend to the spiritual education and development of their children.[23] What was most important to Methodist leaders, in spite of their theological differences, was that a minister had undergone a personal and life-changing conversion and not just an intellectual acceptance of a list of theological truths. This theological evangelical community had strong concerns about the dangers of an unconverted ministry.[24]

The Methodist type of personal and experiential Christianity had an increasing effect on the more formal sects of the Presbyterians and their Calvinist theology. The Presbyterian denomination split into the "New Lights" and the "Old Lights" depending on their participation in these practices of religious enthusiasm. America was quickly moving, according to Rorabaugh, "from the labyrinth of Calvinism . . . into the rich pastures of gospel-liberty."[25] Much of Georgia continued to be heavily influenced by Methodists into the later years of the eighteenth century, when Lucy and John Marks and their young family moved to Georgia (apparently without Meriwether Lewis, who remained in Virginia in the late 1780s).

One of the remarkable cultural effects of the conversion to Methodism by a significant percentage of the population was produced by the stance the church took against drunkenness. Rorabaugh notes that "[a]lthough most denominations had long condemned public drunkenness as sinful, it was revivalistic Methodists who most vigorously opposed alcohol."[26] After 1790, the Methodist church adopted rules that imposed strict limitations on the use of distilled spirits.

Methodist Culture in Early America

By the time of Lucy Meriwether's birth in 1752, there were other important voices within the Methodist faith in America besides the Wesleys. When Lucy was living in either Georgia or Virginia, she very likely came under the direct influence of a talented orator, the Methodist minister Francis Asbury (1745–1816). Asbury, born in England, spent forty-five years in the colonies and early America. This in itself is significant as he was ordained an Anglican bishop by John Wesley at the age of twenty-two and volunteered to travel and work in the American colonies in 1771, traveled an estimated six thousand miles per year from 1780 to the end of his life, and preached to even more parishioners than the miles he traveled. At the outbreak of the Revolutionary War in 1775, he and only one other Anglican bishop remained in the colonies, and Asbury declared his neutrality in the war.

The Revolutionary War laid waste to the membership of the Anglican church in America and also produced other profound cultural changes in America. From 1770–90, the number of American Anglican churches decreased from 356 to 170.[27] There was no longer an Anglican church in an America that was controlled by England-based clerics. Protestant egalitarianism shunned English clerical leadership and yielded control of its churches to American ecclesiastical leadership in both the Anglican as well as the Methodist denominations. That leader was Francis Asbury. After the war, the Anglican church in the new United States became known as the Methodist-Episcopal church.

Statistics on church attendance and growth during the years 1770–90 show that the growth of the Methodist church as measured by the number of churches in existence in America was impressive. In 1770, there were 20 Methodist churches in America, and twenty years later there were 712. If Lucy Meriwether Lewis was a Methodist, as is noted by both historians as well as family members, she was part of a significant movement in early America that identified with the teachings and theology of its founders—John and Charles Wesley, George Whitefield, and Francis Asbury. Although there are some slight differences between the theologies of these leading Methodists, it is fairly easy to outline the theological beliefs of Meriwether Lewis's mother. The decidedly American-flavored Methodist church incorporated other aspects of American culture, such as the growing anti-slavery movement among Northerners, the anti-English cultural sentiment, and negative attitudes toward England-sourced ecclesiastical authority. It is important to note for our story that there is no reason to believe that Lucy Marks differed in her beliefs from her church's opposition to the recreational use of ardent spirits and its view of suicide as an unacceptable means of death.

Suicide: Christian versus Secular Opinions

John Wesley's views on Christian living had more facets than those already mentioned. In England, the act of suicide was considered a felony, an act against both God and the king. But the European Enlightenment had the remarkable effect of lessening the stigma against people who committed suicide. Prior to 1660, only 2 percent of suicides were excused due to "insanity." The rest were considered an act of the will to end life. By 1700, excused suicides had risen to 42 percent, as determined by juries in formal courtroom trials.[28] William Blackstone (1723–80), an eminent British jurist, wrote that suicide was a "double offence: one spiritual, in invading the prerogative of the Almighty, and rushing into his immediate presence uncalled for; the other temporal, against the king, who hath an interest in the preservation of all his subjects; the law has therefore ranked this among the highest crimes, making it a peculiar species of felony, a felony committed on one's self."[29]

In addition to John Wesley's position against drinking ardent spirits, his thoughts on the act of suicide are stated succinctly in his writings. On April 8, 1790, Wesley wrote that he was concerned that the existing laws of England, which considered suicide a felony, did not do enough to deter the potential victim. The extreme laws of England allowed the Crown under some circumstances to confiscate the entire estate of a person who had committed suicide.[30] But a loophole existed in that a trial could be held and the victim found "insane" by a jury, and thus the estate could go to the victim's family.[31] John referenced an ancient Greek practice of hanging female suicide victims naked and in public and added:

> It is a melancholy consideration, that there is no country in Europe, or perhaps in the habitable world, where the horrid crime of self-murder is so common as it is in England! One reason of this may be, that the English in general are more ungodly and more impatient than other nations. Indeed we have laws against it, and officers with juries are appointed to inquire into every fact of the kind. And these are to give in their verdict upon oath, whether the self-murderer was sane or insane. If he is brought in insane, he is excused, and the law does not affect him. By this means it is totally eluded; for the juries constantly bring him in insane. So the law is not of the least effect, though the farce of a trial still continues.
>
> This morning I asked a Coroner, "Sir, did you ever know a jury bring in the deceased felo de se [suicide]?" He answered, "No, Sir; and it is a pity they should." What then is the law good for? If all self-murderers are mad, what need of any trial concerning them?
>
> But it is plain our ancestors did not think so, or those laws had never been made. It is true, every self-murderer is mad in some sense, but not in that sense which the law intends. This fact does not prove him mad in the eye of the law: The question is, Was he mad in other respects? If not, every juror is perjured who does not bring him in felo de se.
>
> But how can this vile abuse of the law be prevented, and this execrable crime effectually discouraged?
>
> By a very easy method. We read in ancient history, that, at a certain period, many of the women in Sparta murdered themselves. This fury increasing, a law was made, that the body of every woman that killed herself should be exposed naked in the streets. The fury ceased at once. Only let a law be made and rigorously executed, that the body of every self-murderer, Lord or peasant, shall be hanged in chains, and the English fury will cease at once.[32]

Wesley clearly outlines his, and thus the Methodist, position on suicide.

Other Protestant Christian commentators' opinions on suicide exist from this era. Caleb Fleming (1698–1779), an English Presbyterian, wrote in 1773 that suicide was greatly "unnatural" and an act of "great depravity."[33] Isaac Watts, a prolific hymn writer, stated in 1726 that suicide was "folly and danger of self murder." He added to his condemnation the opinion that suicide was a shame and disgrace to the victim's family.[34] The Puritan divines Increase Mather and his son Cotton acknowledged "melancholy" as a contributing cause of suicide but condemned suicide and encouraged sufferers of melancholy to seek the help of physicians, friends, and the clergy.[35] Religious leaders were not the only thinkers of that era to provide opinions on suicide. One of the most influential philosophers of all time, Immanuel Kant (1724–1804), wrote that the only morally acceptable suicide occurs when, in certain circumstances, one must be prepared to die in order to live life honorably and "not disgrace the dignity of humanity." He was able to cite only one such example in history—that of the Roman senator Cato the Younger.[36]

John Locke (1632–1704), who contributed to the start of empiricist thinking during the Enlightenment in England and France, was an impressive multitalented individual who was skilled in philosophy, medicine, and science. Locke laid the epistemological foundations of modern science and influenced the thinking brought forth in the U.S. Declaration of Independence, believing that God created humankind and is the ultimate owner of humans' bodies. He argued for a person "not to quit his station willfully."[37]

Both Thomas Jefferson and the Scottish Enlightenment philosopher David Hume wrote in defense of suicide, at least in some circumstances. Jefferson, with his botanical interests, knew of poisonous plants that might be used to decrease the suffering of the terminally ill, and he wrote, "There are ills in life as desperate as intolerable, to which it [suicide] would be the rational relief."[38] David Hume (1711–76), a noted skeptic, wrote that "suicide . . . may be free from every imputation of guilt or blame."[39] Voltaire (1694–1778), in his aggressive stand against French religious and political institutions, avoided making any judgment on the act of suicide, commenting on the fact that the propensity toward suicide is hereditary and often is a matter of fashion as much as anything. He wrote that suicides often resulted from a lack of engagement on the part of the victim and suggested that the remedy for the person who was contemplating suicide was simply to find something to do.[40] It is our position that this judgment on suicide by Voltaire, the very champion of human reason, represents the utter unreliability of human reason.

It is noteworthy that those thinkers who were either openly Christian or who believed in a supernatural being (Wesley, Locke, Kant, Luther) and who had certain moral expectations of human beings and some degree of belief in a divine personal involvement in the affairs of humans were all opposed to suicide. This is not to suggest that they all felt suicide was an unpardonable sin. Some held a compassionate and nuanced view of the subject. Those who were either skeptics of Christianity and/or Deists (Hume, Voltaire, Jefferson) were much more accepting of suicide as either a possible escape from suffering or, in the case of Hume, permissible for any reason whatsoever.

Meriwether Lewis and the Masonic Lodge

As Moulton noted, Meriwether Lewis never seemed to have deep spiritual convictions, at least not any with an orthodox Christian orientation. But his interest in living a productive and what he considered a good life was manifested by his ardent interest in a group active during his era. Lewis was a serious, practicing member of the Masonic Lodge.

Lieutenant Meriwether Lewis, home on furlough from his western Pennsylvania post, applied for induction into his local Albemarle County, Virginia, lodge on December 31, 1796, and was elected into that lodge about a month later in 1797. Within days, he was elected "at sight" as a master mason. It is rather remarkable for a twenty-three-year-old to advance in Freemasonry in such a dramatic and rapid fashion. His association with his comrades in that lodge was remarkably positive. He achieved a higher degree in October of 1799, being "exalted to the sublime degree of a Royal Arch, Super Excellent Mason."[41] After the expedition of 1803–06 and his relocation to St. Louis to assume his duties as territorial governor, Lewis was one of the men who applied to establish the first Masonic lodge in St. Louis. In September 1808, by authority of the Pennsylvania Grand Lodge, Lewis was installed as Master of the new Masonic Lodge No. 111. In September 1809, a month before his death, Lewis relinquished his leadership position to his nemesis Frederick Bates, who became both the head of the lodge as well as the acting governor of the Upper Louisiana Territory during Lewis's absence on his trip to Washington, D.C.

What is the background of this organization, and what are its implications for our story of the death of Lewis? The following is not meant to be an in-depth review of Freemasonry but only a glance at the fundamentals of the organization in order to draw comparisons with the Christian faith of Meriwether's mother Lucy.

The Masonic Lodge evolved from guilds of stonemasons during the Middle Ages. Some lodges developed modern symbolic rites from ancient religious orders and chivalric brotherhoods such as the Knights Templar, some of which were reportedly very anti-Christian, particularly anti-Roman Catholic. From its inception in Europe, the movement encountered considerable opposition from the Roman Catholic church as well as from government officials in various countries as Masonic Lodge members were thought to have beliefs that challenged the authority of the Roman Catholic church as well as the kings of various countries.[42] Although the organization is not an orthodox Christian institution, its teachings include morality, charity, and obedience to the law of the land. According to Noll, "For most upholders of republicanism, it was important that virtue not be defined exclusively as a product of divine grace, but rather as also a product of self-generated, personally chosen, public self-discipline."[43] Such a nonreligious organization would have appealed to those early American men who wished to avoid any type of more conventional, denominational religious organizations. Many of their practices have historically been viewed with suspicion by some outside the group due to the secrecy practiced by the society.

In most Masonic lodges, an applicant for admission is required to be an adult male and to believe in the existence of a supreme being and the "immortality of the soul." Once accepted into the lodge, men are divided into three major degrees of the temple; apprentice, a fellow of the craft, and master mason. As already mentioned, Meriwether Lewis was designated a master mason when he was inducted. His Masonic apron represented his pure heart and the purification of his life. As a master, his apron was a reminder to do no evil to any person. Lewis's apron is reported to have been in his pocket at the time of his death (his Masonic apron is currently on display at the Montana Masonic Lodge Museum in Helena).[44] Masons reportedly wear their aprons at lodge meetings as an emblem of innocence and pride.[45] The images on Lewis's apron represent strength, stability, justice, and restraint of prejudice. The level of master mason generally takes about four to eight months to achieve after the initial petition to a lodge. A master must be in strict compliance with his Masonic duties, pay his dues promptly, and maintain his affiliation with his lodge.

The first grand lodge was founded in England in 1717. The first lodge in America was established in Philadelphia in 1730, and Benjamin Franklin was its founding member. Joining the organization soon became a "social phenomenon."[46] Membership in this popular group particularly appealed to aristocrats in England and to men of "good character" in America. (Interestingly, Thomas Jefferson was never a member of the Freemasons.) Freemasonry was thus a popular and influential force in early America. It was not unusual for men in both colonial and early America to be members of a church (usually of a Protestant denomination) as well as of a Masonic lodge.

According to a high-ranking Mason, Freemasonry does not have an official, internationally applied teaching regarding suicide by its members. Each lodge, based on its location, is a part of a grand lodge, and each grand lodge is sovereign. Individual lodges have their own position on various issues, including how to conduct funeral services for members who may have committed suicide.

A Clash of Worldviews?

Since the story of Meriwether Lewis involves the intersection of the Protestant-Evangelical worldview of Lucy Marks with the personal attitudes of Meriwether Lewis as well as the teachings of the Freemasons, it is helpful to know how the beliefs of the Freemasons were viewed by the Methodist church and, by extension, those who probably influenced the thinking of Lucy Marks. In a June 18, 1773, journal entry, John Wesley critiqued Freemasonry after reading some of their literature: "I incline to think it is a genuine account. . . . If it be, what an amazing banter upon all mankind is Freemasonry!"[47]

An Evangelical and Arminian cleric, Charles Finney (1792–1875), in a scathing editorial on the Masons, stated, "What shall be done with the great number of professed Christians who are Freemasons? I answer, let them have no more to do with it . . . to abandon it." Referring to Christians who continued as Masonic members, he stated, "[T]hey should not be allowed their places in the church."[48] These are rather clear and direct opinions.

The following quotations are from a 1985 Methodist document that specifically addresses how the two organizations view a variety of important issues. The Methodist denomination's twentieth-century views on these issues are probably *more accepting* than were those of John Wesley. This Methodist document soundly criticizes the excessive secrecy of the Masonic Lodge, stating that "[t]he society thus encourages suspicion and lays itself open to charges of corrupt practice which can be neither proved nor disproved." The Methodists further state that "secrecy of any kind is destructive of fellowship" and "[t]he Christian community is an open fellowship."[49]

The Methodists describe the clash of the competing views of the nature of God held by Freemasons and Methodists as follows:

> Freemasons are required to believe in a Supreme Being, sometimes called the Great Architect of the Universe. At various points in Masonic rituals prayer is offered to this Being. Freemasonry claims to draw together those of different religions and Freemasons are required to respect one another's religious beliefs, and this is reflected in the prayers offered. However, the worship included in Masonic ritual seems to be an attenuated form unsatisfactory in any religious tradition. Christians must be concerned that the Supreme Being is not equated by all with God as Christians acknowledge Him, and prayer in craft and Royal Arch Freemasonry is never offered in the name of Jesus Christ. There are documented cases of masonic services in Christian churches in which Christian prayers have been altered to remove the name of Christ.[50]

The most basic tenet of evangelical Christianity and thus of the Methodist church to which Lucy belonged was that people are saved from their sins and will ultimately be accepted by God as a result of God's grace brought about through their faith. This belief is expressed by the apostle Paul in his letter to the Ephesian church: "God saved you by his grace when you believed. And you can't take credit for this; it is a gift from God, Salvation is not a reward for the good things we have done, so none of us can boast about it" (Ephesians 2:8–9 NLT).

The Methodists contrasted Masonic belief with theirs in the following statement:

> Another difficulty about Freemasonry for Christians is the allegation that masonic practices imply salvation by works, through charitable giving and mutual aid. Again, while these elements of Freemasonry can become dominant for an individual, the masonic rituals do not contain any such doctrine.
>
> The case is rather different with the fear the Freemasonry offers salvation by secret knowledge. The suggestion of secret knowledge becomes stronger as one proceeds through the degrees of the society, and becomes explicit in the exaltation rites for the Royal Arch degree. The rites here include a dramatic enactment of the re-discovery of secrets claimed to have been lost. The references to these secrets carry clear implication of a secret knowledge whose possession helps one to obtain immortal life, but there is no explicit reference to salvation and no claim that this is the only way to immortality. Christians believe that the knowledge of the sure way to salvation which includes eternal life, should be freely available to all and must be offered to all.[51]

Other objections from those high within the Methodist hierarchy are mentioned in detail in this document. The Methodist leaders state in conclusion:

> The most serious theological objection to Freemasonry for Christians lies in the name given to the Supreme Being in the rituals of the Royal Arch degree. One of the secrets revealed in this degree is that the name of the Supreme Being

is JAHBULON. It has been suggested to us that this word is a description of God, but the ritual refers to the word as a name of God. The name is a composite, as the ritual explicitly states. The explanation given of the name in the ritual is acknowledged to be inaccurate, but is preserved to bring out the traditional meaning for Freemasonry of the word. The best explanation of the derivation of this word seems to be that two of the three parts, JAH and BUL, are the name of gods in different religions, while the third syllable ON was thought by the composers of the ritual to be the name of a god in yet another religion; modern scholarship suggests they were wrong. In any case, it is clear that each of the three syllables is intended to be the name of a divinity in a particular religion. The whole word is thus an example of syncretism, an attempt to unite different religions in one, which Christians cannot accept. We note that some Christians who are Freemasons withdraw from any ceremonies in which this word is to be used.

. . . [O]n the most generous reading of the evidence there remain serious questions for Christians about Freemasonry, especially theological questions relating to syncretism and the replacement of Christian essentials. Although Freemasonry claims not to be a religion or a religious movement, its rituals contain religious practices and carry religious overtones. It is clear that Freemasonry may compete strongly with Christianity. There is a great danger that the Christian who becomes a Freemason will find himself compromising his Christian beliefs or his allegiance to Christ, perhaps without realizing what he is doing.

Consequently, our guidance to the Methodist people is that Methodists should not become Freemasons.[52]

Putting the Pieces Together

Most murder theorists would argue that no one knew Meriwether Lewis better than his mother, Lucy. They further reason that if the one who gave him birth, raised him, and saw him off on the expedition of the Corps of Discovery refused to believe that he had committed suicide, how could anyone believe that he did? How could someone who had observed him for so many years not have an excellent and accurate view of his character? If one simply considers Lucy as his mother and consciously ignores her beliefs surrounding the many issues involved in this part of the puzzle, one may be able to convince oneself that "Mother knows best" and therefore agree with Lucy that Meriwether was most likely murdered. But, what were the motivating factors and beliefs that likely influenced her insistence that her son was murdered?

If Lucy, as an evangelical Methodist Christian, ever seriously considered or analyzed the belief system of her son, she could not have been happy with his worldview. If we theorize that Meriwether's worldview underwent a change after he entered the army, and particularly since his immersion in the Enlightenment thinking of Thomas Jefferson in 1801, then we can see the great potential for conflict between his view of reality and that of his mother. Methodism during the historical era in which Lucy Marks lived was not a passive, relativistic, "Can't we all just get along?" type of faith. Her faith and practice would have included frequent group Bible study, prayer, and effort to live a sinless life as evidence of her faith, as well as a host of behaviors and attitudes such as helping the poor, sharing her faith with others, being anti-slavery, and not partaking of recreational alcoholic beverages, particularly not in excess. Her religious beliefs were likely central to the way she viewed everything. If she was a practicing Methodist during Meriwether's early life, then without question she would have actively attempted to pass her faith on to Meriwether when he was a boy.

Thomas Jefferson's theological orientation was diametrically opposed to nearly everything that Lucy as a Methodist would have believed about this world and the next. Many of the religious practices that would have been a normal part of Lucy's life were considered by Jefferson to be "fanaticism." Jefferson wrote,

> In our Richmond there is much fanaticism, that chiefly among the women. They have their night meetings and praying parties, where, attended by their priests, and sometimes by a hen-pecked husband, they pour forth the effusions of their love to Jesus, in terms as amatory and carnal as their modesty would permit them to use to a mere earthly lover."[53]

Jefferson did not believe in the same God or Jesus that Lucy and her church did. Jefferson created his own edited version of the New Testament that was in agreement with his humanist, rationalist philosophy. Jefferson did not believe in a miracle-working Jesus. He deleted any references to miracles in his version of the New Testament. Jesus, in Jefferson's mind, was a great teacher, a great man who was worthy of admiration, but he did not heal the sick, raise the dead, make water into wine, or rise from the dead. These orthodox Christian beliefs were not a part of Jefferson's worldview, and he assigned them to the category of mythology, fanaticism, and superstition.

If discussions between Lucy and her son ever took place after Meriwether's early army career, particularly after his becoming secretary to President Jefferson, it is likely that when Meriwether subsequently visited his home, Lucy wondered with some degree of consternation about her son's religious or world views. The fact that Meriwether was a Freemason would probably not have been viewed as positive by Lucy; she probably disapproved of Freemasonry to some degree. She may not have actively opposed his membership and perhaps was ignorant of the specifics of the Masonic beliefs. Many well-respected men in Virginia society were members of a lodge, and it is possible it even seemed positive to Lucy. However, it is also very likely, due to her Methodism, that any ignorance of the differences between her faith and the pillars of truth as presented by the Masonic Lodge did not last very long. Her faith emphasized the study and learning of the Scriptures and interaction with Methodist clergymen, who likely condemned membership in Freemasonry.

One might argue that a significant amount of self-aggrandizing and purification exists within Freemasonry, based on the personal effort required to attain various degrees within the lodge. This personal purification resulting from a member's human effort, without a concurrent change of heart brought about by God, would have provided no comfort to the evangelical Christian Lucy, who could no doubt cite Bible verses that speak of all human-sourced good works as "filthy rags" to God. The Masonic Lodge's requirement that all members must believe in a supreme being may seem to indicate religious thinking, but to Lucy and the Methodists this tenet of Masonic doctrine would have been viewed at best as inadequate and at worst as a false belief. Belief in a supreme being would have carried little or no positive weight when judged by Lucy's religious standards and would have been of little or no comfort to her. She no doubt would have thought of the verse in the book of James that states, "You say you have faith for you believe that there is one God? Good for you! Even the demons believe this, and they tremble in terror" (James 2:19 NLT).

Some might object to our comparison of Christian views on suicide to the beliefs of Freemasonry as Freemasonry is not a "religion." Although in some sense this may be true, as the Masons do not demand adherence to a particular religious doctrine and only require their members to believe in a supreme being, Freemasonry addresses many areas of human behavior, as does organized religion. Their teaching (truth claims) about human behavior, its nature and improvement, the attainment of an eternal reward from the Supreme Being, the nature and name of that Supreme Being, and funeral rituals provided to members could be easily interpreted as "religious beliefs," regardless of their rejection of such an interpretation.

After Meriwether died in 1809, John Pernier, Lewis's servant who was present at the time of his death in Tennessee, traveled east to visit Lucy Marks at Locust Hill. Being fully aware by this time of the report of Meriwether's suicide, Lucy refused to even meet with Pernier and strongly rejected the report that her son had committed suicide.[54] Why would Lucy refuse to meet with Pernier?

Reports undoubtedly had reached Lucy that Meriwether had been drinking to excess, which indicated, as Jefferson expressed in a letter written in 1810, that Lewis had "been much afflicted & habitually so with hypochondriasis. This was probably increased by the habit into which he had fallen & the painful reflections that would necessarily produce in a mind like his."[55] She was no doubt aware of the newspaper reports of his suicide. Lucy's belief system would not have allowed her to accept the report of Meriwether's alcohol abuse. Although the problem was rampant in America in 1809, alcohol use disorder in the nineteenth century was certainly not thought of as a disease as it is today. Alcohol abuse disorder, or even binge drinking without a physical addiction component, would have been absolute anathema to Lucy. She would have been upset by Meriwether's report to her in 1794 of the "oceans of whiskey" that were available to him during his early years in the Virginia militia (see chapter 4). Lucy was no doubt aware of multiple biblical passages about the ultimate fate of drunkards. John Wesley wrote, in his sermon "On Public Diversions," "You see the wine when it sparkles in the cup, and are going to drink of it. I tell you there is poison in it! and, therefore, beg you to throw it away."[56] If that was Wesley's opinion about wine, we can easily imagine what he thought about "ardent spirits." In fact, in 1773 Wesley denounced the process of liquor distillation and called for its prohibition.[57] Lucy could not have possibly accepted with a confident and settled mind the report of Meriwether's suicide, given Christian thinking at that time as expressed in the previously quoted writings of John Wesley and other non-Methodist theologians. If he killed himself, her son was guilty of a very serious personal sin, one that in her mind could never be forgiven. She would have believed as a Methodist that God never overpowers a person's willpower, and if her son had killed himself intentionally, it was a very serious reflection on his soul.

Every student of Meriwether Lewis's life must come to the conclusion that many of his important views were influenced by Enlightenment thinking. If we consider that he held a Deistic and a naturalistic, materialistic view of reality, as did Thomas Jefferson, we may reason that this view of reality in itself did not provide Meriwether with much comfort when, as Moulton put it, "problems mounted and demons set in." When Lewis returned from the frontier in 1806 and enjoyed great adulation and success and then suffered a precipitous loss of status and respect (as he saw it) in subsequent years, he likely thought, "What difference have all my efforts made?" When his Masonic brother Frederick Bates repeatedly attacked him, undermined his duties as governor, and used his political power in an attempt to destroy Lewis, this must have been an overwhelming assault on his psyche. When the vast powers of the federal bureaucracy turned against Meriwether with a degree of aggression that should have been reserved for a corrupt criminal, without question this would have greatly wounded any hope and positivity that remained in Lewis's spirit.

Lewis, by all reliable reports, was a thoroughly honest man, and he no doubt took some pride in that fact. To be accused of being corrupt and/or incompetent would have been a devastating emotional blow. Without the personal religious conviction or reassurance that all would be well regardless of his circumstances and that a personal God took interest in his plight, his positive belief in the benevolence of human reason could have easily evaporated.[58]

Would it have made any difference to our analysis of Lewis's death if Lucy accepted the report of her son's suicide? Absolutely! Her acceptance of the suicide report would have been very strong evidence that Lewis did kill himself. But since Lucy reportedly never accepted that her son died by suicide, is her denial equally as strong evidence against it? Absolutely not. The reasons we cite for her denial are legitimate and profoundly true. The reasons we have provided in detail thoroughly account for her inability to accept the suicide report. The reported suicide of her son was too painful a possibility for her to accept.

We strongly suspect that, as a result of Jefferson's published comments on the death of Meriwether, there was no love lost in Lucy's relationship with this powerful benefactor and mentor to her son. Jefferson's Deism and his denial of everything she likely held dear regarding her faith, coupled with the fact the Jefferson ultimately accepted Lewis's suicide and his suspected alcoholism, must have made a cold chill run down her spine when her thoughts turned toward Jefferson. She was likely confused by the idea that her son had attained such a lofty position within American society and yet had suffered such a mysterious and ignominious death. His fame had come to him as a result of his attachment to Thomas Jefferson. Her son had become the most famous and celebrated man in America upon his return from the expedition in 1806. The following year, American poet Joel Barlow went so far as to propose renaming the Columbia River to honor Meriwether Lewis.[59] Lucy's son's death by his own hand would have been a very bitter pill indeed for her to swallow.

The two philosophical worldviews of Lucy and of her son were in opposition to each other. She wanted to believe the best about Meriwether during his life and was equally as certain regarding how he died. Based solely on her being Meriwether's mother, one must conclude that Lucy's profound sadness was laced with a degree of guilt because in some way she had failed to protect him—and thus failed as a mother.

Meriwether Lewis, a top-tier American hero in 1809, died in an extremely public way. His reported suicide would have reflected very negatively on Lucy's public image as a loving mother, kind and helpful "yarb" physician, and faithful Christian wife and mother. Her son's death by suicide would have been psychologically painful beyond imagination.

Regardless of the potential untrustworthiness of the sources of some of the reports of Lewis's suicide, everyone involved with the story either reported or acknowledged the reports as either factual or believable, from Clark and Jefferson to Pricilla Grinder, John Pernier, Gilbert Russell, John Brahan, Alexander Wilson, William Carr, and James Neelly. Lucy's rejection of the reports could have only been based on her wishful thinking and state of denial.

As a logical extension of Moulton's statement quoted earlier in this chapter, the clockmaker, Deistic, impersonal god of Lewis, Jefferson, and the Enlightenment and the philosophy of Freemasonry could not provide sufficient consolation for Lewis's personal storms. The public adulation, membership in the American Philosophical Society, honorary balls and parties, and appointment as a territorial governor were not enough to sustain Lewis's wounded spirit. In fact, these positive responses to his many accomplishments may have elevated his ego to such lofty heights that when the demons materialized and assaulted his sense of honor, purpose, honesty, and integrity, threatening everything he held dear, the accolades were apparently insufficient to help him resolve his personal crisis. His terrible circumstances and their assault on his mental health were only magnified by his use of alcohol, which only temporarily worked to soothe his soul. He certainly had a very, very long way to fall.

There is nothing in Meriwether's post-expedition life that would have provided much comfort to his mother Lucy's mind after his death. Her view of the cosmos and of what was both fundamental and essential did not corelate with the worldview of her son. To conclude otherwise seems to us to be an exercise in wishful thinking.

Chapter 8
Meriwether Lewis and Malaria: Truth and Fiction

*For every complex problem there is an answer
that is clear, simple, and wrong.*
—H. L. Mencken

There is probably no issue related to the story of the death of Meriwether Lewis that has become such a tangled web as the issue of malaria and its possible role in Lewis's final days. This issue was brought into prominence with the publication of *The Truth About Meriwether Lewis* by Thomas Danisi and John Jackson in 2009. In this work, Danisi and Jackson built a seemingly compelling case that Lewis suffered from a manifestation of malaria during the closing weeks of his life. Numerous assertions of malaria as an explanation of the historical meaning of Jefferson's comment that Lewis had "hypochondriac affections" and their relation to Lewis's health during his final weeks have followed in the wake of the original theory. Clay Jenkinson, in *The Character of Meriwether Lewis*, gave Danisi and Jackson high praise, writing,

> Danisi and Jackson have presented the facts of Lewis's sufferings at the hand of malaria so thoroughly that no future Lewis biographer will be able to ignore their finding or regard Lewis's derangement as exclusively psychological. It is certain that Lewis

was in significant pain as he descended the Mississippi River in September 1809, and that his physical pain was alone sufficient to reduce his mental clarity.[1]

Lewis's apparent use of certain medications has been cited by some Lewis biographers as evidence that he was being treated for malaria, which is another piece of evidence used to support this theory. Given this, it may seem probable from a superficial point of view that Lewis was suffering from a malarial attack just prior to his death. Some Lewis scholars have accepted various aspects of this theory to the extent that it seems to have become a new orthodoxy in the thinking of many historians and Lewis aficionados. In one of my infrequent disagreements with Jenkinson, I (David) conclude that Danisi and Jackson's presentation concerning malaria and Lewis is largely inaccurate. I will dissect this theory one slice at a time. In order to understand this disease, it is necessary to understand the basic biology of malaria.

This parasitic disease, which is obtained by humans through the bite of thirty to forty different species of a female *Anopheles* mosquito, was present in much of America during the Lewis and Clark era. As it still does today, malaria took the lives of thousands of people every year. It is possible, perhaps even probable, that every member of the expedition suffered from its fevers, chills, headache, and weakness at some time during their life. Malaria continues to afflict hundreds of millions of people worldwide and ranks in the top ten causes of death across all age groups. According to the World Health Organization, there were 228 million cases of malaria worldwide in 2018, with over four hundred thousand deaths. Sixty-seven percent of those deaths occurred in children under the age of five.[2] Malaria is probably today the biggest single killer of the world's children. Populations that are affected the most severely are those in less developed countries with warmer climates and poor mosquito control. Although there continue to be reported cases in the United States, malaria was officially eradicated as an endemic disease in the nation in the 1950s. U.S. cases today are found in in people who have visited or emigrated from either Africa, the Caribbean, or other areas where malaria is still endemic.

The organism that causes malaria and is transmitted to its human host via the mosquito is a parasite in the *Plasmodium* genus. This is not a bacterium, like *Streptococcus* or *Staphylococcus*, nor a virus, like influenza or Covid-19. A *Plasmodium* is a one-celled organism that cannot live on its own but requires another species in which to survive. In other words, it is a classic example of a parasite. It was not until 1898 that the life cycle of the malarial *Plasmodium* was established, allowing a more thorough understanding of the disease it causes. It took an additional fifty years to understand the parasite's life cycle within the human body. There are currently five known *Plasmodium* species that cause malaria in humans: *vivax, ovale, malariae. knowlesi*, and the most lethal, *falciparum*.[3]

In the twentieth century, well after the identification of the parasite, various worldwide governmental agencies made repeated attempts to reduce the significant malaria-related death rate. The World Health Organization sponsored programs that treated victims with initially effective medication and also attempted to control the mosquito population with insecticides. These programs cost an astronomical amount of money and, despite their good intentions, were declared a failure by the World Health Organization in 1976. Why did they fail? Because, like many organisms which cause disease, *Plasmodium* developed resistance to medication (chloroquine) and mosquitoes developed resistance to the DDT insecticide. The disease defeated both prongs of the human attack. Successfully addressing this problem and the trillions of mosquitoes that carry the disease is likely impossible.

Although this was not understood during the time of Lewis and Clark, when an infected female *Anopheles* mosquito bites its human victim, it injects into the victim's bloodstream the parasite living in its saliva. This small parasite travels through the human bloodstream and invades the individual's liver cells, where it starts to reproduce. At this stage, the person shows no symptoms (they are asymptomatic). Any time from a week to sometimes a year later, the multiplying parasites within liver cells cause these cells to die and rupture, releasing thousands of new malarial parasites into the victim's bloodstream. At this point, the victim shows symptoms that may include, among others, fever, chills, nausea, fatigue, and headache.

Inside of the human bloodstream, mixed into the liquid portion of the blood, are two major types of blood cells that are produced within the bone marrow. These are the white and red blood cells. Red blood cells (RBCs) are donut-shaped and contain the vitally important molecule hemoglobin. RBCs produce the red color of our blood that we see when we cut our finger. There are about twenty to thirty trillion RBCs at any one time within our bodies. One of the RBCs' chief duties is to carry oxygen obtained from our lungs to the vast number of cells within our body. Every structure in the body is made up of cells, and they all require a source of oxygen. RBCs, with their hemoglobin, provide life-giving oxygen to them. Once the oxygen is delivered to a cell, it is used in the biochemical process of burning glucose and other important functions that allow us to remain alive and healthy. These hemoglobin molecules, after unloading the oxygen, pick up carbon dioxide (CO_2) that has been produced within our cells as a result of burning glucose for energy. The RBCs then return to the lungs, courtesy of our beating heart and circulating blood, and unload the CO_2, which we then exhale. The RBCs then pick up more oxygen in the tiny air sacs of our lungs. RBCs are under constant production within our bone marrow, and these RBCs survive for around 180 days; therefore, at all times we have both younger and older RBCs present within our blood. Remember this fact. It is important in the next several paragraphs.

Symptoms of malaria can vary and can also include symptoms that are not specific or unique to malaria. These may include fatigue, fever, muscle and body aches, shaking chills, nausea/vomiting/diarrhea, labored breathing, headache, and profuse sweating. Severe symptoms of malaria cause by *P. falciparum* (and rarely by the other species), which may lead to death, include central nervous system involvement (cerebral malaria), kidney failure, severe anemia, and respiratory failure. Laboratory findings may include anemia (a low RBC count), with accompanying results that point to kidney and liver dysfunction.

One may ask, "How does the *Plasmodium* parasite cause problems in the bloodstream?"

The forms of malaria that are generally less severe (those caused by *P. vivax* and *P. ovale*) produce milder symptoms because the parasite only attacks RBCs of a certain age, thus only *partially* parasitizing all the RBCs in the person's blood. If a person has twenty trillion RBCs in their blood and only four trillion are infected, then sixteen trillion remain normally functioning RBCs. These two types of *Plasmodium* also produce dormant liver stages that may at a later date become active and produce disease symptoms weeks and years after the initial infection until the body is able to mount an immune reaction to the disease and control the infection.

It is possible to be reinfected with malaria. However, many people in malaria-prone areas of the world develop resistance to the disease and will consequently not develop any symptoms if bitten and infected by a mosquito carrying the parasite. This is significant because it means that malaria is not generally incurable and unrelenting in its symptoms.

The added danger of *P. falciparum*-caused malaria is tied to this species's ability to parasitize *all ages* of RBCs. Thus, all twenty-thirty trillion of the RBCs in a body (both young and old RBCs) are potentially carrying the parasites and will eventually be destroyed when the parasites cause them to rupture. Once the parasite destroys an RBC, the RBC's membrane decomposes. It is believed that the massive numbers of decomposing RBC membranes cause tiny blood-carrying capillaries to clog. These tiny blood vessels normally carry uninfected RBCs that supply oxygen and energy to living cells. When the diseased RBCs rupture and their membranes block the flow of normal blood to an area of the body, this is like trying to drive a thousand cars down a one-lane road. The traffic overload creates a massive traffic jam. So it is within the small blood vessels when trillions of RBCs rupture and their membranes block the flow of blood to various organs. If healthy cells in a person's muscles, brain, kidneys, liver, and other organs cannot get oxygen and glucose from RBCs and the liquid (plasma) portion of the blood, these cells will ultimately malfunction and perhaps even die. If the oxygen and energy deprivation last long enough, the victim will die from multi-organ failure.

It is essential to note, as we go forward in addressing the question of whether Lewis had malaria, that generally the most severe form of malaria, that caused by *Plasmodium falciparum*, does *not* have a dormant liver stage. Once one recovers from *falciparum*-caused malaria, the parasite is out of one's body. One may still be reinfected in the future, however. *P. falciparum*-caused fatal malaria, which causes the symptoms of headache, fever, chills, nausea, and vomiting noted in the less severe forms, becomes fatal because organs needed to keep one alive fail due to a lack of blood and oxygen caused by clogged capillary blood vessels, the result of massive RBC destruction. Cerebral malaria, an invariably fatal version of the disease, is most often found in children, and its effects are profound. Victims of this form of the disease are very sick.

Given this background, let us now look at the question of malaria and the final days of Meriwether Lewis. As already noted, Danisi and Jackson, in their recent book *The Truth About Meriwether Lewis*, formulated a new theory that Lewis's death was related to malaria that gained a good deal of both interest and support within the Lewis and Clark community. The authors expressed the novel idea that Lewis had probably killed himself but, rather curiously, claimed that it was not a suicide. They wrote that Lewis killed himself because he was suffering from malaria—more specifically, a "chronic case" of malaria that was incurable and recurrent.

This theory involves multiple errors of medical interpretation as well as incorrect interpretation of historical terms. Errors in the theory proposed by Danisi and Jackson include

- the misinterpretation of Jefferson's report written after the death of Lewis, citing the presence of "hypochondriac affections" within the Lewis family;
- the misinterpretation of historical nonspecific disease symptoms present within the population as malaria;
- the characterization of the "chronic" nature of malaria;
- the ignoring of specific historical evidence offered by others regarding Lewis's illness during his final days that makes it readily apparent that his symptoms *were not related to malaria* (this evidence includes Lewis's recovery from his reported alcohol abuse at Fort Pickering and Clark's report of his mental condition upon his departure from St. Louis); and
- the misinterpretation of Jefferson's comment that Lewis had fallen into a "habit" that contributed to his death as a reference to malaria, without justification.

Hypochondriac Affections

Thomas Jefferson in 1813 wrote an introduction for the first published edition of the *Journals of Lewis and Clark* and reported that Lewis was the victim of "hypochondriac affections" that he had personally observed in other members of the Lewis family. Jefferson recorded that this hypochondria was, in his opinion, a predisposing condition to the reported suicide of Lewis.[4]

In a creative line of reasoning, Danisi and Jackson tied Jefferson's comments into their case for Lewis's proposed malaria. They maintained that Jefferson's term "hypochondriac affections" referred specifically to abdominal pain resulting from a chronic malarial infection, not to the common meaning of someone who fears illness or has some type of chronic anxiety regarding their health. In addition, Danisi and Jackson used their theory to criticize numerous previous scholars regarding their interpretation of this term. Danisi followed up with another book as well as articles and editorials in *We Proceeded On*, the quarterly journal of The Lewis and Clark Trail Heritage Foundation. In an article in this journal, John and Thomas Danisi write that the numerous reports of Lewis's death by various historical figures "have led most Lewis historians to attribute Lewis's death to suicide as a result of lifelong depression."[5] They then attempt to support their case by citing Stephen Ambrose, Gary Moulton, and myself, stating, "For these historians, Lewis's depression is pathological—in that it is a recurrent symptom of a purely mental disorder of psychoneurotic or psychotic proportions, which is rooted in the early formation of his personality or of his thought processes."[6]

Danisi and Jackson then continue to justify their interpretation of "hypochondriac affections" and to criticize other authors' understanding of it. They quote Jefferson's letter to Paul Allen and Gilbert Russell that mentions Lewis's "hypochondriac affections" and "hypochondria," stating that modern historians have "attempted" to address the "first question using the categories and logic appropriate to modern psychology. But they failed to address the second question in an appropriate way."[7] In their book, Danisi and Jackson had written, "In 1809 American doctors held that melancholia was a mental illness while hypochondriasis was a physical condition with unknown causes. . . . The distinction between melancholia as a mental disease and hypochondriasis as a physical disease would take centuries to unravel and comprehend."[8]

There is absolutely no merit to any of these statements. In simple terms, Danisi and Jackson are proposing that "hypochondriac affections" meant something entirely different when Jefferson wrote it in 1813 than it does today. Their interpretation of the Greek-derived word "hypochondria" as referring to an area of the abdomen just below (*hypo*) the lower ribs (*chondrium*) as an anatomical region is accurate. But the misinterpretation of the term to apply to malaria and particularly to the abdominal pain associated with malaria is obviously an error.

Jefferson's 1813 note was written to Nicholas Biddle, the first editor of the *Journals of Lewis and Clark*. Jefferson wrote that

> Governor Lewis had from early life been subject to hypocondriac [*sic*] affections. It was a constitutional disposition in all the nearer branches of the family of his name, and was more immediately inherited by him from his father. They had not however been so strong as to give uneasiness in his family. While he lived with me in Washington, I observed at times sensible depressions of mind, but knowing their constitutional source, I estimated their course by what I had seen in the family. During his Western expedition the constant exertion which that required of all the faculties of body and mind suspended these distressing affections; but after his establishment in St. Louis in sedentary occupations they returned upon him with redoubled vigor, and began seriously to alarm. He was in a paroxysm of one of these when his affairs rendered it necessary for him to go to Washington.[9]

In an outstanding article in *We Proceeded On*, Lewis and Clark historian Michael Crosby thoroughly repudiates Danisi and Jackson's theory by documenting the historical meaning of the term "hypochondriac affections." Referencing dozens of historical writings, Crosby illustrates their error. Crosby begins by quoting a definition of hypochondriac affections from an encyclopedia written in 1814, hardly a date that reflects a "modern" psychological construct of the term. The 1814 definition is as follows: "Hypochondriac affections. A genus of diseases of the class Neuroses . . . characterized by dyspepsia; languor and want of energy; dejection of mind and apprehension of evil, more especially respecting health, without sufficient cause, with a melancholic temperament."[10]

Several others of Crosby's examples are worthy of note. He writes,

> In 1621 the Oxford scholar Robert Burton published *The Anatomy of Melancholy*, which distilled the essence of ancient and medieval works on "hypochondriac melancholy" and formed a

foundation for future scholars and physicians. Jefferson, whose intellectual interests were eclectic, may have possessed a copy. If not, the writers whose works with which he was familiar were influenced by it. The following is a survey of the medical and popular literature available to Jefferson that would have informed his understanding and usage of "hypochondriac affections."[11]

Crosby then mentions a 1661 work that lists the symptoms as "crudity of the ventricle, pain, stypticity of the belly, flatulency, anxiety, palpitation of the heart, pulsation in the left hypochondrium, dryness of the tongue, difficulty of respiration, and perturbation of the brain, &c." In 1726, Dr. Sir Richard Blackmore wrote, "Hypocondriacal Affections . . . in my Judgment, evidently consist of the irregular and disturbed Motions of the Spirit, and the irritable Disposition of the Nerves." Crosby also notes the transcript of an 1800 coroner's inquest investigating a suicide. The transcript reads that the authorities "were fully justified in their verdict of insanity, as it was obvious that he had for some time labored under an hypochondriacal affection."[12] Crosby documented numerous other specific references to the term showing it has had the same meaning for centuries.

As to whether there is any indication that the term "hypochondriac affections" ever referred to malaria, Crosby wrote,

> Notably absent in the literature is any equation of malaria with hypochondriac affections. In fact, Dr. Gideon Harvey in 1689 cautioned *against* treating hypochondriasis with Peruvian or Jesuit's bark, the 'sovereign' remedy for malaria: ". . . nothing will more certainly kill an Hypochondriac man, or Hysteric woman, in the violence of their returning fits, than the course of bleeding, vomiting, purging and Jesuiting.[13]

If one believes that Crosby's stellar logic and historical documentation are insufficient to prove this point, it might be helpful to consult with one of the medical authorities of that era for their insights regarding this issue. The medical authority of Jefferson's day was, arguably, Dr. Benjamin Rush, who tutored Meriwether Lewis on medical matters when Lewis was preparing for the expedition. In writing about the "hysterical and hypochondriacal states of fever," Rush wrote, "The former is known by a rising in the throat, which is for the most part erroneously ascribed to worms, by pale urine, and by a disposition to shed tears, or to laugh upon trifling occasions. The latter discovers itself by false opinions of the nature and danger of the disease under which the patient labours."[14] Rush is referring to a mental problem manifested in "opinions" of the patient. The patient falsely believes that they are suffering from a disease or is worried that the disease they have is much more serious than it actually is. So, Rush's definition in the early nineteenth century is *precisely* its meaning today. There is no different, so-called modern meaning as suggested by Danisi and Jackson.

In the same lecture, Rush wrote, "Are there certain grades in the convulsions of the nervous system, as appears in the hydrophobia, tetanus, epilepsy, hysteria, and hypocondriasis?"[15] It is clear from this list that Rush categorized hypochondriasis as a nervous system disorder. His usage here also matches the modern association of hypochondriasis with a mental problem or nervous system disorder. Rush again directly associates hypochondriasis with hysteria in his writing about bilious fevers: "The hypochondriasis and the hysteria seldom fail to exchange their symptoms twice in the four and twenty hours."[16] I will not conduct an in-depth study of the word "hysteria." Simply put, it was considered a mental disorder in the early nineteenth century.

Hypochondriac Affections and Abdominal Pain

Did "hypochondriac affections" refer to abdominal pain resulting from a "chronic case" of malaria, as claimed by Danisi and Jackson? The answer is no.

The term "hypochondriasis" was derived from the ancient Greek belief that the seat of human emotions lay in the anatomical area of the abdomen, just below the margin of the ribcage, that was known as the hypochondrium. Thomas Danisi quoted from an 1841 treatise by Dr. Robert Hooper concerning hypochondria to support their abdominal pain theory.[17] Dr. Hooper's nineteenth-century comments are consistent with the ancient Greek belief that the hypochondrium is the source of the emotions. He wrote, "The seat of the hypochondriac affections is in the stomach and the bowels." Hooper observed that, upon autopsy, "[T]he liver and spleen are usually found considerably enlarged" in cases of hypochondriac affections. It is very important to note that Hooper (who wrote his article in a time of relative medical ignorance) was not assigning a causative association between the two organs and hypochondriac affections but was simply making observations of associated findings that physicians in that era made about a myriad of diseases. Since Hooper and his colleagues did not understand much about human physiology and pathology, they made copious observations about associations of various physical diseases and postmortem findings at autopsy. Rush's writings also record nearly endless associations between diseases and environmental and physical findings *without assigning causation to any of the associations*. Hooper was not stating that the "hypochondriac affections" were caused by enlargement of the spleen or liver but that the two conditions were noted to occur together at times. Hooper's statement, when interpreted correctly, reflects the erroneous beliefs of both Hooper and the ancient Greek physicians.

If we assume that Danisi and Jackson's theory is correct and that Lewis's "hypochondriac affection" was not depression and/or a fixation on an imaginary medical condition but abdominal pain associated with a chronic malaria infection and that Jefferson had the same understanding, then Jefferson believed that Lewis's malaria was inherited from his father. Since Jefferson noted that Lewis had probably inherited the disease of hypochondria from his father, did Jefferson believe that Lewis's father suffered from abdominal pain brought on by a chronic case of malaria? If other members of the Lewis family suffered from this disease as well, then we must conclude that they all suffered from inherited abdominal pain brought about by a case of inherited malaria. This is just wrong. Malaria is an infectious disease; it is not inherited.

"Severe Intermittent Paroxysm"

John and Thomas Danisi attempt to equate malaria with other unrelated diseases by arguing that both Lewis and Jefferson suffered from a specific disease (malaria) and incorrectly associating it with a specific symptom—"severe intermittent paroxysm." The only evidence they offer is that Jefferson suffered from periodic headaches and treated himself unsuccessfully with both calomel and barks.[18] In reading Jefferson's description of his headaches, it is clear that they were not brought on by malaria as he did not have accompanying symptoms that would suggest such a diagnosis. His treatment with barks and calomel, as we have already discussed in this book, did not in any way denote a specific diagnosis of malaria as physicians of that era used these substances to treat a myriad of illnesses by physicians of that era. Even a casual reading of the Lewis and Clark journals and Rush's writings shows these medications were used to treat many unrelated illnesses.

Danisi and Danisi then incorrectly equate the intermittent symptom of "severe intermittent paroxysm" with "intermittent fever," one of the nineteenth-century terms for malaria. *Many diseases are intermittent—but not all diseases are malaria. Many diseases have an intermittent fever, but not all such fevers are the result of malaria.*

Diagnosing Malaria in 1809

Danisi and Danisi also misrepresent the state of medical knowledge in Lewis's final year, writing: "He [Lewis] had medical and personal knowledge of the ailments and intermittent diseases because of the treatments that he received from Doctors Benjamin Rush and Antoine Saugrain. He also most likely knew that these sovereign treatments dealt only with the symptoms, not the causes, of such diseases."[19]

There are several problems with this statement. Neither of the medical experts mentioned here, Rush and Saugrain, had any real understanding of any disease process, malarial or otherwise. The germ theory of disease had not yet been accepted, and modern pathology and pharmaceuticals were not available. Since there was no understanding of the actual cause of malaria until the early twentieth century, neither Rush nor Saugrain nor Lewis knew what caused malaria. If they did not know the cause, they certainly had no idea how to cure it. Even if Lewis understood that the medication was only treating the symptoms of the disease and not the source, such knowledge implies that Lewis understood the disease well enough to be able to distinguish between its source and its symptoms. He had no understanding of the source of malaria, so how could he know that he was only treating the symptoms? In other words, Lewis did not know the cause of malaria, so he would have been unable to think about the disease in the way that Danisi and Danisi describe. Physicians of this era knew nothing about the pharmaceutical action of cinchona bark (which contains quinine). If a patient had a fever that occurred during the summer or fall, that came and went every few days and that was accompanied by a headache and some nausea, they were diagnosed with "ague" or an "intermittent fever," and the medical references of that era designated cinchona bark as one of the possible treatments. Again, there is no justification for crediting Lewis, Rush, or Saugrain with such knowledge about malaria and its treatment.

To summarize to this point, Danisi and Danisi are arguing that severe intermittent paroxysm = intermittent fever = hypochondriac affections = malaria. This is the epitome of an illogical and convoluted diagnosis.

Numerous infectious diseases during Lewis's era could have caused "intermittent fevers" (fevers that come and go). Without any microbiology or lab results to confirm a diagnosis, physicians during that era were forced to give names to a "fever," sometimes linking the name of the illness to symptoms or to the location where it was obtained: putrid, bilious, malignant, jail, etc. At that time, fevers were believed to be distinct diseases, not just a manifestation of many different contagious diseases.

Most people today are familiar with the flu and perhaps strep throat, chickenpox, mumps, or measles (specific immunizations have only recently become available for some of these). All of these diseases produce a fever, but the fever is not the disease. The fever is only a manifestation of the body's immune system response to the disease. In Rush's and Saugrain's framework of medical thinking, the fever *was* the disease.

The Chronic Nature of Malaria in Early America

There are a number of misrepresentations of medicine and malaria in Thomas Danisi's *Uncovering the Truth About Meriwether Lewis*. In the first sentence of chapter 13, entitled "Dr. Antoine Saugrain's Treatment of Governor Meriwether Lewis," the text reads, "One of the most fascinating and instructive recent discoveries regarding the life of Meriwether Lewis was his battle with malaria, which in his time was called 'the ague,' an incurable and untreatable disease."[20]

Danisi's labeling malaria as "incurable and untreatable" is not accurate. Although the cinchona bark that contained quinine may have been an unreliable treatment, its unreliability was based on variations in the content of quinine in any given sample of the medication or on using an incorrect dose of quinine. The concentration of any medication used in 1809 was hit or miss since medications were not produced to standards. Even if the pharmacist's preparation of a prescription for the bark was correct, the patient had to take the medication correctly, which was again an uncertain proposition. But if the concentration of quinine in the prescription was adequate and the patient took the medication appropriately, quinine could be effective in ridding the body of the *Plasmodium*. Malaria, even in the early 1800s, was a treatable disease.

Danisi's use of the word "incurable" and his later claim that Lewis's malaria was "chronic" implies that the symptoms of the disease were continuously present or repeatedly occurring over a prolonged period of time. This is misleading for several reasons. Danisi attempts to bolster his claims of a malarial diagnosis in Lewis by incorrectly identifying other diseases that existed at that time as malaria. Numerous infectious diseases share the same symptoms as malaria, and it is inappropriate to diagnose every set of these disease symptoms as due to malaria. Numerous gastrointestinal infectious diseases that were food- and waterborne and were caused by bacteria of the genera *Shigella*, *Escherichia*, and *Salmonella* were common among a population that routinely ingested contaminated water and food. The victims Danisi describes could have just as easily been suffering from one of these unrelated diseases that produce many of the same symptoms as would malaria.

An example of this diagnostic error is found in Danisi's reference to Indian agent John Breck Treat, who, he claims, "succumbed to malaria."[21] Mr. Treat's description of his illness is certainly not specific for malaria. Treat wrote in 1808,

> A few days ago . . . a sudden and very severe attack of the Fever seiz'd me and although it only remained eight or ten days . . . I have . . . constantly . . . been extremely ill; almost the whole time confined to my bed from which I now write this—from the emaciated, and feeble state I now am in, it is extremely uncertain

when I may become convalescent . . . this is the first month of serious sickness which I have ever experienced.[22]

Nothing in this description is specific for malaria.

In medicine, when a patient presents with a series of symptoms, the physician often mentally constructs a differential diagnosis, or a list of all the disease processes that might be responsible for the patient's illness. After hearing Mr. Treat's description, I would construct a differential diagnosis of several dozen different infectious diseases that could produce the same symptoms. Some diseases on that list would, in my professional judgment, be much more likely than the malaria diagnosis made by Danisi.

Danisi repeats this error in the same chapter, such as when he diagnoses malaria based on the report of "camp or putrid fever" that Lewis suffered from in April of 1795. Camp fever and putrid fever are archaic terms for the disease of epidemic typhus, caused by an organism of the bacterial genus *Rickettsia* that is transmitted into the human body by way of the human body louse. This disease was ubiquitous in army camps where poor sanitation resulted in lice-infested soldiers. Other *Rickettsia* species are rather famous as pathogens transmitted by the bite of various tick species that cause Rocky Mountain Spotted Fever and other nasty illnesses.

Danisi is entirely accurate in writing, "The evidence is overwhelming that malaria was a prevalent and formidable disease in seventeenth- and eighteenth-century America." This is followed by another sentence in the same paragraph, however, that is not true. Danisi writes that what Lewis scholars who disagree with him on this issue "fail to appreciate is that once Lewis had contracted malaria, he had it for the rest of his life—it was incurable and untreatable during his lifetime."[23] Danisi may be endeavoring here to bolster his case that Lewis's mental derangement or his indisposition in the final weeks of his life were the result of "chronic malaria" by establishing the idea this unremitting, untreatable, and nearly constant infection with severe symptoms would drive Lewis to suicide. However, the medical reality of this disease suggests otherwise.

It is well established that untreated malaria caused by *Plasmodium ovale*, *vivax*, and *malariae* generally produces an uncomplicated disease picture of a series of recurring chills, intense fever, sweating, and, at times, headache, malaise, fatigue, body aches, nausea, and vomiting. In other cases, particularly in children and pregnant women, the disease caused by these organisms may progress to severe malaria—including cerebral malaria manifested by coma, seizures, severe anemia, and organ failure.[24] The manifestations of malaria that are commonly the most devastating mainly affect young children and are almost exclusively caused by *P. falciparum*.[25]

Victims of malaria often develop a protective immunity following the initial infection, and this can shield the victim from subsequent infections. Victims who are repeatedly exposed to malaria develop antibodies against various stages of the parasite.[26]

Malaria caused by species other than *P. falciparum* may produce chronic infections if the parasites harbor within the victim's liver cells for months to years. But the vast majority of these chronic cases are *without symptoms*; the victims appear to be entirely healthy.[27] The ability of the body to control the parasites at low levels without showing symptoms results from the gradual development of immunity following repeated exposures. This occurs with all forms of malaria. In endemic areas, such as some areas of early America, up to 39 percent of *P. falciparum* carriers remain asymptomatic.[28]

What this means for the malaria victim is that, once infected, their immune system will normally provide the protective effect of either eliminating the parasite and thus the disease or of controlling the number of parasites in the body, thus producing an asymptomatic state. Danisi argues that Meriwether Lewis was chronically ill and mentally deranged due to suffering nearly constant attacks of malaria for many months, with numerous symptoms torturing him on his way back to Washington, D.C., in September and October 1809. This scenario is not likely.

Lewis's Use of Peruvian Bark

Lewis was prescribed a form of Peruvian bark, but it is a significant error to assume that he was therefore being treated for malaria. Peruvian bark was a medication used for malaria in early America, *but it was not prescribed exclusively for malaria*. Dr. Benjamin Rush prescribed the bark for a variety of problems, including intestinal worms, tetanus, painful legs, consumption (tuberculosis), gout, hydrophobia (rabies), and other diseases. Reading through Dr. Rush's essays in *Medical Inquiries and Observations*, it is clear that all of the most popular medications of those days were used for a multitude of unrelated diseases. Thus, the presence of Peruvian bark on Lewis's medication list no more identifies him as having malaria than taking penicillin today identifies one as suffering from syphilis or strep throat. A prescription for bark as proof that a patient had malaria is no proof at all.

Jefferson's Comments about Lewis's "Habit"

Jefferson wrote in 1810 that Lewis's problems had been caused by his hypochondriasis, which was "probably increased by the habit into which he had fallen." [29] Given the context of Jefferson's comments and the reports of Lewis's alcohol abuse prior to his death, of which Jefferson was aware, as well as the correct interpretation of Jefferson's mention of "hypochondriac affections" described in this chapter, Jefferson's reference to the "habit" into which Meriwether Lewis had fallen before his death most certainly did not refer to malaria. He was undoubtedly referring to Lewis's alcohol use and/or his mental state of hypochondria.

Cerebral Malaria's Role in Lewis's Death

Was Lewis suffering from cerebral malaria on his final trip, causing his reported "mental derangement," as Danisi asserts?[30] Cerebral malaria is a greatly feared neurological complication of malaria and is generally caused by *P. falciparum*. It results when parasite-laden red blood cells block the small blood vessels in the brain, robbing brain cells of oxygen and nutrition. This results in swelling of the brain and possibly seizures and coma. The clinical hallmark of this form of malaria is impaired consciousness, with coma the most severe manifestation.[31] These patients can also go into shock and suffer kidney failure, abnormal bleeding, pulmonary edema (fluid buildup in the lungs), and other severe symptoms. Without treatment, cerebral malaria is invariably fatal.

It is nearly inconceivable that Lewis was suffering from cerebral malaria during his last trip to Washington. He would have been extremely sick and would not have taken a boat trip and then recovered within a short time at Fort Pickering on a diet of wine, soon after that resuming his journey on horseback trip across hundreds of miles of dirt roads. Virtually all patients with cerebral malaria are first unconscious and then die; they are often beyond the help even of modern medicine.

The Role of Malaria in Lewis's Death

In closing, I must answer the question of whether Meriwether had malaria during his final days and whether it contributed in some way to his death. It is certainly possible that Lewis could have suffered in the post-expedition years from bouts of malaria. It is also possible that he contracted malaria for the first time at some point after the end of the expedition in 1806. It is reported that he was taking opium tablets, presumably for bouts of malaria, after the expedition. But this does not fall within the malarial picture presented by Danisi and Jackson. Without autopsy results—without any liver or splenic tissue and without any red blood cells for DNA studies to determine if there is any *Plasmodium* DNA within Meriwether's remains—it is impossible to say definitively that he was suffering from malaria. Given his high level of activity during the last weeks of his life, it is certain that he did not have cerebral malaria. At the risk of being repetitive, it is important to keep in mind that in malaria-endemic areas (where people are repeatedly exposed to the malarial parasite), such as many areas of early America, a significant percentage of people who are reinfected with malaria will have no symptoms whatsoever.

It is possible that an uncomplicated form of malaria could have been one of the health-related issues contributing to Lewis's reported mental derangement during his trip to Fort Pickering in September 1809. This possibility is somewhat intriguing. But again, this scenario differs significantly from the one described by Danisi and Jackson. Infections such as malaria are known to worsen the effects of alcohol withdrawal, which by all reports was a significant part of Meriwether's problems during the final weeks of his life. Significant alcohol abuse causes a depressed immunological response to any disease. Without question, there was an entire host of virulent infectious diseases during those days that could have worsened Lewis's overall clinical condition as he made his way back to Washington. These are diseases that would have been accompanied by fever, malaise, and indisposition but that were unrelated to malaria.

After examining the overall clinical and basic science picture of malaria and considering its ramifications on the story of the death of Meriwether Lewis, I believe that malaria could not have been the chief cause of his health problems during his final days. In my medical opinion, the theory that malaria made Lewis kill himself, although it is a novel historical interpretation, is a proverbial house of cards. The entire case is built on a multitude of inaccurate conclusions about the nature of malaria, the incorrect assignment of various nonspecific disease symptoms to malaria, and the ignoring of Captain Gilbert Russell's clear reference to Lewis's alcohol abuse as the source of his illness at Fort Pickering. Cerebral malaria could not have been the cause of Lewis's mental derangement at Fort Pickering because his derangement was reportedly cured by claret wine. The interpretation of some of Jefferson's words as referring to malaria—his description of Lewis's "hypochondriac affections" and the "habit" Lewis had returned to—are transparently inaccurate. Crosby's work on the historical meaning of "hypochondriac affections" has completely eliminated any possibility that this term referred to malaria. The theory of malaria and its relation to Lewis's final days, at least as Danisi and Jackson present it, is without merit.

Chapter 9
Bullets and How They Kill

All bleeding eventually stops.
—Quoted by every surgeon in the history of medicine

One of the few aspects of the death of Meriwether Lewis that is not shrouded in controversy is the fact that he died as the result of one or more gunshot wounds. At this point, the agreement ends and the controversy begins regarding the source of the wounds, the intent of the person or persons who pulled the trigger(s), and the survivability of such wounds. As is true for all facets of this story, historians and others have weighed in with their opinions about the reported wounds and their opinions about others' opinions.

Dr. Eldon Chuinard was the first physician to offer his opinion on the nature of the wounds suffered by Meriwether Lewis. I (David) responded to Dr. Chuinard's opinion with my own explanation in my book *Or Perish in the Attempt*, which briefly described the nature of Lewis's wounds and my case for his reported survival of around two hours. Due to the number of opinions regarding Lewis's gunshot wounds, the confusion and controversy continue regarding the lethality of his wounds. In this chapter, I provide the best medical explanation of the facts as expressed by current experts in the field concerning what we know about gunshot wounds and how we know it.

Reports of razor-inflicted wounds on Lewis's neck and arms appeared in newspaper accounts shortly after his death on October

11, 1809. These reported wounds and the validity of their sources do not change the cause of his death. Lewis died as the result of wounds that caused him to bleed sufficiently to lower his blood pressure to the point that he could not survive. His ultimate death was from *exsanguination*, the medical term for a severe loss of blood. His loss of blood resulted in his organs rapidly failing due to the exhaustion of their supplies of oxygen and glucose. When these life-giving molecules are gone, living organs cease to function and die. The liver cannot do its job of processing food and alcohol by, for example, changing glucose into amino acids. The kidneys cannot filter the circulating blood and control the electrolytes within the body and help to regulate blood pressure and red blood cell production. Heart cells cannot contract properly. Nerve cells cannot conduct impulses. This same sequence of events could be described for every bodily organ. Once he had lost sufficient blood pressure, Lewis would have lost consciousness, and as the bleeding continued, his brain would have ceased to function. It is that simple. The object(s) that caused his wounds—razor, bullet, spear, arrow, or another penetrating object—has no bearing on the ultimate result, which was Lewis's death.

There is a graphic scene in the movie *Saving Private Ryan* in which the medic of Ryan's World War II-era U.S. Army Rangers unit is severely wounded in the abdomen by German machine-gun fire. He is in obvious pain, and his comrades gather around him in an admirable and dramatic but completely ineffective effort to treat his internal wounds. They sprinkle sulfa antibiotic powder on the exterior of his abdomen and apply pressure to the exit wounds on the front of the abdomen where the blood is exiting as a result of his internal wounds. This treatment could never have saved the life of the doomed medic. The only possible fix for such wounds would be immediate surgery, which might be able to identify the source of the internal bleeding and stop the hemorrhaging.

A helpful analogy for this battlefield trauma that I refer to throughout this chapter is as follows. Think of a wooden barrel with a hose inside of it. The barrel represents the external body of a person and the hose represents the blood-carrying veins and arteries inside the body. The water within the hose represents the blood. If someone shoots a bullet through the barrel and the bullet severs the hose, water will start to pour into the barrel and ultimately will go out the hole in the barrel made by the bullet—just as occurred with the wounded medic in *Saving Private Ryan*. A plug over the hole on the *outside* of the barrel (the surface of the wounded medic's abdomen) will not stop the leaking of the hose *inside* the barrel (internal bleeding), which is why putting pressure on the medic's external wound was destined to fail. Today's trauma surgeons and interventional radiologists have multiple tools available to them to stop the internal bleeding from such a wound (and thus plug the hole in the hose).

As we begin to unravel this piece of controversy within our story, we need to understand gunshot wounds and how they kill. Bullets fired from weapons during the era of Meriwether Lewis were made out of lead. Lead is a heavy metal that can be easily melted over hot coals and then poured into spherical molds of differing sizes, where it cools and hardens. Soldiers in the early 1800s routinely made their own bullets.

A weapon's caliber is determined by the size of the ball (its diameter) that it shoots, which is true even for modern weapons. Some data on bullets is expressed in the English system (a 30-caliber bullet is 30/100th of an inch in diameter), but some modern weapons use the metric system (9 mm). The diameter of the projectile reflects the caliber of the weapon. The diameter of bullets in modern firearms can be expressed in either system. The rifles used by the expedition were likely in the 50-caliber range. Their bullets were spherical and measured approximately 13 mm in diameter.

During the 1996 coroner's jury that discussed Lewis's death, firearms expert Lucien Haag testified that several manufacturers of large-caliber (54–69-caliber) black powder pistols were available to Lewis.[1] They all shot spherical balls of lead. These pistols were used for personal protection and were referred to as "horse pistols." Historians and firearm experts, as well as Dr. Glenn Wagner, a contemporary forensic pathologist, believe that Lewis had a "brace" (two pistols) in his possession the night of his death. Lewis reportedly arrived at Grinder's Stand alone, prior to the arrival of his servant Pernier and Neelly's servant. Neelly, prior to his departure from the scene in the hours before Lewis's death, reportedly instructed Pernier not to allow Lewis access to any gunpowder. It is possible that Neelly claimed to have done this to avoid any blame after Lewis's death. At any rate, given the descriptions of Lewis's wounds, it is intuitively obvious that both his pistols were loaded and primed.

Modern firearms are propelled by gunpowder that is contained inside metal casings. In Lewis's time, metal casings did not exist and gunpowder was poured directly into the end (muzzle) of the barrel. The propulsive force was supplied by a controlled explosion of gunpowder within the barrel of the gun, which was ignited by a spark that occurred when a piece of flint, secured in the hammer, hit a piece of metal (the frizzen) and the resulting spark ignited a small supply of gunpowder held in the flash pan. This explosive fire traveled through a pinpoint-sized hole into the barrel and ignited the powder that had been poured into it at the muzzle. This explosion then propelled the spherical lead ball out of the muzzle at a speed somewhere between 800 and 1,200 feet/second. Compared to some modern weapons, which fire bullets at over 3,000 feet/second, this bullet speed is relatively slow. These modern weapons fire high-velocity rounds, whereas the black powder flintlocks of the Corps of Discovery fired low-velocity rounds. The lower killing effectiveness of the flintlocks carried by the expedition is why the men of the Corps of Discovery needed to shoot grizzly bears six to ten times to kill them. Why were so many shoots needed?

The spherical shape of a lead ball is a very poor shape for a bullet compared to a modern-day bullet, which is shaped like a missile. This is due to the spherical shape of the projectile, which, after it is fired, moves through a sea of air that provides friction to the bullet, slowing it down much more than a modern, more aerodynamically efficient bullet. This results in the spherical ball having less kinetic energy at a distance than a modern bullet, which in turn results in decreased ability to wound the target. This is what saved Lewis's rear end (no pun intended) when Pierre Cruzatte shot him with his flintlock rifle. Lewis was probably about fifty yards from Cruzatte; the spherical lead ball lost some of its kinetic energy as it traveled to Lewis and thus had less ability to penetrate Lewis's body and inflict a severe wound. Had Lewis been wounded by a modern missile-shaped bullet, his wound would have been more severe because the bullet would have been moving faster and thus would have contained more energy.

Regardless of a bullet's shape, a significant amount of energy is contained in the lead projectile traveling out of the gun's barrel. If you remember your basic physics, this moving lead ball contains what is called kinetic energy as a function of both its mass and its speed. Kinetic energy is a force contained in a moving body. If you have ever collided with someone when they were running, you felt the force of their kinetic energy at the time of the collision. Thanks to various physicists who developed the equation describing the movement of a body of a certain mass, we can apply this equation to a bullet shot from a gun and calculate the bullet's energy, expressed in "joules." The kinetic energy can be quantified as follows: kinetic energy = 1/2 mass x velocity x velocity (or 1/2 mass x velocity^2).

A superficial look at this equation reveals that the way to increase the kinetic energy of a bullet is to increase its mass or velocity or both. So, a large-caliber lead bullet has more kinetic energy than a small-caliber bullet if the bullets are traveling at the same speed. On the other hand, a bullet that is lighter in weight may possess more kinetic energy than a heavier bullet if the lighter one is going much faster than the heavier bullet. The other important factor, as already noted, is the shape of the bullet. Spherical bullets, after being fired, have less kinetic energy and thus less ability to wound and to penetrate, thus resulting in less collateral tissue damage than a modern bullet of the same weight.

When a bullet enters a living being, it damages the body in various ways. Vincent Di Maio, in his informative book *Gunshot Wounds: Practical Aspects of Firearms, Ballistics, and Forensic Techniques*, notes that

> the concept of a gunshot wound held by most individuals is that of a bullet going through a person like a drill bit through wood, 'drilling' a neat hole through structures that it passes through. This picture is erroneous. As a bullet moves through the body, it crushes and shreds the tissue in its path, while at the same time flinging outward (radially) the surrounding tissue from the path of the bullet, producing a temporary cavity considerably larger than the diameter of the bullet. . . . It is the combination of the crushed and shredded tissue and the effects of the temporary cavity on tissue adjacent to the bullet path (shearing, compression, and stretching) that determines the final extent of a wound.[2]

With low-velocity spherical bullets, the damage is somewhat localized along the direct path of the bullet. If the bullet travels through an organ that contains many blood vessels, it will damage those vessels and cause the blood to leave the damaged vascular system of veins, arteries, and capillaries and either collect within the organ or bleed out into the surrounding tissue. If such a wound occurs within the thoracic or abdominal cavities, blood may accumulate within what is essentially empty space. Such bleeding represents a seriously dangerous situation as this blood is not within the circulatory system and, if severe, contributes to possibly life-threatening lowered blood pressure. If a bullet wound does not produce significant bleeding, then bleeding may not be sufficient to be life threatening. The latter was the case when Lewis was wounded in his buttock by a round from Pierre Cruzatte's flintlock. The flintlock shot a low-velocity round, probably 1,000–1,200 feet/second. Because it was a superficial wound and no organs were involved, most of the bleeding was from a visible source and could be controlled by applying external pressure to the area of the wound until the blood formed clots, which was likely within minutes.

My friend and medical school classmate Dale Carrison, D.O., was the director of emergency medicine at a level 1 trauma center in Las Vegas, Nevada, for over twenty years. Dale has much experience treating gunshot wounds and has offered his insights into wounds caused by bullets of different shapes. He notes that modern-day shotguns, which often shoot numerous small pellets rather than solitary bullets, "make a horrific exterior wound, but don't penetrate deep into the tissue because of the multiple small 'balls' that have a poor ballistic coefficient [ability to overcome air resistance]" and low mass.

As I pointed out in *Or Perish in the Attempt*, if we assume that Cruzatte was fifty yards away from Lewis at the time of this shooting, a mere twitch in his aim that slightly altered the trajectory of the bullet would have sent the 50–60-caliber ball into Lewis's hip, possibly taking out an artery, sciatic nerve, piece of femur or pelvis, or perhaps all of these. Had that happened, Lewis could have died within minutes. A major arterial bleed would have occurred that could not have been stopped by external pressure to the wound—just like the ruptured hose inside the wooden barrel. If you cannot reach the leaking spot in the hose, you cannot stop the leak. If Lewis had lost 30 percent of his blood volume from a wound to an artery or vein, he would have lost consciousness, and at around 40 percent blood loss his blood pressure would have been so low he would have died. He was very lucky to sustain a wound that he recovered from within a few weeks. That day, August 12, 1806, was both a very unlucky and a very lucky day for Meriwether Lewis.[3]

As previously mentioned, modern weapons with their high-velocity bullets produce greater tissue damage compared to the low-velocity rounds in the weapons of the Lewis and Clark era. The bullet's force produces a shock wave, and the resulting increased tissue damage leads to increased potential bleeding. As the bullet travels through an organ, the bullet not only damages the vessels on its direct path but also damages other vessels in the surrounding area via the shock wave that is transmitted into the surrounding tissue through the high concentration of water in the surrounding cells and blood. Water is the vehicle through which the damaging force is chiefly transmitted. The faster the bullet, the more energy it contains and the more damage it produces.

The key piece of evidence, which many murder theorists cite as the *best* evidence against the suicide theory, is that Lewis's reported wounds are inconsistent with his reported survival of about two hours. John Guice (an American history professor) cites the late Dr. Eldon Chuinard, an orthopedic surgeon, as his leading authority supporting his opinion that Lewis was murdered. Guice stated in his testimony at the unofficial coroner's jury held in 1996,

> I would like to point out to you that Dr. Chuinard was an orthopedic surgeon. He was a professor of orthopedic surgery in the Pacific Northwest and in 1991 wrote a lengthy article in a journal called, *We Proceeded On*, which is [the] journal of the Lewis and Clark Trail Foundation. . . . I think if I had to pick a single work to read . . . I guess I'd read that. You know[,] being a medical professor, professor of orthopedic surgery[,] I think he does a wonderful job of destroying some of the arguments for suicide in terms of the fact that he claims that Meriwether Lewis could not possibly have behaved in the manner that Mrs. Grinder said he behaved[,] having been wounded as she said he was wounded.[4]

Guice continues, more emphatically, "Now he [Chuinard] just said it's a medical impossibility for him to have behaved in the manner that she described in one of the letters."[5]

In his article on Lewis's death, Chuinard denied that Lewis could have survived the wounds he had for very long, stating that if Lewis had shot himself in "the breast," his slow death "is totally unbelievable!" Chuinard raised an interesting question. He states, "This second shot would be expected to have killed Lewis instantly, or have disabled him," and then he asks, "What do the supporters of suicide think that this second shot would have done to the heart, lungs, aorta and/or intestines? Certainly Lewis would have been in dire shock and soon have bled to death; or perhaps [been] paralyzed from spinal cord injury."[6]

I want to emphasize my view about this testimony. If it can be shown through the evidence obtained from medical experts that Lewis could have survived his wounds for two hours, then the *strongest* piece of evidence that Guice cites in support of his argument against Lewis's suicide is not valid. Let's take a detailed look at this.

We may interpret the nonspecific term "breast" as meaning somewhere on the chest. If Lewis held a pistol to his chest, with the muzzle aimed at a slightly downward angle as is suggested by the description of the resulting wound, the bullet probably entered his chest, passed through his lung, penetrated the thin, muscular diaphragm, and then possibly wounded his spleen or liver, depending on whether the bullet entered the left or right side of his chest.

Dr. Carrison notes that the degree to which an organ is damaged by a bullet is determined in part by how flexible that organ is. Carrison reports, "I had a patient that was shot in the chest with a .30-06 and didn't even have a pneumothorax [collapsed lung]! Fortunately for him the projectile also didn't hit a rib. If it had hit a rib, the bone would have become a secondary projectile, also doing damage."[7] (.30-06 is a modern-day rifle caliber commonly used to hunt big game animals such as elk and deer.) The significance of his statement is that the wounded lung was so pliable and elastic that his patient was shot in the chest but did not end up with a collapsed lung.

Glenn Wagner, D.O., physician and retired chief medical examiner/county coroner of San Diego, California, has had nearly fifty years of forensic pathology experience in his distinguished medical career. He received his pathology and forensics training in the U.S. Navy and at the National Institutes of Health and is one of the most competent and experienced forensic pathologists in the world today. He has conducted over fourteen thousand postmortem exams in his career, with 25 to 30 percent of them determined to be suicides. Addressing the gunshot wounds of Meriwether Lewis, Wagner stated,

> Some folks felt that a two-hour survival time, which he reportedly had, would suggest that it was not a suicide. I'd have to disagree with that position. Gunshot wounds kill by exsanguination [loss of blood], and it depends on what you hit, how quickly you are going to bleed. Loss of 30 percent [of the volume of your blood] puts you into shock; loss of 40 percent will likely kill if you are not treated medically. The question becomes, If it were a suicide and the first gunshot was a head wound, a graze wound, would he likely have a concussion or a subdural hematoma [bleeding in the brain]? We are talking about a probable 50-caliber ball fired out of a flintlock. He probably had a brace, or two pistols. My guess is that he would probably have great difficulty, if he had a concussion, reloading a single pistol. So, I'm pretty certain that he had two pistols available when this event occurred—if it was self-inflicted. The second one was somewhere over the chest, exiting in the lower back. So, he may or may not have wounded part of his heart. He may or may not have wounded his lungs. But he most certainly got a portion of his liver, stomach, small intestine, and the descending colon . . . and probably the left kidney. Well, of all of those, the ones that are going to bleed the most aggressively are the liver and the kidney. So, he could have very well survived two hours.[8]

Dr. Jerry Francisco, a forensic pathologist, gave the same opinion as Wagner regarding the wounds of Meriwether. Francisco stated,

> There are certain wounds that by their very nature you say that's got to be fatal, and that's got to be fatal within a relatively short period of time. One to the body would not necessarily be fatal rapidly, because it's a function of what organs were damaged

and how rapidly was the bleeding, because the bleeding is going to be the cause of death, and it has to be a large vessel and the bleeding to be rapid for death to be rapid.[9]

What would a modern trauma surgeon have to say about the reported wounds and Lewis's reported two-hour survival? Would they agree with these two forensic pathologists? Dr. Dale Mortenson, a board-certified general/vascular/trauma surgeon who has surgically treated hundreds of gunshot victims during his more than thirty-year career, agrees with Wagner's and Francisco's assessments of Lewis's wounds. Given the reported survival of around two hours, Mortensen observed that the chest and abdominal wound suffered by Lewis "did not hit any major arteries, which doesn't particularly surprise me, as there is a lot of room inside the chest and abdomen for a bullet to pass through and not hit a major artery."[10] If no major artery within Lewis's body was damaged, then there would not have been the uncontrolled and rapid bleeding that would cause the quick death proposed by Chuinard.

If Lewis had suffered these wounds and been rushed to a modern trauma center, his vital signs would have been taken immediately upon arrival in the emergency room. Blood pressure, pulse, respiration rate, temperature, and oxygen saturation would all be obtained in a matter of moments. Given our proposed scenario, Lewis's blood pressure would have been significantly reduced from the average of 120/80 mm Hg. His heart rate would have been significantly elevated, probably 150–200 or higher instead of the normal rate of below 100 beats per minute. This elevated heart rate would have reflected his body's automatic attempt to raise his blood pressure by pumping out more blood into his leaking vasculature (his water hose was leaking inside the barrel).

The initial ER exam would have noted the wounds on Lewis's body, and the first task of the ER physician would have been to try to support the patient's blood pressure by replacing some of the fluid lost through bleeding. Fluid replacement in seriously wounded patients is both an art and a science as aggressive fluid replacement (from normal saline to whole blood) can push the gunshot victim into a fatal situation due to fluid buildup within the lungs.

The sources and extent of the wounds could have been established by an ultrasound, a so-called FAST test (focused assessment with sonography in trauma). This rapid bedside test images the blood surrounding various internal organs as the result of internal hemorrhage. In a healthy person, there is no blood sloshing around inside either the abdominal or the chest cavity. All of the blood in a nonhemorrhaging, healthy person is contained within the arteries, veins, and capillaries.

By this time, the trauma surgeon would already be examining the victim, looking for the entrance and exit wounds and, through interpretation of the FAST imaging, noting any evidence of blood surrounding the spleen, liver, and other areas of the abdomen as well as the chest (see figures 2 and 3). Since the bullet reportedly exited Lewis's body in his lower back, according to Mortenson, "The spinal cord is well protected by the thick bone of the vertebrae, and if the bullet had hit a vertebra, there may not have been an exit wound at all. This is due to the thick bone being a blocking force to the projectile's path. If there was an exit wound, the odds increase that no vertebrae were hit."[11]

If there were any bleeding within Lewis's abdomen, which would undoubtedly have been the case, he would have been taken immediately to the operating room and, as Mortenson put it, "opened up from his neck to his groin." If Lewis's spleen had been damaged, it would be removed to stop the hemorrhaging as this organ is soft and contains many blood vessels; if damaged significantly, the spleen cannot be repaired and must be removed. According to Mortenson, bullet damage to the liver and intestines, if not catastrophic, "can be patched up."[12]

In trauma, there is a so-called golden hour, the first sixty minutes in which the patient has an increased chance of survival if they receive definitive medical care. Mortenson believes there is every likelihood, given the wounds described, that Lewis could have been saved by a modern surgeon had he received prompt care. Mortenson commented, "A trauma surgeon can usually save a life, especially with a penetrating injury like this."[13]

Carrison, too, believes that Lewis's reported survival time of at least a couple of hours is totally within reason. "If he wasn't struck in the aorta or vena cava, or the pulmonary arteries or veins, etc. he may well have survived for some time. This would include a kidney wound as long as it didn't sever the renal artery."[14]

In order to further confirm that the scenario of Lewis surviving for two hours is not only possible but reasonable as well, I presented this case in detail to a fifth qualified source, Anthony Leo, M.D., a board-certified general/vascular/thoracic surgeon in Iowa who has had significant experience in vascular and trauma surgery. Leo was a clinical instructor of Advanced Trauma Life Support for many years. He said he agreed with the previous four opinions in every "jot and tittle." Leo stated,

> Regardless of the specific bullet trajectory, any path that did not injure either the heart, aorta, or vena cava could certainly be expected to produce wounds that would be survivable to a period of two hours. There are multiple trajectories of the described fatal wound that would not have been immediately fatal as proposed by Dr. Chuinard. This is due to the low-velocity projectile and the bullet missing any major vessels.[15]

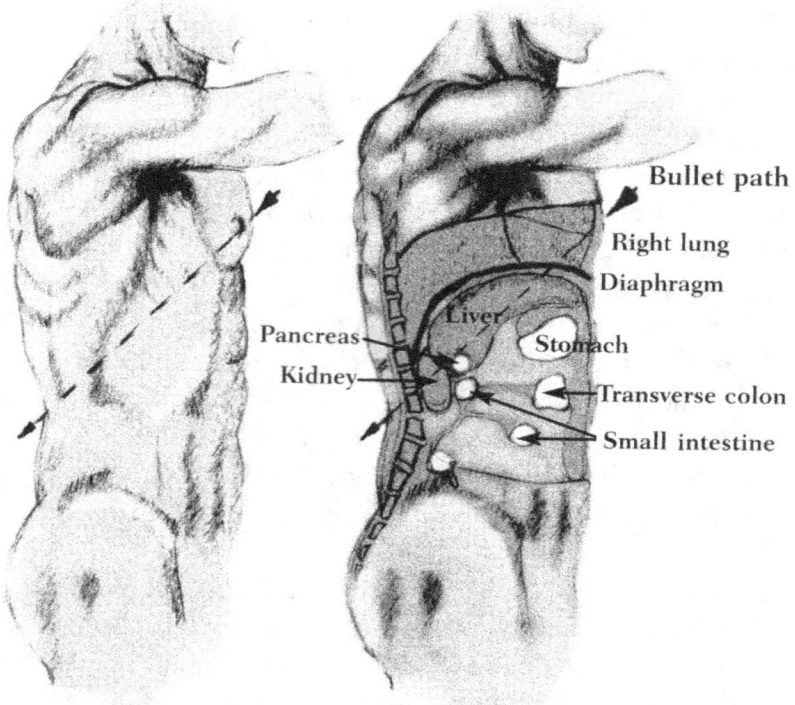

Figure 2. *Lateral Views of Possible Bullet Path through Meriwether Lewis (artwork by David J. Peck)*

Some have noted that Meriwether Lewis was intimately acquainted with his own firearms and was an expert shot. Given his expertise with weapons, how could he have bungled his suicide attempt so badly? The logical and simple answer to this question is that anyone suffering from severe illness, either physical or mental (or, in the case of Lewis, both of these) who is also in a state of alcohol intoxication would not be expected to exhibit efficiency in any motor skill. Lewis could not have walked in a straight line and would not have possessed the more complex motor skills required to shoot a black powder pistol aimed at himself.

A gunshot wound to Lewis's head or scalp was reported by several different sources.[16] Considering that two of these sources were newspaper stories, their veracity is highly questionable. However, Alexander Wilson's letter of May 18, 1810, which was his report on his interview with Pricilla Grinder, gives a more credible description of Lewis's wounds. Wilson notes that Grinder reported Lewis suffered a head wound that she described as follows: "a piece of the forehead was blown off, and had exposed the brains, without having bled much."[17] Given that there was a time lag between the time of the injury and Grinder's observation, I would suggest that such a wound, after tearing off a significant amount of overlying scalp, would have been bleeding profusely. I would also question Grinder's anatomical knowledge and her report of the brains being exposed. However, regardless of the accuracy of her report, such a wound would not necessarily have caused instant death. A tangential wound to the scalp and skull could have resulted in the described wound. I find it more likely that the "brains" that Grinder reported seeing was scalp tissue that was damaged by the superficial bullet wound. But even if Grinder did see some brain tissue, this does not preclude Lewis having shot himself in the torso, either before or after he suffered the head wound.

Any such wound, if it did not penetrate the brain, would cause significant bleeding of the wounded scalp and a possible concussion but would not necessarily cause brain damage resulting in instant death. This is entirely consistent with suicides, as noted by Wagner. The victim often has a last-second reaction and slightly moves the pistol that they are holding near their head, resulting in a superficial head wound.

Carrison reported,

I once had a patient in the E.R. shot in mid-forehead and the bullet went under the scalp and exited the scalp in the occipital [back of the skull] region. Art Linkletter used to say, "Kids say the darndest things," and in my lectures to forensic pathologists I say, "Bullets do the darndest things!" A low-velocity bullet grazing the head may have no consequences other than causing a minor wound in the skin/scalp.[18]

The question continues to be, What would a forensic pathological exam reveal about the reported wounds? The answer, of course, is complicated by the fact that the body of Lewis has been buried for two

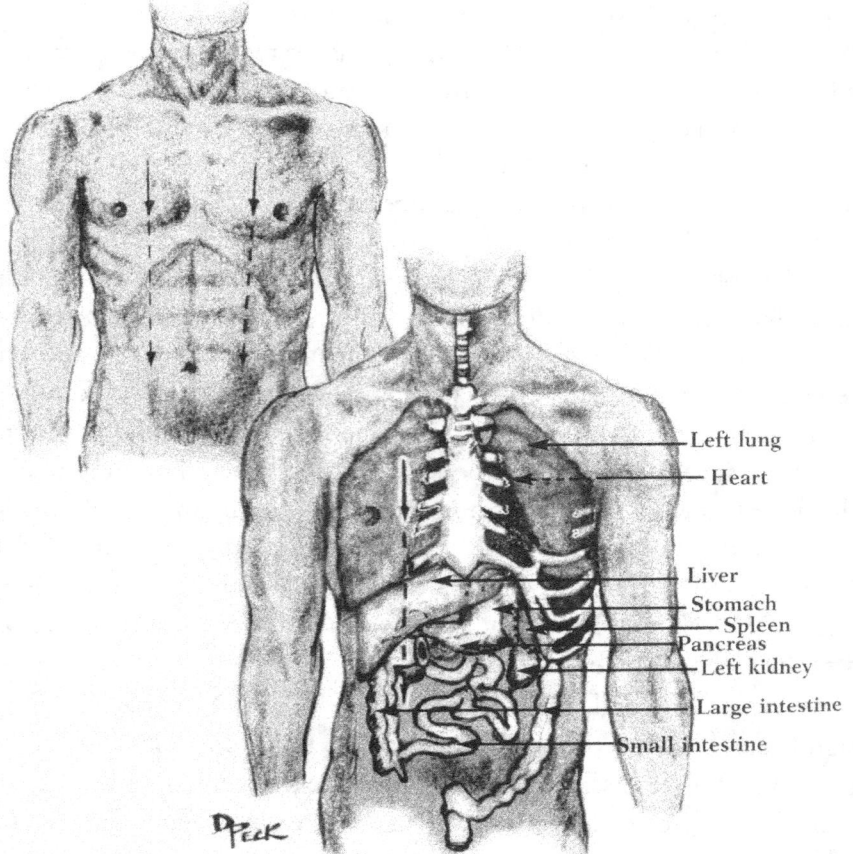

Figure 3. *Frontal View of Possible Bullet Paths through Meriwether Lewis (artwork by David J. Peck)*

hundred-plus years. The best material to study in any forensic examination is generally either bone or skin. Since this chapter deals specifically with gunshots, what could be found on Lewis's bone or skin remains that would add evidence to either the murder or the suicide scenarios?

The presence of any "stippling" or "tattooing" of the skin would indicate that the shot fired was at close range and thus was a potentially self-inflicted wound. This effect is produced from the burning powder that is blown out of the barrel during the ignition of the powder charge. In a self-inflicted wound, the muzzle has to be positioned somewhere between the length of the victim's arm and in direct contact with the body. The firing would produce stippling or tattooing on the victim's skin. If the muzzle were held directly against the body, the entrance wound would be similar to Gilbert Russell's report of Lewis's body: the "edges of the entrance wound are seared by the hot gases of combustion and blackened by the soot of the gunpowder. This black soot is *embedded* in the seared skin and cannot be completely removed either by washing or by vigorous scrubbing of the wound."[19]

In addressing the possibility that Lewis suffered a head wound, Wagner stated, "If the gun was held close, regardless of whether he held it or someone else did, there would likely still be powder burns and lead wiping on the skull itself, regardless of the presence of any tissue. Now if there is tissue on the skull it will be present there but that might require scanning electron microscopy or some more specific means of analysis."[20]

The microscopic arrangement of soot around an entrance wound can tell a pathologist a great deal about the gunshot. If the weapon's discharge was in direct contact with the body, the pattern of tattooing is dense and concentrated. If Lewis was holding the weapon when it was fired but it was not in direct contact with his body, the tattooing effect would vary depending on the distance of the muzzle from his body. The presence of tattooing does not automatically indicate suicide, just that the gun's discharge occurred in close proximity to the surface of Lewis's body. Someone other than Lewis could have fired the shot at close range, and this still would have produced stippling.[21]

Soot is arranged irregularly around an "angled-contact" shot when one edge of the barrel is in contact with the skin and the other edge allows for soot or powder to escape the barrel. Soot residue can also produce a fan pattern on the skin, quite different in nature and implication from other wounds. Without going into more detail regarding the intricacies of forensic pathology, a detailed microscopic exam of a body may reveal a great deal about a person's death. As Wagner reminded me in our conversation, "The dead have a story to tell."[22]

Chuinard's opinion that Lewis did not commit suicide based on the reported two hours Lewis survived after being shot, according to all available medical knowledge, is not supported by the opinions of modern-day trauma surgeons, an experienced trauma-level emergency room doctor, or forensic pathologists. Chuinard's anti-suicide theory is not supported by the opinions of Drs. Wagner, Francisco, Mortensen, Leo, and Carrison. These are not different opinions on a medical condition that might have multiple legitimate explanations. If a patient is diagnosed with a strep throat, multiple appropriate antibiotics are available to eradicate the infection and physicians may argue about the most appropriate antibiotic. But Lewis's wounds and their survivability, and whether they might have been self-inflicted, are not that type of medical scenario. If one physician's opinion states that Lewis could not have survived the reported suicide wounds and other expert physicians state that he could have, both opinions cannot be correct. Those who side with Chuinard's opinion are in disagreement with the experienced professionals we consulted who are very well acquainted with these types of injuries, both their treatment as well as how they kill their victim.

If our five medical experts are correct, the chief argument that many murder theorists cite against the suicide theory is false and thus is off the table. Lewis's survival of his wounds for a couple of hours cannot be legitimately used as proof that he was murdered.

We have now concluded our review of most of the medically based subjects surrounding Lewis's death and some of the theories that have been proposed to explain his death. The following three chapters cover the psychological issues involved in Lewis's life. This material is not easy, but these chapters offer a new set of ideas to consider in evaluating what happened to Meriwether Lewis in the final years of his life.

Chapter 10
Understanding Mental Health and Meriwether Lewis

Mental health affects every aspect of your life. It's not just this neat little issue you can put into a box.
—Shannon Purser, actress and mental health advocate

*I*n our study of the life and death of Meriwether Lewis, my (Marti's) chief contribution is the analysis of his personality. In chapter 2, we provided a general chronological overview of the life of Lewis and described some of the major events he experienced at every stage of his development. But, we offered little commentary on the meaning or significance of these events in shaping his personality.

Many authors have published their interpretations of Lewis's character and personality. Some have suggested that Lewis suffered from a mental illness, such as bipolar disorder/manic depression (Stephen Ambrose in *Undaunted Courage*), Asperger's syndrome/autism spectrum disorder (Stephenie Ambrose-Tubbs in *Why Sacagawea Deserves the Day Off and Other Lessons from the Lewis and Clark Trail*), posttraumatic stress disorder (PTSD; David Nicandri in *River of Promise*), and depression/anxiety/"hypochondriasis" (Thomas Jefferson). Howard Kushner, a historian of medicine and neuroscience, has some familiarity with psychoanalytic theory and has offered a psychologically minded description of Lewis in his book *American Suicide*. He cites depression and alcohol abuse, as well as emotional conflicts related to unresolved grief over the deaths of his father and stepfather, as contributing factors in Lewis's death.[1]

All of these authors contribute unique perspectives from various disciplines (e.g., American history, history of science, and literature), but to our knowledge the only in-depth view ever presented of Lewis's psychological makeup by a licensed mental health professional is that of Kay Redfield Jamison, a psychologist who expresses her view that Lewis committed suicide in a chapter in her book *Night Falls Fast: Understanding Suicide.* In a courageous sharing of her own life-long struggle with bipolar disorder (manic-depressive illness), she offers her opinion that Lewis suffered exclusively from depression and *not* from the frequently cited condition of bipolar disorder.

To their credit, these authors have made insightful observations in their writings about the personality of Meriwether Lewis. Although the views on Lewis's mental life offered by these non-mental health professionals are valuable explorations of Lewis's personality, some of these perspectives have not provided much understanding about *how* his behaviors fit together to form his personality and how they would be interpreted and understood if a modern-day professional diagnosis were employed to more precisely capture the state of his mental health. Given that some Lewis scholars have speculated that he suffered from mental illness, addressing the professional diagnostic process seems fundamental to achieving our goal of providing a psychological profile of Lewis.

In addition to my training as a clinical psychologist, I completed eight years of postdoctoral training in adult psychoanalysis. In *psychoanalytic psychotherapy*, the patient meets with their therapist once or twice per week. *Psychoanalysis* is a relatively more intensive version of psychoanalytic psychotherapy. The patient/analysand meets with their psychoanalyst three to five times/week for several years. My extensive training (which included coursework as well as my own psychoanalysis) allowed me to use this process to help my patients explore their personality in greater depth with the goal of gaining insights that would, I hoped, help them to achieve their fullest potential and deal more effectively with the realities of their everyday life.

All forms of psychotherapy (which typically take place at a frequency of at least once per week) consider how thoughts, feelings, and behaviors interact on a conscious level. What differentiates psychoanalytic therapy and psychoanalysis from other forms of treatment is that psychoanalytic methods place an emphasis on *unconscious* thoughts, feelings, and behaviors that we are not even aware of that can—and do—influence and motivate us. Psychoanalysts, who spend years of immersion in this form of in-depth exploration, are in a unique position to understand the complexities of the mind and how the mind affects behavior. Moreover, this training and experience make it possible to look at the reported behavior and statements of an individual and, much like a trained eye can determine how the surface currents of a river reveal its underlying structure, determine how this may reflect their underlying personality structure. This leads to a coherent holographic (3-D) picture of a person that can be viewed from all sides.

As clinical psychologists, Dr. Jamison and I operate under a professional code of ethics that does not permit us to diagnose the presence of any psychological or mental health condition without having personally met an individual and formally assessed them, and it is not my intention to do so now with Lewis, someone whom I never met and who died over two hundred years ago. However, there is a provision that endorses what I intend to do here in that our ethics code states, "When, despite reasonable efforts, such an examination is not practical, psychologists document the efforts they made and the result of these efforts, clarify the probable impact of their limited information on the reliability and validity of their opinions, and appropriately limit the nature and extent of their conclusions or recommendations."[2]

I provide in this chapter a very basic understanding of how current-day psychologists might conceptualize Lewis's personality dynamics from a comprehensive psychoanalytic perspective. Considering his life experiences, how he described himself through his writings, how others who knew him described him, and what we know about the way he lived his life, I apply a contemporary psychological perspective to the entirety of his life and offer some impressions that I think provide the best fit for describing him psychologically and emotionally. I do so with the caveat that there are limitations to how reliable or valid these ideas can be, given the impossibility of assessing Lewis today. Some may agree or disagree with my conceptualization, but I have given careful thought and consideration to this process and have brought my background and training to bear on my conclusions.

A Brief History of Our Understanding of Mental Illness

Lewis lived his life during an era of great change in the diagnosis and treatment of mental illness. Ancient theories about what caused mental illness included the influence of evil spirits as well as an imbalance of four bodily humors.[3] These eventually gave way to more "enlightened" explanations of physical and mental illness. In the late 1700s, the renowned French physician/neurologist Philippe Pinel (1745–1826) became an early advocate for the humane treatment of the mentally ill and insisted that people suffering from mental disorders be released from the chains that many of them had worn for thirty to forty years. Pinel's chief contribution to the treatment of mental illness came from his belief that excessive exposure to social and psychological stresses, as well as heredity and physiological damage, all played roles in the development of mental disorders. He encouraged an approach to treatment that included friendly, personal contact with patients and a discussion of their difficulties coupled with a practical program of activity.[4]

During Lewis's time, Dr. Benjamin Rush, deemed by many the father of American psychiatry, applied his belief in the inflammation of the circulatory system as the source of many diseases to explain the origin of mental illness. Rush's novel treatment using his "tranquility chair" was meant to decrease the flow of blood to the brain, thereby decreasing any inflammation there. Although this treatment was destined to fail from the start, his Enlightenment-based belief that mentally ill patients should be treated like any other physically ill patients heralded improved psychiatric treatment in the early United States.

The increased understanding of mental illness by the medical community in the nineteenth century led to identification of those who suffered from various mental problems being labeled on U.S. Census forms as either "insane" or "idiotic." The term "feeble-minded" was added in the early twentieth century to account for mentally ill people who caused social problems within their communities.[5] What all these early simplistic systems failed to recognize was the myriad of behaviors and physiological problems that result in a broad spectrum of mental illnesses.

More effective psychiatric treatment methods slowly gained favor in the United States during the nineteenth century, but the academic understanding of mental illness had little insight into the extent of mental pathologies. Dramatic progress was made in the field of neurology, however, with giants such as Jean-Martin Charcot (1825–93) in Paris contributing discoveries in pathology and neurology. Charcot is renowned for his serious investigation of hysterical symptoms—the perplexing variety of physical complaints such as numbness of a body part (e.g., an arm or a leg) without any discernible physical cause—and the use of hypnotism in the treatment of hysteria.

A quantum leap forward in the understanding of both the human personality and the treatment of mental illness came through the work of the Austrian physician Sigmund Freud. Freud studied under Charcot in Paris in 1885–86. During that time, he attended Charcot's lectures in which Charcot demonstrated hypnosis on hysterical (i.e., overly dramatic or melodramatic in character) patients. In the 1890s, Freud, who was trained as a neurologist, started to develop his groundbreaking work on mental illness.

Freud revolutionized the field of psychology/psychiatry with his theories on mental life and the influence of unconscious processes operating within human beings. Freud's theories on the workings of our minds, and his treatment method called psychoanalysis, were referred to in his day as "the talking cure." As odd as it may seem to us today, the practice of just sitting with and listening to and talking with a patient had never actually been tried before in just the way Freud suggested. His work changed the concept of mental illness by including an expanded array of conditions and terms for these conditions that went beyond a simplistic understanding of people as either sane or insane. Previously, such as during the era of Lewis, the only patients identified with mental illness were those who were obviously psychotic (out of touch with reality) or who had severe problems with their ability to think coherently.

Many different schools and techniques of psychotherapy exist today and form the majority of psychological treatments practiced by mental health professionals. These include cognitive behavioral therapy (CBT), dialectical behavioral therapy (DBT), and eye movement desensitization and reprocessing (EMDR). These methods have all evolved from the psychoanalytic orientation that originated with Freud.

Some of Freud's theories and practices have been retained and others abandoned in the light of evolving neurobiological research and our increased understanding of how neurotransmitters work within the brain to produce healthy functioning of the body and the mind. In addition to talk therapy, modern-day psychoanalysts may recommend the use of medications that target various deficiencies of the brain's neurotransmitters.

A Modern View of Personality

Because I evaluate some of the behaviors of Meriwether Lewis, the reader must have a working knowledge of how I will accomplish that task. Without some framework in which to place my observations, the reader will not understand the process, and this and the next chapter may sink into the abyss of "psychobabble." The psychological concepts and terms presented in this section involve some abstractions. Unlike in physical medicine, where lab results and X-rays can be physically observed, a challenge in understanding mental health is that emotions and thoughts are not things that can be seen, and therefore they may be somewhat difficult to grasp. To apply the knowledge gained in this section, it is important to understand some of these concepts. These include the idea that there are broad levels of personality organization as well as several personality types and that different defenses are used against emotions by different types of personalities. The final concept I will present is that people experience both internal and interpersonal emotional conflicts.

The issues related to the term "personality" have far more meaning and significance to mental health professionals than they have to the general public. We have all heard of people with outgoing or extraverted personalities as well as people with the opposite condition, introverted types. Other personality characteristics of people have been given common labels such as bullying, understanding, and having good intuition. There is a current cultural phenomenon of people with rather remarkable self-absorption becoming famous for no particular individual merit or accomplishment and being followed on social media just because they are famous. This phenomenon has allowed the technical term "narcissistic" to make its way into the lexicon of the general public.

In some ways, the determination of personality type is facilitated by the simple identification of various behaviors. If a person treats others with little or no consideration for their feelings and does not care if the feelings of others are injured in their interactions, then these personalities may be identified as having narcissistic patterns. If these behaviors are consistent and severe, the person is said to have a narcissistic personality disorder. Personality-disordered people exhibit deeply engrained patterns of impaired functioning that affect the quality of their own lives as well as that of people with whom they interact. These types of personalities, although only formally described in modern times, were without question also present during the days of Meriwether Lewis.

Everyone in the world has a personality style, and everyone could be placed into one of three groups that describe how their brain processes reality and the way they interact with the world around them. The three major categories, or levels of personality organization, are (1) psychotic, (2) borderline, and (3) neurotic to healthy.

Psychotic individuals are not in touch with reality. These individuals may display various forms of thinking that do not reflect reality. Some believe that they are receiving special personal messages through a television broadcast, while others may believe that the CIA is monitoring their thoughts. Some line their windows with aluminum foil in their efforts to keep UFO-based aliens from reading their minds. During David's first two years of medical school, I worked at a residential treatment facility for individuals who had been diagnosed with chronic and severe psychotic disorders such as schizophrenia. I conducted individual therapy sessions and co-led therapy groups of eight to ten members with this population of psychotic patients twice a day for two years. I had the opportunity to observe very closely the symptoms manifested in these individuals and to assess their mental functioning. Patients who are psychotic can benefit greatly from modern medications, which may allow them to perceive reality more clearly. One phenomenon I observed over and over was how relatively normal and in touch with reality they behaved when they were taking their antipsychotic medication—and how quickly their psychotic symptoms returned (e.g., hearing voices, having delusions) when they stopped taking it. Talk therapy with these patients can be challenging, but fortunately strides have been made in this regard in the decades since I worked with people with psychosis.[6]

Individuals who operate at a borderline level of functioning, as the name implies, fall between the neurotic and psychotic levels of classification. Borderline personalities generally greatly fear being abandoned or rejected. They require relatively more consistent and stable personal life circumstances than someone considered neurotic as a severe emotional trauma in their lives would be more likely to have a more profound and destabilizing effect on them than it would on a neurotically organized individual.

People who operate at a neurotic level in their personality functioning are in touch with reality. If it is Monday and they live in California, they will be aware of these facts. Conversations with neurotics are usually pleasant and informative. But due to some of their personal beliefs about themselves and others, and their resulting behaviors, neurotics may experience problems in their lives. Some neurotics may experience periodic anxiety or depression in response to common but negative life circumstances. Some neurotics may treat others with disdain and contempt; they have little concern about how their behaviors affect other people. Some neurotics may go through life with seeming ease and accomplish great things. The degree of impairment in the functioning of a neurotic (or psychotic) individual can range from mild to moderate to severe. As human beings, we all may function at different levels, and sometimes under great emotional stress we may fluctuate between levels. This is the human condition.

Some confusion regarding psychological terminology has appeared within the Lewis and Clark literature. For example, Richard Dillon states, in his biography of Lewis and in defense of his position that Lewis was murdered, "If there is such a person as the anti-suicide type, it was Meriwether Lewis. By temperament, he was a fighter, not a quitter. . . . Sensitive he was; neurotic he was not."[7] As I will explain later, defining the term "neurotic" as mental health professionals define it, I think Lewis could definitely be described as operating at a neurotic level of personality organization.

Modern-Day Assessment and Diagnosis of Mental Illness

Mental illness diagnosis today is based on the presence of certain behaviors and characteristic ways of processing reality. In the 1890s, mental and physical illnesses were all classified together in 1893 with the publication of the manual titled *The International Classification of Diseases* (ICD). By the time Freud died in 1939, this manual had undergone several revisions as more and more diseases were recognized over the years.

By the early 1950s, mental health professionals felt the need for a classification system specifically for mental illness diagnoses. In 1952, the American Psychiatric Association published the first edition of the *Diagnostic and Statistical Manual of Mental Disorders* (DSM), which described about sixty disorders based on abnormal psychology and had a psychoanalytic theoretical orientation. The DSM is now in its fifth edition (2013) and contains 265 diagnoses of mental disorders. It is considered the authoritative diagnostic guide by mental health professionals in the United States today. Mental health descriptions in the twenty-first century have progressed far beyond the three categories—insane, idiot, and feeble-minded—of over a century ago. In the DSM-5, diagnoses are listed in a total of nineteen categories (e.g., neurodevelopmental disorders, schizophrenic, autism spectrum, other psychotic disorders, bipolar and related disorders, depressive disorders, anxiety disorders), and for any particular diagnosis to be considered accurate, specific criteria must be met for the presence of certain symptoms that correspond to that diagnosis.

It is very important to be able to identify the particular symptoms corresponding to particular diseases as well as to consider the complexity of the personality of the person with the symptoms. Originally, the DSM was created with this concept in mind because its theoretical foundation was embedded in the psychoanalytic tradition. However, over the years between 1952 and its most current edition, there has been a movement away from its psychoanalytic foundation toward a relatively more symptom-focused description of mental illness.

By 2006, the psychoanalytic/psychodynamic community (i.e., those who emphasize unconscious processes in their treatment/therapy with patients) became concerned that the prevailing DSM had lost the complexity of the person behind the symptoms. They remedied their concern by publishing their own manual, the *Psychodynamic Diagnostic Manual* (PDM), now in its second edition (2017). This manual addresses both the symptoms of various mental illnesses as well as the personality of the person underneath their symptoms. In other words, the PDM-2 "highlights the importance of considering who one is—rather than what one has."[8] In chapter 12, I provide more detailed information about the PDM-2 as it provides the framework I use to create my psychological profile of Lewis.

There are similarities between the DSM and PDM. The DSM lists symptoms and criteria that need to be met for a specific diagnosis to be made, while the PDM looks, in addition, beneath the surface of the symptoms. The PDM considers factors contributing to the presence of the symptoms, taking into account the complexity of the mental life of the person exhibiting the symptoms. For our purposes, it is relevant in addressing a possible diagnosis of Lewis as having major depressive disorder. In the DSM-5, for a diagnosis to be made of major depressive disorder, "Five (or more) of the following symptoms have been present during the same two-week period and represent a change from previous functioning; at least one of the symptoms is either (1) depressed mood or (2) loss of interest or pleasure."[9] A total of nine criteria are then listed to choose from, including fatigue or loss of energy and insomnia or hypersomnia (difficulty in the ability to fall asleep or stay asleep vs. sleeping excessively) occurring nearly every day.[10] I explain how the PDM-2 makes diagnoses in ways that are similar to and different from the DSM-5 in chapter 12.

In addition to the dimension of levels of personality organization (i.e., psychotic, borderline, and neurotic), a dimension of types of character organization also exists. Noted psychologist/psychoanalyst Nancy McWilliams, co-editor of the PDM-2 and author of two definitive textbooks on personality structure and diagnosis, identifies these types as psychopathic (antisocial), narcissistic, schizoid, paranoid, depressive and manic, masochistic (self-defeating), obsessive and compulsive, hysterical histrionic, and dissociative.[11] She describes how the dimensions of levels of personality organization interact with the types of character organization. For example, a depressive character type (or any other type) can be organized at a psychotic, borderline, or neurotic level (e.g., a depressive-psychotic vs. a depressive-borderline vs. a depressive-neurotic). What defines the level for any specific character type depends on the defenses the person uses to cope with their thoughts, feelings, and beliefs.

The concept of defenses is very important to understand when considering Lewis's psychological functioning. Simply explained, defenses represent ways Lewis adapted to the circumstances he encountered in his life. Although sometimes viewed as maladaptive or pathological, defenses are actually the processes people learn to use early in their lives as the best solution they could find at the time to cope with what they perceived to be dangerous or threatening situations. What is the purpose of a defense? According to McWilliams, "The person using a defense is generally trying unconsciously to accomplish one or both of the following: (1) the avoidance or management of some powerful, threatening feeling, usually anxiety but sometimes overwhelming grief, shame, envy, and other disorganizing emotional experiences; and (2) the maintenance of self-esteem."[12] This concept of defenses is critical to understanding Lewis's behavior during his life and is explained further in chapter 12.

As mentioned earlier in this chapter, what distinguishes psychoanalysis and psychoanalytic psychotherapy from alternative methods of treatment is that psychoanalysts believe that thoughts, feelings, and behaviors all interact with one another and exist below our level of awareness but nevertheless influence our reactions. In fact, these thoughts and emotions may influence behavior more profoundly precisely because the person is unaware of their influence. One can see the results of these subconscious influences on many occasions in Lewis's life.

During Lewis's lifetime, young men in the South were trained to respond to personal insults by being assertive and defending their honor. During his court-martial, Lewis noted that his life was not worth living if his honor was lost. This attitude did not originate in his interaction with Lieutenant Elliott in 1795. These attitudes were so well incorporated into the very fabric of Lewis's personality since his early childhood that by the time of the perceived insult from Elliott, Lewis's subconscious reaction was automatic and reflexive, producing both tears and some type of strong emotional reaction that led Elliott to file his charges. These feelings came on so abruptly and strongly for Lewis that he was unable to control them.

We see this type of response fairly frequently during the expedition. Lewis inflicted explosive verbal and physical assaults on several Native American men who mocked him for eating dogs, took (stole) an oar mount out of a fire Lewis had set to destroy everything he did not want to fall into the hands of the local tribes, stole his dog Seaman, and stole a horse and some equine-related gear. These feelings are also evident in Lewis's leaving the Jefferson peace medal around the neck of a dead Blackfeet man. I share the view of my colleague Calvin Colarusso, M.D., a psychiatrist and psychoanalyst who has written numerous books on child, adolescent, and adult development, that the basic foundations of our lifelong development are established and built within the first few years of our lives.[13] All of Lewis's strong emotional reactions during these incidents arose from his deeply ingrained belief that he had developed in childhood based on his Virginia gentry upbringing. This cultural indoctrination, based on a plantation owner/slave master mentality, most likely fostered the perception of himself as superior to others. In addition, Lewis's army career as an officer and then a high-ranking government official in Jefferson's inner circle greatly reinforced his view of himself as more powerful and important than others. It is understandable that, given such an inflated sense of his own importance, Lewis could not tolerate any perceived insults from anyone.

I disagree with Nicandri in his assessment of these behaviors as evidence that Lewis suffered from posttraumatic stress disorder. Nicandri states that

> Lewis had at least two traumatic experiences, defined diagnostically as a real or perceived threat of physical injury or death or similarly horrifying circumstances, during the course of the expedition. The first was when he stared down a grizzly that attacked him near the Great Falls of the Missouri westbound, and the second was the fatal skirmish with the Blackfeet on the return trip.[14]

Nicandri cites these events as possible precipitating factors that led to Lewis's unraveling emotionally during the spring of 1806 and ultimately to his decompensation into depression, drinking, and eventual suicide.

Lewis's well-demonstrated "undaunted courage" was legendary. I do not believe he necessarily experienced the two events Nicandri cites as traumatic. For the ordinary individual, these might have been experienced as such, but for Lewis, who on multiple occasions displayed "ice water in his veins" responses to dangerous situations, his reactions to these threats were those of a man who had mastered his fear with the ultimate in self-confidence. He exhibited (1) calm in his response to Private Windsor's potentially lethal circumstances when the private dangled off a cliff above the Marias River with the very real possibility of falling to his death or serious injury, (2) cold military efficiency in his responses to the Teton Sioux in September 1804, and (3) a cool emotional response after being shot in the rear by Cruzatte in August 1806. In the two events cited by Nicandri, he likewise exhibited mental toughness in the face of physical danger that would qualify him as a U.S. military "special operator" of 1806. People such as Lewis are not affected by circumstances that would leave many of us emotionally frazzled. One may see this same personality in modern days in multiple careers. Emergency doctors frequently deal with bleeding and emotionally distraught people with detached coolness. From the days of his childhood until the days along the Columbia and Missouri Rivers, Lewis's rapid changes in mood were always associated with either perceived slights to his honor or some mildly foolish act on the part of an enlisted man, never with any threat of physical danger to himself.

There is an additional nuance in the behaviors that Lewis displayed toward the Columbia River Indians and the Blackfeet. Lewis felt bad or humiliated on all these occasions, and he dealt with these internal feelings by trying to make the outside source of the insults feel the painful emotions that he felt. He projected his painful feelings onto the source of the insult as he could not tolerate feeling them within himself. Lewis's culture taught that the proper defense against such emotional slights was a physical fight—either with fists or in a legally sanctioned duel. Elliott insulted Lewis. The historical record states that Lewis responded with tears, demanding "satisfaction" from Elliott, which resulted in his court-martial trial. Of course, Lewis was consciously aware of his anger and hurt in these circumstances. However, he was not able to articulate his feelings that the accusations by Elliott were making him feel bad inside, so he defended against them by projecting them out of himself and into Elliott so that Elliott would be the bad guy and not Lewis. Lewis was undoubtedly not sufficiently self-aware to be able to analyze all this. The capacity for such self-analysis was not part of the male gentry in early American culture.

The final important concept in this chapter is the difference between internal and interpersonal emotional conflicts. Internal (intrapsychic) conflict occurs when a person has competing thoughts that conflict with one another. An illustration of this would be the conflict between two ideals within one's conscience. We might think of this as a "should vs. should" conflict. Lewis might have experienced such an intrapsychic conflict in his belief that Jefferson wanted him both to complete his journals as well as to be an effective governor of the Upper Louisiana Territory. When he began to fail at both tasks, this would have created a significant conflict for him and lowered his self-esteem. Given his penchant for wanting to do things perfectly, getting feedback that he was not doing either task well must have been a significant source of emotional pain for Lewis. Such an intrapsychic conflict would understandably result in feelings of depression and the potential desire to self-medicate with alcohol, at least temporarily, to eliminate the painful emotions. All of these circumstances likely damaged his sense of himself as honorable. By this point, we know what type of outcome this scenario produced within the mind of Lewis. But Jefferson and other federal government officials were not weak or helpless Native Americans who could be bullied with physical beatings and threatening tomahawks. Lewis was left to suffer blows to his honor from these powerful governmental officials to which he had no effective, honor-saving response.

Emotional conflicts also occur between individuals in their interactions with one another (interpersonal conflicts). To use an experience in the life of Lewis as an illustration, let us consider the very contentious relationship he had during the last year and a half of his life, while serving as governor of Upper Louisiana Territory, with his assistant Secretary Frederick Bates. The stimulus or emotional trigger that sparked the interpersonal conflict between Lewis and Bates in the ballroom at the Masonic Lodge in June 1809 was Bates getting up and leaving when Lewis sat down at the same table as Bates.

This followed a series of events over the previous year and a half, after Lewis had assumed the governorship of Upper Louisiana Territory, that had left him feeling so frustrated and angry that his assistant had undermined him at every turn that the two men apparently had a conversation before the ball in which they had agreed that they would behave civilly with each other in public despite their diametrically opposed views on many policy matters. Following this conversation, we have only the written description by Bates of what transpired at the ballroom table. If accurate, Bates was sitting at a table when Lewis entered and sat down at the same table. Bates reported that he then rose and moved to another table. This response incensed Lewis, who felt so insulted that he left to find Clark (see chapter 2). According to Bates, Clark came to assist Lewis, and Clark's actions may have narrowly averted a duel between Bates and Lewis.

In his own mind, Lewis considered himself a person of high integrity, responsibility, reliability, and discipline. Lewis likely believed that he was a great guy. In the mind of Bates, however, Lewis was a rigid, incompetent superior who deserved to be removed from his position of authority. He likely viewed Lewis's behavior at the ball as very rude and condescending. Lewis was outraged that his honor was being offended and his reputation impugned by someone who not only was his subordinate but who also did not share Lewis's own view of his greatness and superior social rank. We can observe that Lewis might have experienced an inner conflict. On the one hand, he saw himself as a respectable and respected leader (deserving of being treated as a person of value and as someone who valued all human beings) and, on the other hand, he felt so outraged that he wanted to kill another human being. We might consider that his mental compromise to resolve this conflict was to enlist the aid of his trusted friend William Clark in an attempt to prevent himself from acting on his possible impulse or wish to kill another human being (whose life he presumably respected). We can clearly see here how Bates's action of getting up from the table triggered a very intense emotional reaction in Lewis—this interaction between two people served as a spark that ignited a fire within Lewis, whose sense of himself differed so dramatically from the belief that Bates held of his superior. Hopefully, this example helps to illustrate the idea that what was operating within the mind of each individual (internal) influenced what happened between them (interpersonal).

These definitions and examples of basic psychological terms and concepts provide a foundation for the psychological profile of Lewis I create in chapter 11.

Photo Section

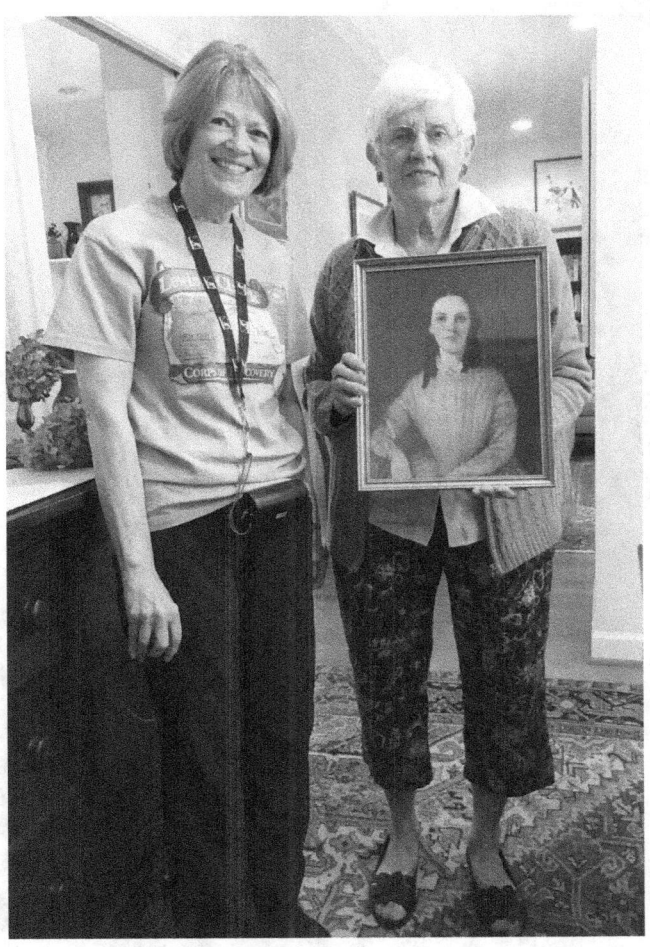

Marti Peck with Jane Lewis Sale Henley, Meriwether Lewis's four-times-great-grandniece, with painting of Jane Lewis, Meriwether's sister and Jane Henley's four-times-great-grandmother.

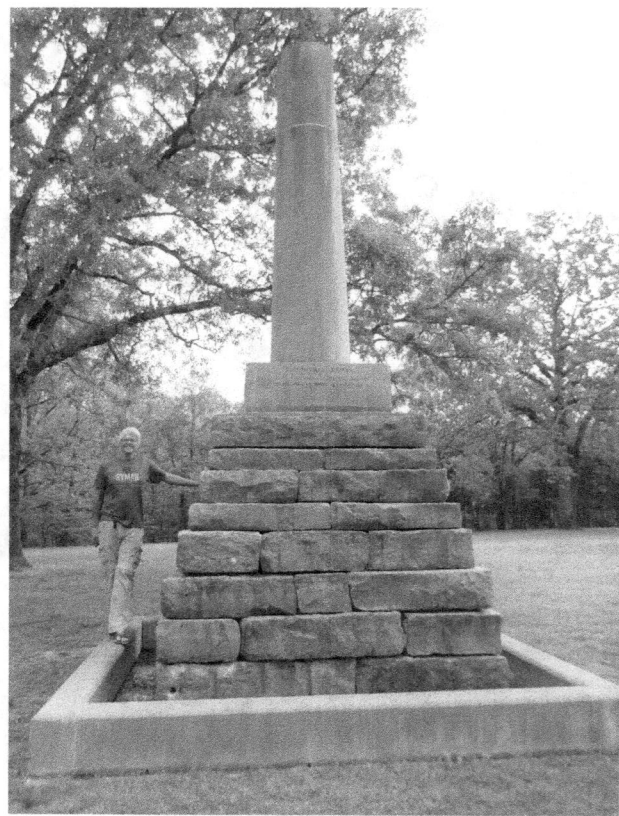

David Peck at the Meriwether Lewis memorial near Hohenwald, Tennessee.

Jane Lewis Henley and David Peck explore the Warner Hall cemetery, resting place of some Lewis ancestors.

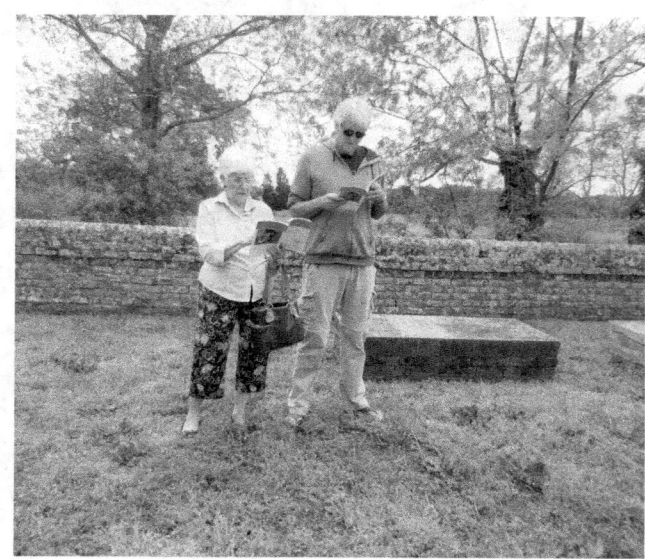

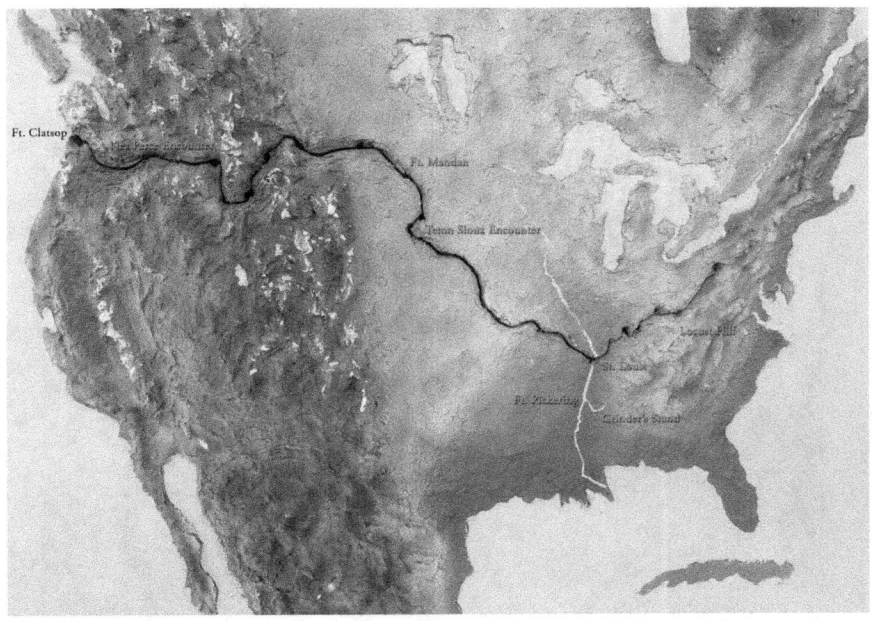

The overall route of the Lewis and Clark Expedition of 1803–1806 beginning in Pittsburgh, Pennsylvania, in the east and extending westward to near present-day Astoria, Oregon.

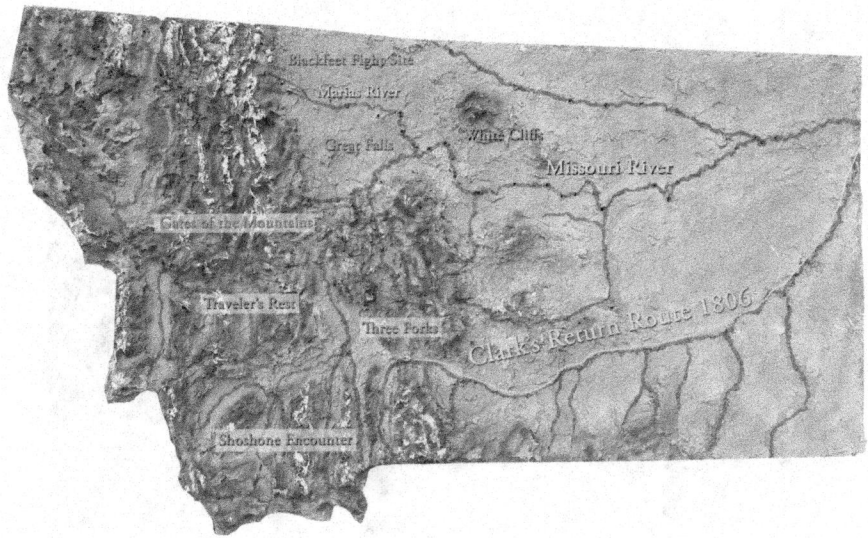

Important sites of the expedition in Montana.

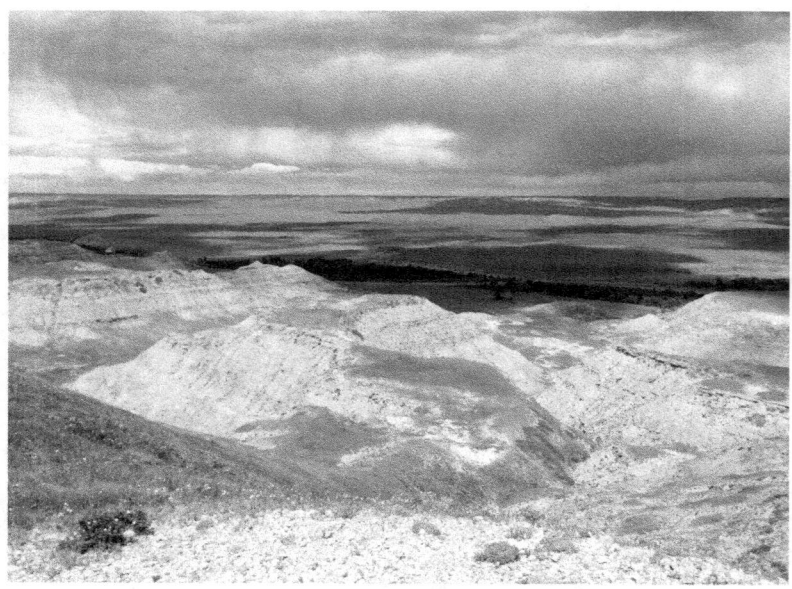

Two Medicne River, site of the deadly encounter with the Blackfeet men. Actual campsite is thought to be near the tree in the middle of the photo, just in front of the trees along the Two Medicine River.

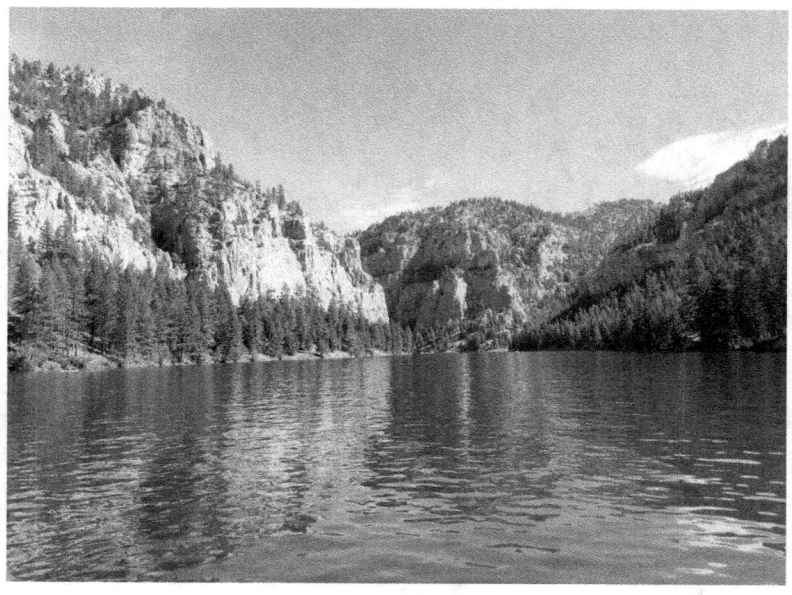

Gates of the Mountains near Helena, Montana, is one of the beautiful areas named by Meriwether Lewis.

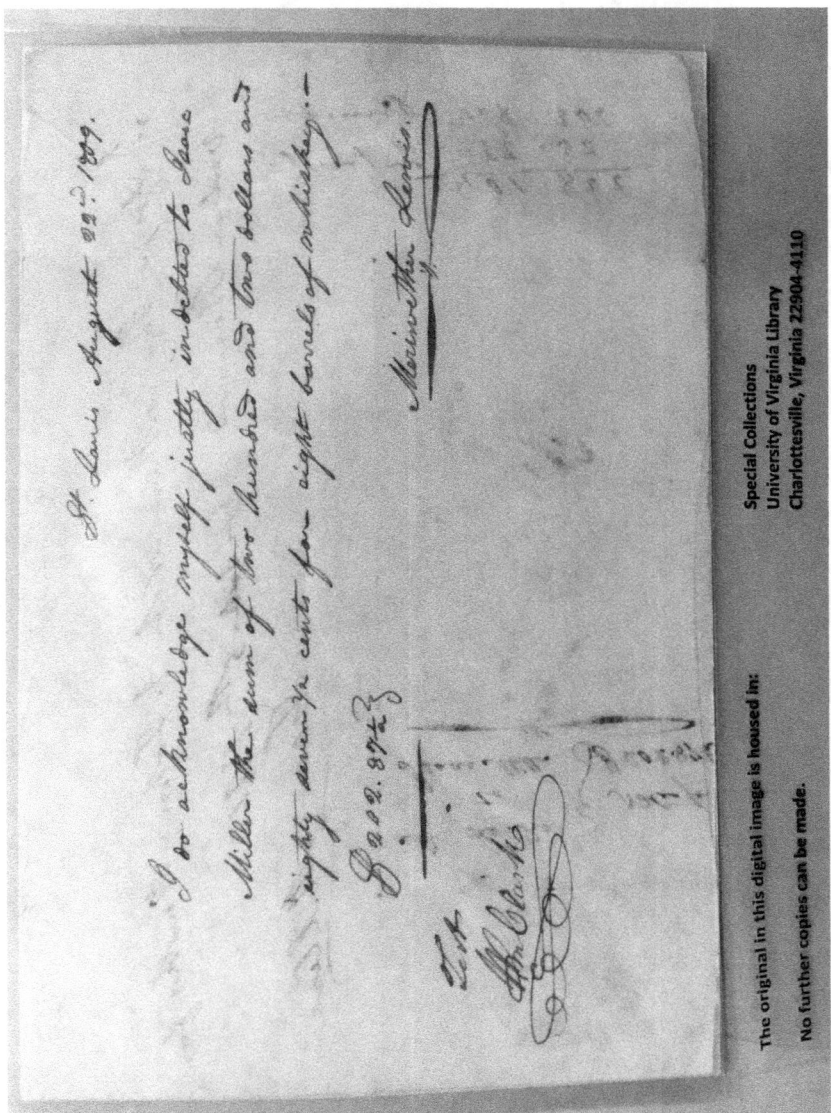

Meriwether Lewis's IOU for purchase of eight barrels of whiskey in 1809.

Chapter 11

A Psychological Interview of Meriwether Lewis

You are not your illness. You have an individual story to tell. You have a name, a history, a personality. Staying yourself is part of the battle.
—*Julian Seifter, M.D., Harvard Medical School*

In my (Marti's) work on this book, perhaps the most important of my efforts is to provide a psychological profile of Meriwether Lewis. In order to create this profile, I conduct a series of three fictitious interviews as a way to bring you into much the same process I would go through in conducting an initial assessment in my office. These imagined interviews are (1) with Lewis a couple of weeks before he travels to Washington from St. Louis to protest the War Department's denial of payment of the vouchers he had submitted, (2) with William Clark (a "collateral" session) one day after my interview with Lewis in order to get the perspective of someone who knew Lewis well, and (3) with Lewis during his stay at Fort Pickering on his way to Washington within two weeks of his death. During my interviews with Lewis, I invite you to sit in as an unseen observer while I "talk" with him about his life. By observing the process I would use as a clinician through these imaginary consultations, I hope an understanding will unfold about how the information he provides—as well as the way and manner in which he provides it—helps me to gain insight into how his mind works and to develop a portrait of his personality. In presenting the material in this manner, I am attempting to give you a sense of how it might be to see him and listen to him through the eyes of a clinician who does this most days of her life.

In reality, there was no such thing as psychotherapy in 1809 as we know it today, and even if it did exist, it would be highly unlikely that a military officer like Lewis would agree to come into a psychologist's office for such an interview. Even in 2021, there is still some stigma attached to military personnel who seek mental health treatment. With this disclaimer, I assume that Lewis self-referred for the initial consultation at the encouragement of his good friend William Clark.

The topics that I would hope to cover in the initial interview include his presenting problems and concerns, what triggered them, and what steps he took to try to solve or cope with the problems, as well as how these problems might be affecting his functioning and handling of everyday tasks, work, health, self-esteem, relationships, legal matters, and finances. I would ask him about symptoms he was experiencing, such as sleep problems, eating difficulties, fatigue, depression, and anxiety. Some of these important issues, if not actually stated in the historical record, are strongly implied.

Other areas of interest would be his current and past history of suicidal and homicidal behavior, his marital status, and his academic and work history. Information about his family of origin; social support system; racial, ethnic, and religious background; his own as well as his family history of medical and mental health conditions; and his alcohol, drug, and medication use would also be important for me to know. Although many of the exact details of Lewis's life are forever unavailable, some of what he would report in his answers to my questions can be reliably inferred from the circumstances of his life, his position in the culture and times in which he lived, and his membership in the Masonic Lodge, as well as through direct quotations of his words in the historical record.

What Lewis tells me and how he says it constitute what is referred to as a mental status exam. For example, I would observe aspects of his speech (was it pressured? hesitant?), his behavior (calm? tense?), and his attitude (cooperative? belligerent?). I would also consider his appearance (was he neatly groomed? disheveled?), his emotional state (did he appear to be depressed? irritable? sad? frustrated? frightened? tearful?). Both the content and process of his thoughts (did he express them clearly or inarticulately?) would be important clues in my analysis. As Lewis relates his story, these are some of the important factors I would observe.

Although these interviews are fictional, you should not assume that Lewis's contribution to them is entirely fabricated and inaccurate. In creating the content of these interviews, I have incorporated reports that Lewis wrote regarding both his experiences and his feelings. I have added words or phrases where necessary to produce a more conversational transcript. Some of Lewis's replies include his own words from the journals and/or reasonable implications of those established events. As noted, I paraphrase some historical material, but I identify direct quotes by placing them inside quotation marks. I have also given the sources of some (but not all) of the information Lewis provides in the interviews.

In reality, the material I have presented in interview #1 would likely unfold over the course of three to four sessions, with elaboration of further detail possible. For the sake of brevity, I have included it all as occurring in one rather dense session. It is also possible that Lewis might not have been as open in disclosing information to me as I have presented in these interviews. I have portrayed a sense of relative openness to ensure that the facts we know about Lewis's life are covered.

Interview #1: With Meriwether Lewis, August 18, 1809 (Lewis's thirty-fifth birthday), St. Louis, Missouri

The procedure I typically follow in conducting an initial interview with a new patient, and what I have done with Lewis, is to ask him to fill out my informed consent form for treatment. This lets him know that everything he talks about with me will be kept confidential and that I will not share any information about him without his written authorization (which might seem ironic to the reader since I share information from his interview here; however, this is the only way to illustrate what an interview is like). I will also assume that he understands, from our going over the form together and my answering any questions he has about it, that there are certain exceptions to confidentiality and that I would be mandated by law to break it if he lets me know that he was a danger to himself or others or if he reported child or elder abuse to me.

Therapist (T): Governor Lewis, please come in.... [After both are seated] Please start wherever you'd like and tell me more about what brings you in today.

Commentary: I'm encouraging him to speak freely and tell his story in any way he would like.

Lewis (L): I am involved in a most distressing situation. I just received a letter from the federal government, the War Department to be exact, that is calling into question not only my abilities as governor of this territory but my honesty as well. In many ways, it is a preposterous situation. My best friend William Clark thought it would be helpful if I came in to talk to you. He is concerned about my state.

After all that I have accomplished in my career, including successfully leading an expedition with my friend Clark from St. Louis to the Pacific Ocean and back, I can hardly tolerate this insult to my honor and reputation! Under President Jefferson's administration, I served as his private secretary in the President's House for about two years before I went on the expedition. After the expedition, President Jefferson arranged with Congress for my appointment here, as governor of this Upper Louisiana Territory, and throughout the entire expedition and my work here in St. Louis, which I took up about a year and a half ago, I have had the unwavering support of the president and his complete confidence in my competence to perform the duties that were assigned to me.

Since this past March, when President Madison came into office, the unwavering confidence placed in me as governor has changed. President Jefferson's administration reimbursed all the financial vouchers I submitted for administrative expenses for over a year since I took up my position here, but now the current administration has begun refusing payment for expenses incurred from projects President Jefferson explicitly gave me orders to carry out! President Jefferson asked me—in fact, *ordered me*—to return Sheheke-shote, the Mandan chief, to his home 1,600 miles up the Missouri River. Clark and I were able to convince the chief of the importance of his visiting Washington on our return trip from the Pacific, and he agreed to return with us to visit Jefferson in 1806. This was not my idea—it was President Jefferson's idea—and he made it a priority for me to return the chief to his home near Fort Mandan.

The first attempt to return the chief failed due to the Arikaras' attacks on the party. Now we are ready once again to attempt to accompany the chief and his family back up the Missouri. This effort has required a good deal of planning and money to accomplish. Secretary Eustis has refused to pay the bills that I signed for, even writing that our group taking the chief home had no "object & destination"![1] Where does Secretary Eustis believe them to be traveling? A letter I received on July 15th from William Simmons, with President Madison's approval, states that my expenditures for outfitting the group of one hundred forty men required to return the chief "has not been honored."[2] Some in the territory are even accusing me of financially benefitting from this attempt. Now that Mr. Madison is president, he and his Secretary of War Eustis have informed me, in a most insulting way, that not only will the vouchers for this trip not be paid but I will be expected to pay these expenses to the Treasury and War Departments out of my own personal finances. "I call my God to witness"[3] that I have never cheated the government out of one penny. So many men to whom I owe money are now coming and asking me—me personally—for payment. Of course, I do not have sufficient cash to cover all these expenses. This means I am going to have to sell seven hundred acres of land I bought here and deplete my bank account in order to cover these debts! These protested bills "have effectively sunk my credit; brought in all my private debts, amounting to about $4,000."[4]

What is more, my assistant, Frederick Bates, has undermined me at every turn since I took over my position a year and a half ago. Prior to my assuming leadership, he served as acting governor until my arrival here in March of 1808. He has insulted my honor, and I believe he slanders me and speaks ill of me to others behind my back. I do not trust the man at all—in fact, I would not be surprised if he is acting in ways to remove me from office. My only recourse is that I am going to have to go back to Washington and attempt to clear my name. If the government doesn't pay for these vouchers, I will be financially ruined. I have reported on all these issues to my trusted friend Clark. It seems that I am at the mercy of the government's intentions.

Commentary—In this fictitious conversation, Lewis has addressed important issues that I would have explicitly asked him about if he had not already addressed them ("When did these problems begin?" or "When did they get worse?") in order to determine the duration of the problem/symptoms. It would be one matter if these were life-long, long-term problems and another if the problems developed recently. Because he is describing a more recent onset, I am forming the impression that he is facing a crisis situation and that my focus needs to be on helping him manage an acute crisis rather than a chronic condition.

T: How very distressing all this is. Your honor and credibility are being questioned, and you are now also having all these financial difficulties . . .

Commentary: I am focusing on his feelings, expressing empathy, and attempting to create an atmosphere in which he will feel safe to continue providing more details of his narrative.

L: I have often tried to talk with Bates and get him to cooperate with me, which is his duty, after all, as I am the governor of this territory and his superior! None of my efforts have worked. Most recently, he and I had a conversation in which we agreed that we disagree about everything and that we would speak to each other only when we had to—about business-related matters—but then he disrespected me again after that understanding.[5]

T: Can you tell me more about that?

L: Well, after our discussion, this past June there was a dinner and ball that was held at the Masonic Lodge here in St. Louis—following the procession to celebrate the Festival of St. John the Baptist. This is a very important event for members of the Masonic Lodge, and I am the leader of the Lodge here. When I entered the ballroom, feeling it important to treat others, particularly Masonic brothers, with respect, I sat down at the same table as Bates, who is also a Mason. He immediately rose and left the table! What an insult! I was so incensed at this impropriety that I sent a servant to get Clark to speak to Bates about his insulting behavior and my desire to confront him then and there. My friend the general was very concerned and wanted to keep us apart at that point because he was probably afraid that I might challenge Bates to either a fight or a duel. Both Clark and I tried on two separate occasions in the days after this incident to approach Bates to see if we could attempt some kind of reconciliation, but he would have none of it. He insisted that it was *his* honor that had been offended and that *he* was the injured party.[6] It is beyond my understanding why my fellow Masonic brother, who is not supposed to act in this manner, is behaving like this.

T: You really felt like you were the wounded party here, from what I am understanding. . . . Have you ever had any other experiences like this during your life?

Commentary: I am still trying to focus on the emotions he is having about this experience in the hopes of establishing a positive therapeutic relationship and helping him to feel safe to open up even further about his concerns. It seems entirely reasonable, given the reports of Clark, that Lewis's emotional state would be one of depression. If so, Lewis's facial expression would probably be very somber, with his eyes cast downward and his whole body slumped forward.

L: [silence] . . . Yes, I . . . yes—but undoubtedly one of the worst—probably *the* worst, was early in my army career when I was an ensign and stationed under General Anthony Wayne in Greenville Ohio. I had just turned twenty-one, and my superior, Lieutenant Joseph Elliott, accused me of bursting in on his dinner party and in a drunken state challenging him to a duel. I did go to his house and ask to speak with him, but how he presented the circumstances was just not true. I indicated that I was seeking "satisfaction" in my encounter with him, but he misinterpreted my use of the word as meaning I wanted to fight him with weapons to get "satisfaction" and resolve a conflict between us in this manner. He brought charges against me for behavior unbecoming an officer, and a court-martial was ordered. The trial went on for several days, and I served as my own defense attorney. I denied his accusations as nothing he was accusing me of was true. I called witnesses who testified as to the absurdity and falseness of these charges, and in the end I was acquitted of all charges with honor. This was a very, very distressing time for me, and all this could have derailed my career in the army.[7]

My honor as a man is the most important thing in my life. "It is very disagreeable to hobble through life with a broken reputation. I conceive the duty of every man to connect intimately [intimately], their life and reputation by all possible ties, to the end, that when the one makes its exit the other may also."[8] As you can see, my entire reputation and character were at stake then. If I don't have my honor and good reputation, what do I have? But I felt vindicated because after that matter was resolved, there turned out to be a silver lining in the cloud. Of course, I could no longer stay and work with Elliott in the same location, so I was reassigned to Lieutenant William Clark's Chosen Rifle Company, where I served under him for about nine months. That's when we really got to know each other. Fortunately, he could see my potential for leadership in my service under him, and I had such high respect for him as my superior. I thought of him immediately when I considered who I wanted to accompany me on the expedition as co-commander, and he has been my very loyal friend ever since. After that, I just kept getting promoted in rank, from ensign to lieutenant to captain.

That court-martial could have easily ruined my reputation and career—I still feel so angry every time I think about it!

T: This sounds like it was a very difficult and painful experience for you, and I can see why this experience for you as governor would bring up similar feelings as that court-martial experience—there certainly seem to be many similarities between them, especially of your honor being questioned. From what I am understanding, you have spent your entire adult life in service to your country, and to have your sense of duty and patriotism doubted like this now must be unbearable for you.

Commentary: I am now developing an even stronger impression of how insulted and outraged Lewis feels whenever his honor or integrity are brought into question.

L: It is absolutely insufferable . . . I can hardly believe this is happening to me now . . .

T: Yes, of course, you feel very angry when you have been insulted. I am wondering if there might be even more experiences you've had when you've felt this way?

Commentary: I am wondering about the pattern of this behavior, how strong the pattern might be, and under what circumstances it might be triggered.

L: Well, what comes to my mind right now when I think about it . . . is once, on the expedition . . . it was on the return trip from the Pacific Ocean when we encountered some Indians who repeatedly stole our supplies. They took tools, blankets, nearly anything that was within their grasp when they found an opportunity. "They were the greatest thieves and scoundrels"[9] I ever met. They even stole my dog, Seaman. . . . That was an outrage so insupportable that I sent three of my best men out after those thieves with orders to shoot them if they did not return my dog. Fortunately for them, they released the dog when they discovered my men descending upon them. That dog is very important to me—he came with me through the entire trip—he is a Newfoundland, a very large dog, and I often took him with me when I went ashore along the Missouri to collect plant specimens and to hunt game for our meals. Although he is a large dog, he is very docile, which impresses everyone, including the many Indians we met along our path.

Another day, around that same period of time, "while at dinner an Indian fellow very impertinently threw a poor half starved puppy nearly into my plate by ways of derision for our eating dogs and laughed very heartily at his own impertinence; I was so provoked at his insolence that I caught the puppy and threw it with great violence at him and struck him in the breast and face, seized my tomahawk and showed him by signs if he repeated his insolence I would tomahawk him, the fellow withdrew apparently much mortified and I continued my repast on dog without further molestation."[10] We did eat dog meat at times during our journey, and this was this Indian's way of making us the target of his rudeness. This was an act from a savage that I could not let go unanswered. After all these thefts by these people and then to be so ill-mannered—it was more than I could endure. Not all of the Indian tribes were like this—some were very kind and helpful to us. The Shoshone and Salish tribes sold us the horses we needed to cross the mountains to get to the Pacific . . . but I had had enough with these particular Indians along the Columbia River who repeatedly stole our property.

Probably the worst case of deceitful behavior by Indians was when . . . also on the return trip . . . Clark and I had split up the party. I headed toward the Great Falls over a shortcut revealed to us by our New Perce guides. Clark took most of the party and headed overland toward the three forks of the Missouri and beyond to the Yellowstone River. Once my party had crossed the mountains via the shortcut, we descended onto the plains near the Great Falls of the Missouri. I took three of my best men and traveled north to the Marias River. I was making a reconnaissance of this river to determine the source of its waters and if they came from the north or the west. This was in late July of 1806. I knew this area was the homeland of the mighty Blackfeet nation as we had heard of their dominance from other tribes we encountered. Many tribes were afraid of them, and our young Nez Perce guides who brought us back over the great mountains warned us about them. During our reconnaissance of the area, coming back along a branch of the Marias River, we unexpectedly came upon a party of about eight Blackfeet Indian men on horseback. Since the Shoshones and Nez Perce had warned us about the danger of this tribe, I believed them to be "a vicious, lawless and rather an abandoned set of wretches."[11]

I tried my best to indicate to the young Blackfeet that we wished to be friendly and accommodating toward them. I gave one of the fellows a peace medal that President Jefferson had provided for us for occasions just like this in order to show our good will toward them and our wish for friendly relations. We ended up camping and smoking tobacco with them overnight at a place called the Two Medicine River. George Drouillard communicated my speech to them with his hand sign language. It is a long story, but suffice it to say, on the morning of the twenty-seventh of July, at daylight, the Indians got up and crowded around the fire while I was asleep. Joseph Field, who was on post, had carelessly laid his gun down behind him near where his brother was sleeping. "One of the indians—the fellow to whom I had given the medal, slipped behind Fields and took his gun and that of his brother unperceived by him. At the same instant two others advanced and seized the guns of Drewyer [Drouillard] and myself."[12] Joseph saw an Indian running off with his gun. Joseph called to his brother Reuben, who chased down the Indian, wrestled his gun away and stabbed the fellow in the chest. He ran about fifteen steps and fell dead.

With our small party being located about one hundred miles from the nearest help, we all had to act quickly and decisively! We engaged the thieves in battle, and I ended up shooting one in the stomach. The fellow I shot fired on me, and I felt the wind from the bullet as it passed my head. The other Blackfeet made a successful escape.

Of course, we had to take leave of that area in great haste after that incident because we knew we would be pursued once other members of the tribe were informed by the young men who escaped. So, we rode with great dispatch out of the area—we rode for nearly twenty-four hours, only taking breaks to rest a bit and give our horses a rest—until we reached the Missouri River and joined up with some of the party in the canoes on the river. It was all quite a potentially fatal situation . . . but those Indians trying to take advantage of us, especially after all of our good faith efforts to show we wished to be on friendly terms, to turn on us like that . . . I was not plagued with doubt regarding my actions against those Indians. Before we rode away from that fight site, we threw some of their bows, sheaths, and arrows and some of their other possessions into the fire, but I left the peace medal around the neck of the dead Indian so that when their fellow tribesmen found them "they might be informed who we were."[13]

Commentary: I am noting at this point there have been several instances in which it appears clear to me that Lewis's anger upon experiencing insult could be explosive to the point of threatening an assault or committing homicide. I also am aware that he is an army officer and that killing people in the course of his duties, particularly given the circumstances of this event, would be considered normal behavior.

T: Can you tell me more about what you have tried to do to deal with all of these stressors you are encountering in your work as governor?

Commentary: I am wondering about his problem-solving abilities, and I also want to learn more about any solutions he may have already applied to solve the problems he is reporting.

L: I just keep trying to do my job every day. These disputes between the settlers here, wanting to push forward and claim more land for themselves, and the Indian tribes whose lands the settlers are trying to claim, are a constant source of tension for me to have to resolve. I have been trying my best to negotiate compromises between them, but sometimes I have been forced to engage military force in order to make sure that situations don't escalate. It has been impossible for me to sit down and prepare the journals of the expedition that Clark and I completed in September of 1806. It has now been three years since the end of the expedition, and I have not completed that very important task. Mr. Jefferson has been such a good friend, mentor, and advocate for me, and he has been asking me repeatedly when am I going to get this done. I feel some reproach from him, and it is my reputation with him that is suffering as a result. I feel so badly about the fact that I have not been able to meet his request. Jefferson tells me that his reputation with world leaders is being harmed by my lack of progress on this book. I feel so overwhelmed, and the pressure of getting the journals done has just added to the many vexations from which I am suffering.

T: You said you were planning to go to Washington. When do you plan to leave for your trip?

L: I am hoping to depart by the end of this month or early September. I am going to have to put my affairs in order so that things run smoothly in my absence. "I shall leave the Territory in the most perfect state of Tranquility which I believe, it has ever experienced."[14] My very close friend Clark, who lives here in St. Louis and is serving as my chief Indian agent, is going to have to help me prepare guarantees for all my creditors who are expecting to be paid.[15] The government is disputing some of Clark's bills as well. It looks like I am going to have to hire a couple of attorneys and authorize them to hold my property as security for debts I owe until I can get these problems settled in Washington.[16] I am going to have to get these vouchers in order and pack all the necessary supplies to take with me on the keelboat down the Mississippi to New Orleans and then on to Washington.

T: Yes, I can see that you will have a lot to do to prepare before you leave and that it all must feel very overwhelming.

L: It is all so intolerable! It is really a troubling situation. I have done nothing but work hard to serve my country my entire adult life, and to be turned against so utterly and completely like this is an outrage. I have no other choice but to return to Washington and defend my record and the financial vouchers I have requested from the government—it is my reputation and honor that are being questioned!

T: Your anger is so understandable under these circumstances . . . you must feel so hurt and betrayed.

L: I can't begin to tell you how vexed I am about all of this . . .

Commentary: At this point in the interview, any competent psychologist would ask a new patient, especially one in an acute crisis situation, questions to assess their risk of attempting suicide or homicide. Lewis has provided information to me thus far that indicates he has a history of difficulty managing his angry feelings, so these issues appear essential for me to know immediately. Since any responses Lewis would have given to my questions about any thoughts, intentions, and/or plans to hurt himself would be purely speculative, I will leave his response blank as to his response about self-harm but will present the questions I would have asked Lewis in this interview.

T: I'm wondering if you have been having any thoughts about hurting yourself now or if you have made any attempts to hurt yourself or have made a plan to hurt yourself?

L: [intentionally left blank]

T: Are you having any thoughts about hurting someone else or made any attempts to hurt someone else, or do you have any plans to hurt someone else?

L: I am not a murderer. My honor has been offended to a terrible degree, but I am a past member of the U.S. Army and I am the leader of our local Masonic Lodge. It is not within my nature to murder anyone. But I have considered a duel to reestablish my honor. There is always a duel available.

Marital Status/Family and Social Support

Commentary: I always want to assess a person's marital status, which provides a lot of information about their personality. Are they married?

Single? Never been married? Married but widowed? Divorced? Each of these states can reveal different experiences and different responses to these experiences.

T: Are you married? Single?

L: I am single—I have never been married.

T: Are you in a romantic relationship now?

L: No.

T: Have you ever been in any romantic relationship, or relationships, that you would consider to be serious ones?

L: Well, not really . . . I've always been so busy with other pursuits. It's hard to have to pursue a wife when you're in the army, which was the case when I was twenty to twenty-six years old. It's not like I haven't seen many handsome women whom I have considered good candidates to become Mrs. Lewis.[17] And, after President Jefferson asked me to become his private secretary in the President's House, I spent two years there with him. It was as if the two of us were like church mice there most of the time.[18] Although he had a lot of dinner parties, and I met a lot of interesting people, there really was very little opportunity for me to meet any ladies there.

Then, after that, I was on the expedition for three years—no chance for any romantic relationship then, except for having sex with some Indian women. Some of the tribes offered Clark and me their women and were quite offended when we refused. But once I returned and was in Philadelphia a couple of years ago, doing some preparation work to publish the journals we kept on our voyage to the Pacific, I really was ready to look for a wife. I socialized there with my good friend Mahlon Dickerson, and I was interested in three or four young ladies while I was there, but nothing ever came out of those relationships.[19] In early November 1807, I was back in Albemarle County with my family, and I wrote a letter to Mahlon about how determined I was at that point to find a wife and get married.[20]

On the trip out to St. Louis, my brother Reuben and I stopped at the home of my good friend Clark's future father-in-law in Fincastle,

Virginia. We arrived there at the end of November; Clark was getting married in January 1808 to Julia, and, of course, I wanted to attend the wedding. I met a girl there who I think would have been the closest prospect for a wife I ever came to, at least on my side. Her name was Letitia, and she was sixteen at the time and the daughter of a very respected military officer. She was one of the most handsome women I had ever laid eyes on, and in our conversation, I expressed to her my wish to call upon her. I do not know if I came on too strong, or what might have happened, but within two days, I got word that she had left town to accompany her father to Richmond. I felt disappointed. She would have been everything I think I would have wanted in a wife—she was beautiful, and she came from a very respected family.[21]

About seven months later, I got word from one of my friends that Letitia had married. It was to a man I had known since boyhood—"he is a good tempered, easy honest fellow . . . both his means and his disposition well fit him for sluming away life with his fair one in the fashionable rounds of a large City. such is the life she has selected and in it's pursuit I wish she may meet all the pleasures of which it is susceptible."[22] He is a fine fellow, and now she gets to live in a more cultural center, like Richmond—I guess that was her desire. I have sometimes wondered whether the thought of living more on the frontier, like St. Louis, is what really disagreed with her, as well as other women, too. I do imagine this contributed to the difficulties I have encountered in finding a wife. Now I just consider myself to be "a musty, fusty, rusty old bachelor."[23]

T: I want to be able to help you as much as I can, and in order to be able to do so, I would like to get more background from you, if I could, at this point. Is that OK with you?

L: Yes, OK. . . . What do you want to know?

T: Well, perhaps we could start at the beginning, and you could tell me where you were born and raised?

L: Well, I was born in Albemarle County, Virginia, near Charlottesville, and I pretty much lived there on my family's plantation until I was twenty and joined the military.

T: Can you tell me about your family?

L: Well, there is my mother, who is essentially running the plantation now and has done so with help since I left home. My father died when I was five. He was a lieutenant in the Virginia militia and then a soldier in the Continental army during the Revolution. I don't remember him very well because I was so young and he was away fighting a lot of the time after I was born, but my mother and relatives tell me that he was a brave patriot and that he had been home on leave in the fall of 1779 and was returning to the front when he tried to cross the Rivanna River on horseback. They told me that the river was swollen because of the autumn rains and that his horse was swept away, but he managed to swim to the other side and got himself to Cloverfields—that is my mother's ancestral home. But he died of pneumonia there within days and is buried there. I have a lot of uncles on both my mother's and father's side of the family who helped to raise me—a lot of them were officers in the military too, so I have had a lot of good role models.

T: I see. . . . Do you have any siblings?

L: Yes, I have a sister three years older than me, Jane. She is married, and she and her husband live in Virginia. Then I have a brother three years younger than me, named Reuben. My mother remarried within about six months after my father died, and she and my stepfather have two children—so I have a half brother, John, who was born when I was eleven, and a half sister, Polly, who was born when I was fourteen. I really love all of them and consider all of them to be my brothers and sisters, pretty equally.

T: Can you tell me more about your relationships with your family members?

Commentary: I am wondering what the quality and nature of these relationships are like. Is he close to them? Estranged? Close to some and estranged from others? How often does he have contact with them? etc.

L: My mother is a pretty strong and resourceful woman—she is the yarb doctor of our county [herbal medicine doctor]. She rides around and tends to people with her "simples" [herbal remedies] when they're sick. She taught me a lot about these when I was growing up, taking me out and teaching me the different plants and what could be used for which ailments—this really came in handy for me when I was on the expedition. It was my responsibility to gather plant and animal specimens during the trip, and I used some that I had brought with me in our medicine box, but I also gathered a lot of new plants that I had never seen before in my life.

T: It sounds as if you really admire your mother . . .

Commentary: I want to verify if my understanding is accurate that he feels a positive emotional attachment with his mother.

L: Yes, I really do. My mother is strong-willed and resourceful—in this manner I guess I take after my mother. I wish I could see my mother and all of my family more often, but I have always visited them as much as I could when I was on leave in the army and before and after the expedition. I write letters to my mother to keep in touch with her, and I keep in touch with all of them by letters as much as I can. I've been so busy here for the past year and a half, though, that I feel a little guilty that I have not written to my mother more often.[24]

T: Can you tell me more about Jane?

L: Jane is about four years older than me. She is married and has eight children. She had my niece Sarah just a few months before I left Albemarle County in 1807. Her husband has tried some business ventures but has not had a lot of success with them . . . unfortunately.[25]

T: And Reuben?

L: Reuben and I have always been close. He is thirty-two now. He traveled out here with me to St. Louis so that he could start working in the fur trade industry. That is quite a lucrative business these days, with westward expansion really opening up, especially after our expedition. He helped to organize a fur trading company and is now a partner with several other individuals in it.[26]

My half brother, John Marks—he is twenty-four now. I really think of him and my half sister Mary—we call her Polly—as just like Jane and Reuben. Like I said before, I care about them all, and I am most concerned for their welfare. I do not know for sure what John and Polly are doing right now. Mary is twenty now. I am not sure if John has returned to Philadelphia to study medicine—I wrote to my mother this past December to ask her about this. I am concerned about how he is going to support himself there and if he has enough funds to get by. I really want him to get a good education.[27]

T: Oh? Why is that?

L: Well, when I was seventeen—my mother and Reuben and John had moved down to Georgia with my stepfather when I was twelve, and I stayed in Albemarle County and my maternal uncle William and paternal uncle Robert were appointed to be my guardians. I had three different tutors between the ages of twelve and seventeen.[28] When I was seventeen, I got word that my stepfather had died, and my mother requested that I travel down there and help move them back to Virginia, so I decided to quit school then, and I went down to Georgia about three months before I turned eighteen and moved them all back to Locust Hill, the plantation where I was raised. I always wished I had been able to go on to college, but once they were all back, and with me being the oldest son (I had inherited the estate, although my mother had dowager rights), I really knew I needed to help her run the plantation, so that is what I worked at until I joined the Virginia militia, when I was twenty. But I really did want to go on to college and would have continued my education as it had been going along, under my tutor at that time, if my stepfather hadn't died. But my mother was really anxious to get back to Virginia, so I quit school and had a carriage built at Mr. Jefferson's estate—Monticello—it was only a few miles from where we lived. So, I guess you could say I was the dutiful son and headed down to Georgia that spring, helped her pack everything up, and brought her, Reuben, John, and Mary, who was only three at the time, back up to Locust Hill.

T: Can you tell me about your family's background?

L: My Lewis side of the family is Welsh, and the Meriwether side is from England. Both sides emigrated from those countries when Virginia was in the early stages of colonization—as far back as the mid-1600s. I would have to say that I am a member of the gentry because my relatives were large land-holding families, having been granted tracts of land by

King George II, and these tracts were among the largest in the early colonial days of Virginia. I am very proud of my heritage—I was raised to value virtues like duty to my country from an early age. A lot of my relatives were military officers, of course, including my father.

T: And what about your religious or spiritual beliefs? Can you tell me about them?

L: I am a member of the Masonic Lodge and have moved up its ranks quite quickly since I first joined, after enlisting in the military. The Masonic Lodge believes in a supreme being, although unlike some religions we do not insist that Masonic members hold to any particular religious dogma. During my time with President Jefferson, we discussed some of these topics of religion. He supports, as I do, people's right to believe about these things as they see fit and as agrees with their conscience. My mother is a Methodist and is quite serious about her beliefs, many of which seem to conflict with mine. Methodists oppose using ardent spirits and drinking in general. Methodist beliefs are much more exclusive than the beliefs of Masons. President Jefferson believes that a great deal of the current religious fervor in the United States represents fanaticism, but he nevertheless supports those who choose to believe such things. But, as I love and respect my mother, I allow her to believe what she desires. I believe we will all someday die and receive our reward from the Supreme Being.

T: I see. . . . Can you tell me more about what it was like for you growing up? What, for example, is your earliest memory?

L: I do remember when my father died, but not a lot about it . . . I was only five, but I know all my relatives told me what a hero he was, how brave he was in fighting to create our country. I do have more clear memories of a time when I was seven that really made an impression on me. The Revolutionary War was still going on, and there was a very cruel British officer that rode through Albemarle County, destroying everything in his path! Everyone was terrified of him. Stories I've heard as I grew older, that I really didn't understand at the time, are that this Tarleton was on his way to capture members of the Virginia Legislature, including Jefferson. But Jefferson got tipped off and fled Monticello and managed to escape into the surrounding hills. But this "butcher" as some people called him, and his Green Dragoons traveled over the land of three of my relatives' plantations. At one, he forced some of my relatives to feed his men breakfast, and he even made his headquarters at another one of them. When he reached Charlottesville, he raided the town, burning goods and county courthouse records and stealing firearms.[29] It was a very frightening experience for me—we must have hidden out, but that part is hard for me to remember, exactly what we did to protect ourselves from him. This is what really made me despise the British, what they were doing to our friends and families and all of our property. My dislike of the British was increased during my time with the president as he does not like their way of life either.

T: Can you tell me more about growing up, after that very frightening experience?

L: I spent a lot of my time hunting in the forests—I really liked to do that. I still remember how, when I was eight, I'd go out into the forest with my dog, even in the dead of winter, and I would hunt. I just didn't seem to mind the cold and dark of winter or the heat of summer. . . . I found it all very exciting. I guess that is how I developed my expectation to be an explorer—it just seemed to always be in my blood. As early as when I was sixteen, I remember dreaming of being part of an exploring party and traveling to the unchartered Western frontier.[30] Being able to lead the expedition from 1803 to 1806 was the culmination of my greatest expectation and desires . . . those years were the highlight of my life. I can't even begin to explain to you all of the amazing adventures and wonderful things we discovered and witnessed on that journey. The day we left Fort Mandan and set out westward toward the Pacific Ocean I viewed our party "with as much pleasure as those deservedly famed adventurers [Captain Cook and Columbus] ever beheld theirs; and I dare say with quite as much anxiety for their safety and preservation." This "voyage which had formed a da[r]ling project of mine for the last ten years of my life, I could but esteem this moment of my departure as among the most happy of my life."[31]

When I was young, I also spent a fair amount of time learning about the herbs and "simples" from my mother. She sometimes took me out into the forests and such and showed me the different herbs that grew there and explained to me which ones would go into the concoctions of medicines she put together to treat different illnesses. That education from her, along with what I learned from Dr. Rush in Philadelphia before the expedition began, really helped Clark and me treat a lot of the medical situations we encountered on our trip.

I have always been interested in a lot of things—I especially like geography. When I was a teenager, I had three tutors who taught me about mathematics, geography, natural sciences, and practical matters of mapping the area through which we traveled and taking celestial measurements to help establish our latitude and longitude. I always liked botany, and I particularly liked gathering and collecting specimens during the expedition. I collected over three hundred plants and animals that were new to science.

My tutors were all men, and although I don't really remember my father, and I know I had my uncles to help guide me as I grew up, I think I really missed having a father to mentor me. Mr. Jefferson kind of took me under his wing—I really looked up to him as a father figure. He was our neighbor—in fact he always ordered his cured hams from my mother—he thought those were the best ones there were. And he invited me to come over and read any books I wanted from his library, and he and I seemed to share a lot of the same interests. We would talk about these things together, especially when I worked for him in the President's House in Washington.

T: You've experienced a lot of losses in your life—your father, and then maybe we could say your mother, in a way, when she married your stepfather so soon after your father died. Then, when you were twelve, when she, your stepfather, Jane, and Reuben moved down to Georgia, what was that like for you?

L: Well, I think I did feel like I'd been left on my own more than I would have wanted to be . . .

T: What effect to you think these losses have had on you?

L: That's a good question. I'm not sure I've ever really thought about that a lot, but I guess they would have had effects on me.

T: How would you describe yourself as a child? And how would you say that other people would describe you who knew you well?

Commentary: I am wanting to get some idea of Lewis's self-concept as well as to see how consistent or inconsistent this perception is compared to reports by others who have observed his behavior.

L: I have always considered myself to be a hard worker and always very physically tough. I was raised to have strong values when it comes to being honest, responsible, and reliable. I think other people—my family, my friends—would probably say that I am pretty determined, that once I set my mind to something, I really stick to it . . . and want to accomplish what I set out to do. I think some people might see this as a fault in me and would call me obstinate. I've heard a lot of people say that they see me as being able to be calm under pressure and that they find that quite remarkable about me.[32]

T: Oh? What makes you say that?

L: Well, probably the best example I can give you is the time, on the expedition, I recall that it was June 14, 1805—during those days when I had first witnessed the sublime spectacle of the Great Falls of the Missouri River. I was out by myself near the Great Falls exploring the area and became hungry and shot a buffalo. "While I was gazeing attentively on the poor anamal discharging blood in streams from his mouth and nostrils, expecting him to fall every instant, and having entirely forgotton to reload my rifle, a large white, or reather brown bear, had perceived and crept on me within twenty steps before I discovered him, in the first moment I drew up my gun to shoot, but at the same instant recolected that she was not loaded and that he was too near for me to hope to perform this I before he reache me, as he was then briskly advancing on me; it was an open level plain, not a bush within miles nor a tree within less than three hundred yards of me; the river bank was sloping and not more than three feet above the level of the water; in short there was no place by means of which I could conceal myself from the monster untill I could charge my rifle; in this situation I thought of retreating in a brisk walk as fast as he was advancing untill I could reach a tree about three hundred yards beloe me, but I have no sooner turned myself about but he pitched at me, open mouthed and full speed, I ran about eighty yards and found he gained on me fast. I then run into the water . . . the idea struck me to get into the water to such depth that I could stand and he would be obliged to swim, and that I could in that situation defend myself with my espontoon; accordingly I ran haistily into the water about waist deep and faced about and presented the point of my espontoon, at this instant he arrived at the edge of the water within about twenty feet of me; the moment I put myself in this attitude of defence he sudonly wheeled about as if frightened, declined the combat on such unequal grounds, and retreated with quite as great precipitation as he had just before pursued me."[33] That was a close call—but, I'll tell you, I never forgot to make sure of my surroundings or to reload my gun again.

I've told a lot of people that story, and I know it really was a close call, but I guess it is a good example of my ability to somehow be "cool under fire." That was required so many times during the expedition. . . . I could tell you more stories like that. It is just something about me; I'm not sure how to explain it. I just don't get scared like other people. Once one of the fellows was about to slip off a cliff to his death, but I calmly assured him that he was in no danger at all. Of course, that was not the case! But if I lose my confidence as a military leader, who will be able to have confidence in me? I just talked him through the steps to regain his foothold and climb back up to safer ground, and he was fine. I don't really think of myself as particularly brave, but I've heard a lot of people tell me they think I seem to be fearless. . . . I really don't see this as anything extraordinary.

Now that I think about it, maybe an effect on me of all those losses we were talking about earlier might have been that I felt like I was alone and had to make it on my own and become very independent and self-sufficient in a lot of ways. Like when I would go hunting by myself when I was very young. I think that gave me a lot of confidence, like, "Yes, I can make it on my own; I'll be OK." Maybe those losses made me feel insecure in some ways, so I felt like I had to prove to myself that I was strong and could accomplish a lot of things. I can see how on a lot of occasions I took risks that maybe other people wouldn't—maybe just to prove to myself that I'm not a weak person. It is very important to me to be both strong and brave, and it's important to me that other people see me this way, too.

Medical History

T: I'd like to ask you some questions about your physical health to get a better understanding of this area of your life. First of all, do you have any physical discomforts or conditions that you are dealing with now? If so, what are they?

L: At the present time, I am very distressed about several things. The stimulation to my system that these thoughts are having is not having a good effect on my health. Some friends of mine have told me that I look "indisposed." I feel indisposed. I suppose I should explain to you how I know these things.

During my time I spent in Philadelphia in 1803, I had the most extraordinary opportunity to come under the tutelage of Dr. Benjamin Rush. Dr. Rush is a friend of President Jefferson's and has spent many years learning about the state of animal life and the causes of health and disease. He explained some of this to me during our days together, and I have always tried to use his ideas both during the expedition and in my own life as well. Dr. Rush is an amazing man and an excellent observer of many of the issues of health-related phenomena. He told me himself that his ideas may not be entirely correct. He once told me that "my errors, like the bodies of those who fall in forcing a breach, will serve to compose a bridge for those who shall come after me, in our present difficult enterprise."[34]

Dr. Rush explained to me that a healthy life results from the balances of nervous stimulation. He said that in order to be healthy, the human body must have balances of motion, heat, sensation, and thought. He compared the healthy human body to both a seashore and waves. Both the shore and the waves are moved by the stimuli acting on them . . . in the case of the shoreline, the waves; in case of the waves, the wind. Every part of the human body possesses different degrees of what has been called excitability; one's nerves, the stomach, the muscles, the bladder, and the brain. All of these have the ability to respond to stimuli. Stimuli may be a needle for the nervous system, food in the stomach, a weight for the muscles, and urine in the bladder. Stimuli are necessary for life, just like air is to a flame. The human body is kept alive and in motion by the constant action of stimuli upon it. Air, light, food, sound, exercise, pleasure, smells, heat—all of these things serve as stimuli to a healthy body. This is what accounts for life. Dr. Rush explained to me that in addition to these stimuli, alcohol, opium, and other medications may supply some stimulus to an underexcited system or correct some state of overexcitation. His practice of bloodletting is the best example of this principle. All of these stimuli ultimately act on the blood system and may put it into spasm, which causes a state of disease. Bodily passions and emotions, according to Dr. Rush, have profound effects on health. He said that hope, love, and joy are excellent for health, like a "flame gentle and pleasant, like oil perfumed with frankincense in the lamp of life."[35]

I have always been a positive and hard-working person. Dr. Rush warned me that "violent and irregular actions of the passions tend to wear away the springs of life."[36] All of these stimuli may ultimately cause a severe problem within our blood vessels, causing them to spasm. That is why he stated that bloodletting was so vitally important in treating a disease. Removing some blood helps the blood vessels to relax and thus restores a state of health.

There were many more things that Dr. Rush did not have time to explain to me about medicine during those days in Philadelphia. My younger brother, John Marks, wants to study medicine under Dr. Rush at the University of Pennsylvania, and I am very supportive of his efforts to do so.

Forgive my ramblings about what Dr. Rush has taught me, but to answer your question, my thoughts about my situation as governor have stimulated my mind and my passions to such a degree that I fear for my health. I do not sleep well at night. All of my investments and my personal honor are threatened to be lost because of the actions of the federal government.

My happiest memory was the day we set off from Fort Mandan in the spring of 1805. These days now are the opposite. These days are filled with anger, disillusionment, and disgust for those governmental people who do not trust me and have essentially accused me of being a traitor to my country. When I spoke with my friend Clark and told him of all of my current problems associated with this governorship, he was very unhappy.

T: Have you ever had any serious accidents, illnesses, or hospitalizations?

L: The most severe accident I had occurred during the last months of the expedition. We had to hunt for our food, so Pierre Cruzatte and I went away from the Missouri River to stalk some elk. We separated and were approaching a gang when suddenly I felt a tremendous pain in my thigh area. I had been shot. I feared we were under attack from some Indians, so I retreated with the utmost pain and difficulty back to the canoes. The men assaulted the area where I was shot but found only Cruzatte. He was the one who shot me! The pain involved was terrible. One day, after we reunited with Captain Clark's group, Clark had to treat my wound by packing it with cloth so it would not abscess. The pain was so great I fainted. Part of this time I spent lying on my stomach in one of the canoes. But within a few weeks, I was returned to a state of health and was able to walk and even run a bit.

Other than that accident, I have had a number of diseases that are common among my fellow Americans. On the expedition, many of the diseases were manifest by diarrhea, sometimes with fevers, various skin problems, and Louis Veneri [syphilis], which some of the men caught after having sex with the Indian women. I have had some of these problems as well. Much of it was related to the food we ate. We went for several weeks without much to eat while crossing the Bitterroot Mountains and then gorged on camas bread and salmon. I was so sick and in such pain in my stomach that I just lay on the trail for extended periods of time. Many of the men had the same problem. Other than that, I believe that I have been very healthy throughout my life. As I mentioned before, my mother Lucy was an accomplished herbal doctor back in Virginia and used her "simples" as remedies for illness. Her type of medicine was somewhat different than that of Dr. Rush, who learned his medical practice at a university. He learned from Dr. Redmond for several years in Philadelphia and then traveled to Scotland to the University of Edinburgh for his medical school training. His education and knowledge are second to none.

T: Can you tell me what medications you are currently taking, and for what conditions?

L: Well, my doctor here in St. Louis is Dr. Saugrain. He has prescribed several different medications for me to rebalance my system. One of these is the bark of the cinchona tree. We took that along during the expedition. Dr. Rush explained to me that this can be used for many different illnesses. It is good for ague, but Dr. Rush also uses it for worms, typhus fever, tetanus, and even sore legs.[37] I used the bark once on a rattlesnake bite of Private Fields. I remember it bit him on the 4th of July on our way north along the Missouri River. We applied a poultice of the bark and he got well. At times, I have taken opium, which Dr. Rush told me would benefit me by "invigorating the whole system." Dr. Rush also told me that mercury, although effective against syphilis, "appears to act as a universal stimulant" and is "most useful when it excites a salivation."[38] Of course, that means that the best treatment effect when using mercury occurs when the patient salivates. Other medications I have used have caused me to vomit or sweat. All these things are putting my system back in balance.

Substance Abuse Assessment

T: I'd like to ask you some questions now about your current alcohol and drug use. I know you've told me something of your use of opium already . . . what about alcohol? Do you drink alcohol?

L: Well, yes, I do drink ardent spirits, usually whiskey. In my neighborhood in Virginia, it was a common thing for young men in their early teens to drink spirits, and I also did so when I joined the militia and into my days with the U.S. Army, before I went to Washington. I even wrote to my mother after I joined the militia, telling her about how well the army was taking care of us with "oceans of whiskey and mountains of beef."[39] Essentially, everyone in the army drinks whiskey. It is part of army life. The only people I have ever seen who do not drink whiskey are Methodists and Quakers as their religion tells them it is sinful to drink ardent spirits for recreation.

The use of ardent spirits as a possible problem first came up for me when I was an ensign. As I told you before, about the court-martial, I had that commanding officer who insulted my honor when I went over to his house, and he accused me of "being intoxicated" on that day, but I was not drunk.

I remember the day during the expedition I made some "punch" out of a little whiskey that was remaining in July of 1805. This most unusual event happened near the Great Falls when very large hailstones, seven inches in circumference, fell all around us. I gathered some of them up and iced some of the last of our whiskey and made myself some punch.

Dr. Rush explained to me that ardent spirits are a very strong stimulant remedy for many illnesses but warned me that the indiscriminate "practice in the use of stimulating remedies, the most popular of which is ardent spirits," can be dangerous. Dr. Rush said that people often try to use these medicines to combat their "debility and indisposition."[40] Dr. Rush says that debility or weakness is often a sign of an oncoming disease. Rush said that if anyone on the expedition is suffering from debility or indisposition, he would be much better off to rest, fast, and take a gentle purge or a weak diluting drink . . . this would be safer than to use ardent spirits as a stimulant. Dr. Rush was very much against the use of ardent spirits for drinking for nonmedical uses. He told me that it was a good stimulant but I could also use it to rub the men's feet in the morning to fight off the effects of cold.

T: What do you mean by "indisposition"?

L: Well, that just means that I am feeling ill. Sometimes the doctors do not know what is wrong with me. I know this for certain, as I had to be a doctor on many occasions during the expedition. I had to look at the symptoms of the sick person and try to figure out which medicine to give. When Private Field was bitten by the rattlesnake, I made a poultice of Peruvian bark and he got well. My doctors do exactly the same thing with me. I take different medications that supply stimulation to my debility and my indispositions.

T: How much do you drink, and what?

L: I usually drink whiskey. Recently, I purchased eight barrels of whiskey from Isaac Miller in St. Louis. Some of that supply was for Clark as I have purchased whiskey previously for him. Lately, since all of this trouble is upon me, I feel debilitated, and some have said that

I am "indisposed." So, I use whiskey as a stimulant for my system. It always works to make me feel better.

T: In a typical week, how many days would you say that you have four or more drinks?

Commentary: I am asking about this particular number because, according to the Alcohol Use Disorders Identification Test, the most widely used alcohol screening instrument currently used in the world, if a male drinks four or more drinks/day, this is considered alcohol abuse. Two drinks/day (a drink is either one glass of beer or wine or one one-ounce glass of hard liquor) is considered the maximum amount of alcohol a man should drink in order for alcohol abuse to be ruled out.

L: I really don't know. I drink enough whiskey to make me feel better. I don't go to work intoxicated. In this city, nearly everyone drinks quite a lot and quite frequently.

T: Are there any other medications you use, in addition to opium?

L: Dr. Saugrain has given me several medications in the recent past, like quina quina a form of bark. This is used for lots of reasons and for many diseases. Like I've already told you, I even used this excellent medication to treat a rattlesnake bite during the expedition. Dr. Rush uses it for lots of diseases.

T: How much opium do you use per day or per week?

L: Well, again, Dr. Rush told me that opium is a tremendous stimulant to the system and he uses this medicine for a number of diseases. I use it when the doctor thinks that I need it. I wrote down a recipe for making opium tablets for use for typhus or "nervous symptoms." I keep this recipe handy in case I need it. It contains opium. If I use that medication, I take one of the pills every night at bedtime. This makes me sleep most of the night. But, I cannot help but notice that the opium is such a powerful stimulant to my system that it affects my ability to think. It relieves any nervous symptoms, but it changes my thinking. That is undeniable.

T: Do you feel you need to cut down on the amount of drugs or alcohol you use?

Commentary: I am asking this question to assess whether or not Lewis subjectively thinks he has a problem with alcohol or drug use. If he states that he thinks *he has a problem, this would be quite a different matter than if he states that he doesn't think he has a problem at all. Individuals who abuse alcohol are notorious for denying that they have any problem with their alcohol use, even though other family members or close friends, if questioned, would typically state that the individual does indeed have a problem.*

L: I don't know. I use these things to feel better. The whiskey always works at helping me to feel better . . . at least for a while. If the doctors who treat me use these things, I think they are probably good.

T: Do you use tobacco? How much? How often?

L: Yes. I smoke tobacco and I inhale snuff up my nose. We smoked a lot of tobacco with various Indian tribes during the expedition. They always looked on this practice as a sign of good will. The smoke is believed to be healthful and beneficial for our bodies. I remember one Indian fellow who inhaled it deep into his body and kept it in as long as he could in order to get the full measure of benefit from it. It struck me as kind of interesting . . . enough so that I wrote about it in the journals of the trip. It was a sad day when we used up the last of our tobacco supplies. Many of the men were very unhappy about this loss of tobacco.

Mental Health History

T: Have you ever been physically, sexually, or emotionally abused, or mistreated as a child? For example, did anyone ever touch you in a way that made you feel uncomfortable? Or hit you so hard it left bruises?

Commentary: Any response Lewis would give to this question would be purely speculative, so I will leave his response blank. I record it in order to let the reader know that this is a question I would ask any new patient in the course of an initial consultation.

L: [intentionally left blank]

T: Do you have any history of depression or anxiety in your family?

L: Well, some of my relatives have had some "hypochondriac

affections." This means that some of the family either fear an illness or have some type of discomfort within them that is manifested by worry. This of course contributes to feeling indisposed, which, if this indisposition is sufficiently severe, requires some medicine to counteract it.

T: Governor, all of this background that you have given me has been very helpful for me. Is there anything else you would like to add that you think would be important for me to know about you that we haven't talked about?

L: Not that I can think of at the moment, but I know my friend Clark is very worried about me. He told me that he would like to talk with you too—he thought that might be helpful.

T: And how would you feel about that? Would that be OK with you?

L: Yes, that would be fine.

T: OK. As we talked about at the beginning of our session, in order for me to be able to talk with him, I will need to have you sign this written authorization form giving me your consent to do so.

[Lewis signs the form, and we end the session with the understanding that we will meet again before he leaves for his trip to Washington and that I will work with him on constructive ways he can manage the stress he is experiencing.]

Interview #2: With General William Clark, August 19, 1809, St. Louis, Missouri

T: General Clark—please come in. Thank you for meeting with me. I understand from the governor that you are very concerned about him, and he has signed a release giving his consent for me to speak with you. Please start wherever you'd like.

C: Yes, I appreciate the opportunity to be able to speak with you about Governor Lewis. I am very, very worried about him. He has been such a close friend for many years now, and I have never seen him in such a state of distress before . . . at least not to this degree. I am sure he told you that he and I led a large party of dozens of men, and our interpreter Sacagawea, to the Pacific Ocean and back for a period of three years. We encountered many life-and-death situations that he faced with the utmost bravery and calm under the most dangerous circumstances you could imagine. He has spent his entire adult life in service to his country, and, as he probably told you, with this new presidential administration coming into office this past spring, these War Department officials are refusing to reimburse the vouchers he has submitted to them.

This is a very grave situation for him because it is forcing him to have to pay these debts out of his own finances, and he is becoming undone by it all. The government is refusing payment of my vouchers as well, and I also plan to leave here and go to Washington myself to protest this very unfair treatment of both of us. But I will be taking a more easterly route, and he will be heading south first, to New Orleans. But we both plan to straighten out this terrible mess. His financial straits are much worse than mine, though—all of his creditors are now flocking in at once. I have been trying to help him with his financial situation by retaining two lawyers to handle his land titles. My situation is also bad, but I have extended family members with whom I have made land investments, and they are understanding of my predicament at the moment and ready and willing to wait to see things resolved. Also, I have a wife, but poor Lewis—he does not have these supportive backups.[41]

T: Yes, thinking he is facing financial ruin if all these funds are not covered by the government is very worrisome.

C: Yes, it is. Governor Lewis is under such pressure from so many that, based on our visit recently, I fear that the weight of his mind will overcome him.[42]

I have known my dear friend for many years and love him dearly. It defies comprehension that the same government that trusted, valued, and appreciated his service has suddenly turned on him and almost accused him of dishonesty and impure motives. I know his character, and there was never a more honest man in Louisiana "nor one who had pureor motives than Govr. Lewis."[43] If he had not spent his entire adult life engaged in the most conscientious service he has, this might not be so upsetting. But he has dedicated himself so completely and in such patriotic ways for his country, and I think it is understandable that he is taking this very, very hard. It is, after all, his reputation that is being questioned here. So unfair . . .

Interview #3: With Meriwether Lewis, September 28, 1809, Fort Pickering (in present-day Memphis, Tennessee)

Commentary: Lewis left St. Louis to begin his trip to Washington on September 4, 1809. On September 15, he arrived at Fort Pickering in such a state of ill health that he had to be carried on a stretcher. For this consultation, it will be assumed that Captain Gilbert Russell, the commanding officer of Fort Pickering (about three hundred miles south of St. Louis), had requested that I come to this location to assess Lewis in his debilitated condition, based on the strong concern Captain Russell expressed to William Clark back in St. Louis about Lewis's health and safety. (Note: No actual evidence exists that Russell dispatched any message to Clark from Fort Pickering in September 1809. My assumption is for the purpose of creating a fictitious interview with Lewis while he was at this location). Upon my arrival, I learn from Russell that the boatmen aboard the vessel that Lewis was traveling in with Pernier, his personal valet, along with other crew members, had informed Russell that after leaving St. Louis they had stopped in New Madrid (in present-day Missouri about 250 miles south of St. Louis). Pernier informed Russell that Lewis had asked him to witness the signing of his last will and testament, in which he left all of his earthly possessions to his mother, Lucy Marks. The boatmen also informed Russell that Lewis had made two suicide attempts before arriving at the fort, "in one of which he had nearly succeeded."[44] Russell informs me that he has placed Lewis under house arrest so that he will not be permitted to leave and has also put him under the care of the surgeon's mate, W. C. Smith.[45] My interview with Lewis begins in a room in Russell's quarters, after Lewis had been at the fort for two weeks. He was planning to leave the following day, September 29, because he was feeling much better.

T: Governor Lewis—how are you? I understand that you arrived here a couple of weeks ago, and I came as quickly as I could, at Captain Russell's request. I understand from him that he dispatched a message to General Clark and is very concerned about you and your health. Tell me what has happened since we last met in St. Louis.

L: I am feeling much better than I did when I arrived two weeks ago. It's been a difficult journey—the weather has been very hot. I was drinking very heavily on the boat, so after I arrived, Captain Russell withheld all hard liquor from me, allowing me to have only some claret and a little white wine. I do feel embarrassed about the condition I was in when I first arrived here, from drinking so heavily. But now, after several days, I am feeling much better, and I am determined "never to drink spirits again, or use snuff again."[46]

T: Governor, I was informed by Captain Russell that Pernier told him you had written a last will and testament when you stopped in New Madrid, on the way down to the fort here. Is that correct?

L: It's true—I did have my servant witness my signature on this document, and I left all of my possessions to my mother. I just wanted to make sure that if anything happened to me before I got to Washington, all my belongings would be taken care of. Since I have those valuable journals with me from the expedition, which I then plan to take on to Philadelphia to see to their publication, I didn't want to take any risks that anything would get lost.

T: I understand . . . but what do you think might happen to you before you get to Washington? I was also told by Captain Russell that the boatmen told him you had tried to take your own life on two occasions between the time you left St. Louis and when you arrived here at the fort? Did you write the will now because you are thinking about killing yourself?

L: I was drinking heavily while on the boat, so I really wasn't in my right state of mind. Because I have been feeling so distressed, when I was on the boat I was feeling very hopeless about my future. I really feel bad about all that now, but I can assure you, as I said before—that will not happen again. I do not intend to drink again, so I believe I am ready to continue on with my journey to get all of these financial problems straightened out with the government and then to proceed on with the publication of the journals in Philadelphia. I know I have a lot to look forward to in my life, and I can see that clearly now since I am not affected by the ardent spirits. I want to bring my mother out to St. Louis to live, and I still hope that I will be able to find a wife. I think I will be fine now, and I intend to continue on with my trip tomorrow morning.

Commentary: I have strong doubts that Lewis will maintain his sobriety after leaving Fort Pickering, despite his best intentions. It is very common for individuals who struggle with alcohol abuse to make declarations that they know they will never drink again. Without strong social support and rehabilitation efforts—none of which Lewis has at this time—relapse is highly likely.

On September 29, 1809, Lewis left Fort Pickering accompanied by Major James Neelly, Neelly's servant, and Lewis's servant Pernier, traveling overland toward Nashville. Seven days later, on October 6, Neelly and Lewis left the Chickasaw Agency for Nashville, needing to stop there for a couple of days due to Lewis's continued illness (and what I believe was a probable relapse into drinking alcohol again, despite his best intentions to abstain). They left for Nashville along the Natchez Trace. Two horses were reportedly lost on October 9 or 10, and Neelly went in search of them while Lewis proceeded on. Lewis arrived at Grinder's Stand, a country inn along the Natchez Trace, in the early evening of October 10, 1809. Early in the morning of October 11, gunshots were heard, and later that morning, Lewis, at the age of thirty-five, died of gunshot wounds, reportedly to his head and either his chest or abdomen.

Chapter 12

A Psychological Profile of Meriwether Lewis

*We are such stuff as dreams are made on, and
our little life is rounded with a sleep.*
—William Shakespeare, The Tempest, Act 4, Scene 1

You may object to my (Marti's) analysis of Lewis's behaviors and personality by the application of psychological principles based on a modern understanding of human behavior. You may feel that judging the behavior of a person who lived in 1809 by the standards of the twenty-first century is not legitimate. We believe that line of reasoning is in error, for the following reasons.

Lewis's behavior and his emotional issues with anger, frustration, disappointment, depression, and betrayal were the same for him as they are for any of us living today. The emotions and interpersonal and intrapsychic conflicts brought about by the negative behaviors of Lewis himself and others in his life have not changed in human beings across time periods.

We are not judging behaviors that may have been accepted in the culture of the early nineteenth century but would raise eyebrows today. For example, in Lewis's time many thirty-something-year-old (or older) men married young teenaged girls; to judge them by the social mores of today would be an error. Such behavior may not have caused any intrapsychic or interpersonal mental pain that affected a person's life negatively because it was accepted in the culture as normal behavior.

On the other hand, judging the drinking habits of many Americans in the early nineteenth century as very harmful, even though they were generally accepted by that culture as normal behavior, is entirely legitimate. People suffered from and sometimes died from the effects of alcohol abuse in 1809 in exactly the same way they do today. The negative effects of excessive drinking produced the very same societal, intrapsychic, and interpersonal problems, despite their acceptance in Lewis's culture. The same can be said of the culturally accepted behavior of fighting a duel. Despite Lewis's acceptance of this method of resolving an interpersonal conflict, it was a bad idea—bad then and bad now.

My (Marti's) analysis using the terminology and principles of modern psychology not only assigns labels to these issues but also helps to explain and understand them. Human actions, emotions, and issues of personality development, although perhaps somewhat different in their essence or quality in the late eighteenth century, produced the same types of outcomes in Lewis's generation as they do now. Lewis developed great self-confidence because he performed independent activities that promoted confidence in his abilities, such as hunting with his dog in the dead of night as a child. Modern children develop self-confidence by learning to play a sport or master a musical instrument. The vehicle used to develop self-confidence was different in Lewis's day, but the resulting personality characteristic is the same. Children who were physically abused in 1800 grew up with the same emotional problems as those who are abused today. These transcendent psychological principles are why I believe my analysis of Lewis's personality in the following paragraphs is legitimate.

My detailed analysis of Lewis's psychological profile utilizes the respected 2017 edition of the *Psychodynamic Diagnostic Manual* (PDM-2), which is based on clinical knowledge, process-outcome research, and empirical studies and examines an individual's personal psychology in a highly systematic, scientific manner. This approach is of value largely because other authors have created rough impressions of Lewis and/or have focused on one element of his behavior or symptoms without integrating it with the larger picture. First, I address the three categories in the PDM-2, and then I put all of them together to produce Lewis's psychological profile.

The PDM-2 is organized according to three categories, which are called *dimensions*.

Dimension I—Personality Syndromes (P Axis). This dimension takes into account the level of personality organization (i.e., psychotic, borderline, neurotic, healthy) as well as the types of styles possible within any given level (e.g., depressive, obsessive-compulsive, narcissistic, etc.).[1] The task force who developed the PDM placed this dimension first in the PDM system "because symptoms or problems often cannot be understood, assessed, or treated without an understanding of the personality patterns of the individual who has them."[2]

Dimension II—Mental Functioning (M Axis). This dimension provides a *microscopic* examination of a person's mental life and a way to describe their abilities that contribute to their personality and "overall psychological health or pathology."[3] Such capacities include how accurately the person observes themself and others and how they establish and maintain relationships, process information and experiences, and regulate and express their emotions.

Dimension III—Symptom Patterns: The Subjective Experience (S Axis). This dimension examines symptoms and how they may be organized into *clusters* or *patterns* with the intent of better understanding any difficulties the patient is experiencing in either their personal or professional life or both.[4]

The following is my analysis of how these categories apply to Lewis.

Personality Syndromes (P Axis)

This dimension addresses the *predominant* personality style that best characterizes an individual. It is relatively rare that any one individual can be viewed as fitting into one pure style since there is often some degree of overlap between different styles. Also, there is some crossover within this grouping as every person is unique. To use the metaphor of a tapestry, a personality is composed of many threads that are interwoven to form the complete image they produce, and factors such as genetic predispositions, early life experiences (including neglect, abuse, and traumas), natural temperament, cultural background, and early attachments (or lack of them) create a pattern that forms a unique person. Just like snowflakes, no two human beings are alike.

Most of the personality syndromes described in the PDM-2 are easily understandable by laypeople and mental health professionals alike, so I will not define them in detail since they are relatively self-explanatory. Instead, I will list them to provide a context for the one I believe best describes Lewis. Much like choosing from a menu of food items, you will then be able to see specific items from the list that I apply to Lewis. Obviously, not all of these syndromes apply to Lewis. These syndromes are as follows:

- Depressive (includes hypomania—highly energetic—and masochism—seeming to be drawn to pain and suffering)
- Dependent
- Anxious (avoidant and phobic)
- Obsessive-compulsive
- Schizoid (withdrawn)
- Somatizing (highly concerned about one's health and body)
- Hysteric or histrionic (flamboyant/dramatic)
- Narcissistic (self-centered)
- Paranoid (highly fearful)
- Psychopathic
- Sadistic
- Borderline (generally marked by strong fluctuations in mood, behavior, and self-image, leading to relationship problems and impulsive behavior)[5]

I would describe Lewis as having features of a depressive personality, but the style I think depicts him the best is the obsessive-compulsive personality style (this is not the same as obsessive-compulsive disorder). The PDM-2 describes individuals with this specific style as

> emotionally constricted and regimented. They prefer to operate as if emotions were irrelevant and to defend against threatening emotions and desires through rigidity, regimentation, and intellectualization. They tend to be excessively concerned with rules, procedures, order, organization, schedules, and so on, and may be excessively devoted to work and productivity to the detriment

of leisure and relationships. Central to obsessive-compulsive psychology is resistance to feeling 'out of control.'[6]

The PDM-2 identifies key features of this personality style as including central preoccupations or concerns, emotions (and ways of defending against their feelings so as to not feel them), characteristic beliefs about themselves and others, and genetically ingrained patterns.[7] There are multiple illustrations of each of these attributes in the historical record of Lewis's life. One preoccupation of individuals with the obsessive-compulsive personality style involves either submission to or rebellion against controlling authority.

Sometimes individuals can find very satisfying matches between their natural inclinations and the professions they choose. They may go through their entire lives relatively smoothly because their personality characteristics are very adaptive for their work. For example, a small child who likes to do math problems and pays great attention to details might grow up to be an excellent accountant, a career in which these skills are required to do a good job. Lewis's choice of a career in the military may be an example of how this principle worked well for him. A soldier's life is filled with following orders, rules, and regulations, and Lewis seemed to thrive in this milieu. By November 1794, young Meriwether had proven himself to be so adept at military life that he was promoted from private to a commissioned ensign in the Virginia militia. His emotional satisfaction at this important life moment can be felt in his statement, "I am quite delighted with a soldier's life."[8] His strong need for control coupled with his strong intellectual ability also help to explain his rising in the ranks to become a U.S. Army captain.

Some may ask, "If Lewis had OCD and was so preoccupied with getting things accomplished that needed to be done, then why wasn't he more diligent about writing journal entries while on the expedition and then getting them published more quickly after the journey ended?" To answer this question, it is necessary to understand similarities and differences between possessing an obsessive-compulsive personality *style* and having an obsessive-compulsive *disorder* (OCD), which may or may not overlap.

According to the PDM-2, an individual possessing an obsessive-compulsive personality *style* has such a deeply embedded and long-standing need for rigid control and perfectionism that these traits of overconscientiousness and inflexibility often create difficulties in their interpersonal relationships. The historical record contains sufficient documentation, as previously discussed, to conclude that Lewis possessed characteristics of this style.

In the *disorder* (OCD), the emphasis is on the presence of *obsessions* and/or *compulsions*. *Obsessions* are repetitive, unwanted, and intrusive thoughts, images, or urges such as wondering whether you locked the front door when you leave the house. *Compulsions* are *behaviors* engaged in to get rid of the obsession, such as returning home to check whether the door was locked.[9] In OCD, symptoms focus on a specific theme. For example, an obsession with a fear of germs leads to repetitive hand washing in order to get rid of the fear of germs. I have never seen any documentation that Lewis struggled with distinct obsessions and/or compulsions as I have just defined them. The absence of such documentation does not necessarily mean he did not suffer from them; he may have. But, it is not correct to assume he had OCD.

During the expedition, Lewis had multiple responsibilities and did not have to justify his decision to leave the writing to Clark. He could very conscientiously collect his plant specimens and describe them in painstaking detail in his characteristically obsessive-compulsive way while leaving the writing to Clark. (Some authors have proposed that Lewis did keep more comprehensive journal entries during the expedition but that they were lost, and this scenario must be considered as well.) Once he was faced with preparing the journals for publication, he likely felt much more pressure to accomplish this task than he did during the expedition, when he was in total control of how he spent his time. Preparation and editing of the journals was a far more daunting task than simply keeping up with his journal entries. When faced with the complexity of editing the journals while at the same time attempting to fulfill his duties as governor and attending to his mounting problems with the federal government, he was unable to accommodate them all effectively.

In his book *The Character of Meriwether Lewis*, Clay Jenkinson comprehensively addresses several explanations of Lewis's failure to publish the expedition journals. He offers busyness with competing tasks, the presence of a mental illness, punishing others by withholding communication, his low self-esteem/insecurity, and Lewis's characteristic arrogance as possibilities, all of which he theorizes can be distilled down to a "failure to communicate."[10] I concur that it is likely that some combination of all these reasons enter into the picture of Lewis's procrastination—writer's block, resistance, or whatever other term we want to use to convey the idea that Lewis simply did not get this job done.

My view on this matter is slightly different from Jenkinson's, however, in that I believe we are always communicating. The real question is, are we communicating verbally or nonverbally? Even silence communicates different things to different people for different reasons. We might think of Jenkinson's thesis of Lewis's "failure to communicate" as the symptom. Underneath the symptom, if we could put words on his behavioral response of inaction and silence, he might be communicating different things to different people—as well as communicating a number of different things at the same time. We know his silence generated strong feelings of frustration, irritation, confusion, and disappointment, particularly in Jefferson. Jefferson expressed such sentiments to Lewis in his letter dated July 17, 1808, after not hearing from Lewis for ten months. Jefferson wrote, "Since I parted with you in Albemarle in Sep. last I have never had a line from you."[11]

Other expressions of Jefferson's disapproval undoubtedly added to Lewis's disappointment in himself, making it even more difficult for him to engage with Jefferson, the father figure whose approval Lewis desired. We can infer that this was likely the case based on the somewhat reprimanding tone of two of Jefferson's letters during the last months of Lewis's life. Jefferson scolded Lewis about his lack of communication in a letter dated August 16, 1809:

> I am very often applied [asked] to know when your work will begin to appear; and I have so long promised copies to my literary correspondents in France, that I am almost bankrupt in their eyes. I shall be very happy to receive from yourself information of your expectations on this subject. Every body is impatient for it.[12]

In another letter dated August 24, 1809, Jefferson wrote, "I am uneasy, hearing nothing from you about the Mandan chief, nor the measure for restoring him to his country."[13] Given how soon Jefferson wrote these letters before Lewis's departure from St. Louis on September 4, as well as the slowness of mail delivery, it seems likely that Lewis never saw these letters.

In addition to the long gaps between his journal entries during the expedition, Lewis wrote less often than previously to his mother, siblings, and friends during the last two years of his life.[14] If we could put words to his withdrawal, perhaps Lewis was communicating nonverbally his sense of inadequacy relative to Jefferson. Lewis may have been thinking, "How in the world can I ever write an acceptable account of an expedition that took place over nearly three years to the president of the United States and the man who wrote the Declaration of Independence?" Such anxiety about being able to measure up to Jefferson's expectations would surely have given Lewis pause. At the same time, his silence could be interpreted as a passive-aggressive way of expressing his anger to Jefferson: "How dare you scold me after all I have done for you!" and/or "I'll show you for putting me in an impossible bind of expecting me to govern an entire territory and publish these journals. Each one of these tasks is a full-time job in itself. I just won't write them!"

Last but not least, let us not forget the number of significant losses Lewis had experienced earlier in his life and the effects they had had on him. When we feel abandoned by someone, we may "take in" or internalize the person who abandoned us, which is sometimes referred to as "identification with the aggressor." Abandonment experiences during his developmental years by several family members could have impacted Lewis's self-esteem. He might have viewed himself as someone worth abandoning. There is a level on which Lewis could be perceived to be abandoning many of the people he consciously professed to care about the most. He would not have wanted to consciously "own" that he, a person who was abandoned, was doing the same hurtful thing to someone else. His projection of this "badness" can be seen in a comment to his mother in his letter to her dated December 1, 1808. In the letter, Lewis implies that he has hurt feelings over not having received correspondence from his half-sibling and brother-in-law: "What is John Marks and Edmund Anderson about, that they do not write to me?"[15] It is noteworthy that he made this comment *after* apologizing to his mother in the same letter for not having written to her in such a long time. Once Lewis became aware of feeling bad or guilty, he then felt the need to project it out of himself and into someone else to help himself think he was not so bad for being a negligent letter writer.

Lewis's obsessive-compulsive *style* also helps to explain why, once he was out of his military lifestyle and into the role of an administrator with Bates as his assistant, who questioned his authority at every turn, Lewis had great difficulty adapting to such a different work situation. Unlike in the army or on the expedition, where he gave orders and they were followed without question, his ingrained expectation that his orders would be followed was not always met. This would result in Lewis experiencing a sense of being "out of control," and he would react very strongly—as we know he did on numerous occasions. The degree of Lewis's inability to adapt to a life with relatively less rigidity and regimentation, as he was forced to do as a governmental administrator in St. Louis, is attested to by Bates, who wrote to his brother Richard, "How unfortunate for this man that he resigned his commission in the army: His habits are altogether military & he never can I think succeed in any other profession."[16]

David Nicandri, in his work *River of Promise*, notes that Lewis started to emotionally decompensate during his months on the west side of the Rockies from September 1805 into early June of 1806. Nicandri disagrees with Stephen Ambrose's assessment that Lewis returned to St. Louis in September of 1806 emotionally intact, and he also believes that Lewis's demise was fueled by posttraumatic stress disorder after his return to civilization.[17] I disagree for a variety of reasons. The first is because the roots of Lewis's personality were formed during his childhood, and some of his issues showed themselves long before the problems Nicandri describes in 1805–06. Lewis's behaviors toward Lieutenant Elliott that led to his court-martial early in his career resulted from the same personality traits that led to the behaviors that Nicandri cites as evidence of posttraumatic stress disorder in 1806. Nicandri's assessment of Lewis as suffering from posttraumatic stress disorder is similar to a blind man describing what an elephant looks like by feeling only its trunk. To appreciate the personality and emotional issues that led to Lewis's problems, one must look at his entire life. His classmate and cousin Peachy Gilmer described Lewis as having a "martial temper" during his childhood.[18] A member of Jefferson's cabinet made observations about Lewis's high level of confidence, which he worried might result in bad judgment during the expedition.[19] Attorney General Levi Lincoln commented that Lewis would be much more likely, "in case of difficulty, to push too far, than to recede too soon."[20] It is obvious that certain behaviors of Lewis were a common thread woven into the tapestry of his entire life.

As the PDM-2 notes regarding obsessive-compulsive individuals, "Central to an obsessive-compulsive psychology is a resistance to feeling out of control."[21] The occasionally harsh physical environment of the expedition, particularly the five months of rainy weather in 1805–06, when coupled with the many difficulties related to Lewis's command of the expedition (difficulties navigating the springtime Columbia and finding food, having sick expedition members, being attacked by the Blackfeet, suffering a serious gunshot wound), in addition to the interactions with natives who violated his personal ethos, mostly likely led to his feeling out of control. Lewis assaulted several Indians for various reasons, as already covered. These temporary negative circumstances, rather than being the fuel for posttraumatic stress disorder, caused the obsessive-compulsive but highly self-confident Lewis to feel out of control. When these circumstances disappeared, so did his sense of feeling out of control. When he arrived in St. Louis in September of 1806, he had left the Columbia's difficulties in the past. The Blackfeet had been "taught a lesson" by Lewis's leaving the peace medal on the body of the Blackfeet man he had killed, and Lewis's gunshot wounds had healed. Lewis had cheated death on several occasions. For a man of Lewis's extraordinary self-confidence, there was likely no emotional baggage carried over from these events. His self-confidence was, in fact, likely even stronger than before the expedition.

I believe Lewis experienced his court-martial earlier in his military career as more traumatic than his narrow escape from a grizzly bear he encountered near the Great Falls of the Missouri. Just like beauty, trauma lies in the eye of the beholder. What one individual might interpret as traumatic might not be perceived as such by a different person. We must remember that it was always the insults to his reputation by other people rather than physically dangerous situations that evoked the strongest emotional reactions in Lewis. Given Lewis's nerves of steel in situations that the average person might consider terrifying, it seems more likely, based on how often they encountered bears and Lewis's nonchalant description of his encounter with the grizzly bear near the Great Falls, that he was affected by the experience and concerned but was relatively nonplussed by this and other encounters he had with these enormous animals (e.g., "these bears being so hard to die rather intimidates us all; I must confess that I do not like the gentlemen and had rather fight two Indians than one bear").[22]

In reality, grizzly bears probably bothered Lewis far less than Bates's provocations. To this point, while I do agree with Nicandri's conclusion that the distressing events that occurred on the return trip in the Columbian region added to the accumulation of stress that no doubt increased as the journey progressed, I disagree with his overall conclusion that Lewis suffered from posttraumatic stress disorder based on his close encounters with the "white bears" and the Blackfeet.

Both David and I have witnessed this type of matter-of-fact reaction in current and former members of branches of the U.S. Special Forces. They have told us stories that drop our jaws regarding the dangerous situations they have faced. Yet they report to us that all of these situations are a normal day at work and that their previous training and experiences allow them to go to bed at night and promptly fall asleep. Lewis was an equally cool character.

Lewis's life moved forward relatively smoothly as long as he was in control; the moments in his life when he felt he was "losing it" were the ones that unbalanced him, such as his court-martial, the time Bates insulted him and Lewis probably came close to having a duel with him, and the federal government's refusal to reimburse him for his financial commitments. The avalanche of circumstances that befell him during the last few months of his life had to have been the most intense of his entire life; he was faced with financial ruin, the loss of his good reputation, and the loss of support and valuing of his adult life of dedication, patriotism, and service to his country. There can be no doubt that Lewis must have felt more "out of control" then than he ever had before. His desperation to get to Washington and fight back against the injustices he faced in order to regain control over his life cannot be overestimated.

One could argue that *any* person who faced similar circumstances would feel betrayed, hurt, and angry, as Lewis felt, and that any reasonable person would have wanted to take the steps that he did to regain control of his life—and this would be true. The fact is that *different personalities react to any given set of circumstances in different ways*. Evidence of this can be found in William Clark. Clark's personality has generally been characterized as level-headed and even-tempered. It could be said that Lewis was very fortunate to have found such a tried-and-true friend as his co-captain for the voyage to the Pacific. Clark recognized his friend's talents and strengths, valued and appreciated Lewis, and always treated him with the greatest respect. When Lewis got upset, Clark could help calm him down, as evidenced at the Masonic Lodge Ball in June 1809. Clark also had submitted vouchers that the government had denied, and, like Lewis, he set out for Washington in an effort to make things right. But Clark's reaction appeared to be much more measured, no doubt accounted for by the fact that he had the social support of a wife and family members with whom he stayed along the route. In addition, it is vitally important to recognize that Clark did not have an obsessive-compulsive personality style and thus did not require order and control in his life to the extent that Lewis did. Without Clark's presence, Lewis had no one to soften the blows on his journey to the capital city from the day he left St. Louis until the day of his death.

Lewis was fortunate to have encountered Captain Russell at Fort Pickering to help nurse him back to health, but this support was necessary but *insufficient* to sustain him throughout the entire journey. In fact, after they left Fort Pickering, Agent Neelly probably enabled Lewis's relapse into alcohol abuse. According to the historical record, Captain Gilbert Russell reported to Jefferson that Neelly was essentially responsible for Lewis's death: "This Agt. being extremely fond of liquor, instead of preventing the Govr from drinking or keeping him under any restraint advised him to it & from every thing I can learn gave the man every chance to seek an opportunity to destroy himself."[23]

Dr. Benjamin Rush, in his writings, cautioned against the premature discharge of a mentally deranged patient who had seemingly returned to sound mental health. However, Captain Russell was without a doubt unaware of Rush's teaching on this situation. In addition, Lewis's apparent return to normalcy at Fort Pickering did not signal a return to solid mental health. Lewis's mental state when he left the fort was just a step away from a relapse into alcohol abuse, depression, and despair brought on by a lack of positive emotional support and Neelly's harmful influence.

The PDM-2 reports that people with an obsessive-compulsive personality style

> fear that their impulses, especially their aggressive urges, will get out of control. Most obsessive thoughts and compulsive actions involve efforts to undo or counteract impulses toward destructiveness, greed, and messiness. Because guilt over unacceptable wishes is severe, the conscience of a pathologically obsessive-compulsive person is famously rigid and punitive. Self-criticism is harsh; such individuals hold themselves (and others) to ideal standards. . . . They are scrupulous to a fault, but may have trouble relaxing, joking, and being intimate.[24]

While I would not describe Lewis as *pathologically* obsessive-compulsive, I would say that he had strong *tendencies* toward these characteristics, and this may help to at least partly explain his difficulty in establishing the long-term, intimate relationship with a woman that we know he longed for. These personality characteristics are exactly what made him such a good naturalist. Observing and describing dozens of various plant and animal characteristics would feel very gratifying to an obsessive-compulsive personality. When one reads about all that Lewis accomplished in his life, it is difficult to dispute his obsessive-compulsive style. Lewis was a very hard worker, very disciplined, and paid great attention to detail. Again, great attention to detail is required in an astute naturalist, expedition organizer/leader, and army paymaster.

The reason why my diagnostic impression is that Lewis had tendencies of a depressive personality is that individuals with this style can be described as "chronically vulnerable to painful affect [feelings], especially depression, guilt, shame, and feelings of inadequacy."[25] Depressive personalities are characteristically highly self-critical (similar to obsessive-compulsive personalities), even though in reality they may have accomplished a lot.

We see some evidence of both of these personality types in Lewis's journal entry on his thirty-first birthday:

> This day I completed my thirty first year, and conceived that I had in all human probability now existed about half the period

which I am able to remain in this Sublunary world. I reflected that I had as yet done but little, very little indeed, to further the happiness of the human race, or to advance the information of the succeeding generation. I viewed with regret the many hours I have spent in indolence, and now soarly feel the want of that information which those hours would have given me had they been judiciously expended. but since they are past and cannot be recalled, I dash from me the gloomy thought and resolved in future, to redouble my exertions and at least indeavour to promote those two primary objects of human existence, by giving them the aid of that portion of talents which nature and fortune have bestoed on me; or in future, to live for mankind, as I have heretofore lived for myself.[26]

Keep in mind that Lewis up to this point had provided service to his country by joining the army at age twenty, been promoted to the rank of captain by age twenty-six, and working for two years as the private secretary to the president of the United States. When he wrote this entry in August 1805, he was in the middle of co-leading a very important expedition across the North American continent. Any realistic evaluation of such a person would hardly echo Lewis's harsh self-criticism of living a lifestyle of "indolence" or laziness. Lewis's view of himself represents a distortion of the objective reality of his life, yet it is not unusual for people with obsessive-compulsive and depressive styles to experience the emotional reality that they have failed. Lewis was expressing this thought on his birthday: "I *feel* like I have failed." Lewis's self-perception is consistent with the depressive style in that he seems to hold himself to unrealistic standards.

Jefferson, who knew Lewis well and probably thought of him in some ways as the son he never had, provided a view of Lewis that fits with this depressive style and points as strongly and clearly as seems possible to the presence of a genetic predisposition for anxiety and/or depression in Lewis in the often-quoted biographical statement he sent to Paul Allen, who published the first edition of the journals. On August 18, 1813, which would have been Lewis's thirty-ninth birthday, Jefferson wrote,

Governor Lewis had from early life been subject to hypocondriac affections. it was a constitutional disposition in all the nearer branches of the family of his name & was more immediately inherited by him from his father. they had not however been so strong as to give uneasiness to his family. while he lived with me in Washington, I observed at times sensible depressions of mind but knowing their constitutional source, I estimated their course by what I had seen in the family.[27]

Jefferson explained his belief that Lewis did not display any depressive symptoms during the expedition due to "constant exertion which that required all the faculties of body and mind, suspended these distressing affections."[28] But when Lewis assumed a more sedentary position as governor in St. Louis, the affections "returned upon him with redoubled vigor and began seriously to alarm his friends."[29] Jefferson was not physically present to observe Lewis's behavior in St. Louis, so we cannot know for certain how he came to this conclusion. Perhaps it came through William Clark, who had visited Jefferson at Monticello after Lewis's death to discuss the publication of the journals. Clark most probably expressed to the former president his concern about Lewis before he departed from St. Louis. Or, Jefferson might have been influenced by Lewis's friend William Carr, who wrote about Lewis's "imprudence" and his leaving St. Louis with his governorship in tatters.[30] Carr's written opinion is in stark contrast to Lewis's report in his August 18, 1809, letter to Secretary of War William Eustis that "I shall leave the Territory in the most perfect state of tranquility which, I believe, it has ever experienced."[31]

With so much to keep Lewis's mind busy from 1803–06, there would have been little chance for depressive thoughts to take root and grow into significant problems. This is consistent with modern psychological knowledge that satisfying and pleasurable activities may supply a person with some relief from depressive symptoms. There is also validity to the idea that physical exercise has a beneficial effect on depressive symptoms. Such activity results in the release of endorphins, hormones that act on opiate receptors in the brain, leading to a reduction of pain and an increased sense of well-being.

Every person has tendencies of self-centeredness or *narcissism*. Typical behaviors of people with a primarily narcissistic style include the easy berating of other people, explosive anger at people whom they perceive as inferior to them (sometimes referred to as narcissistic rage), and the necessity to always be right. Narcissistic personalities are often very invested in either achieving or maintaining a high social status. They invest a lot of energy in defending their wounded self-esteem by either devaluing or idealizing others. Sometimes the terms "narcissistic vulnerability" or "narcissistic injury" are used to describe the degree of sensitivity a person has when they perceive that they have been scolded or criticized. This phenomenon and narcissistic behaviors are repeatedly evident in Lewis, such as when his honor or authority was questioned or he suffered insulting behavior by Elliott, various Native Americans, Bates, Eustis, Simmons, and Madison. Lewis felt instantly and deeply insulted and wounded whenever this happened.

Although Lewis exhibited aspects (beliefs, thoughts, feelings, and behaviors) of each of these styles, my evaluation based on the parameters of the PDM-2 is that Lewis possessed a predominantly obsessive-compulsive *style*, with depressive and narcissistic *tendencies* within this style.

Mental Functioning (M Axis)

In the PDM-2, twelve categories of basic mental functioning are described to help clinicians "capture the complexity and individuality of each patient."[32] In making my diagnosis of Lewis's mental health, I am not simply putting my hand in the proverbial hat and pulling out random conclusions about Lewis. Research has identified empirically based methods that can be used to assess each of these capacities. The PDM-2 provides a rating scale for each capacity, with a 5 representing the highest level of functioning within that capacity and a 1 the lowest. When all these twelve components are given a score, a range of scores from 54–60 indicate a *healthy* level of functioning; scores between 40–53 indicate a *neurotic level* of functioning, followed by *borderline* (19–39) and *psychotic* (12–18).[33]

Where does Lewis fall within this axis?

The first capacity addresses how we process our experiences and learn how to adapt and cope with them. Accomplishing this requires that we pay attention to the information we take in, organize it in some way in our minds, and remember it. This process is very much influenced by how strongly (or not) our emotions are triggered by any given situation. For example, we could watch video A, of blue-and-green-striped fish swimming serenely around a beautiful and colorful coral reef, and feel very calm inside. Later, when asked what we saw, we could probably describe the images accurately and likely recall that we also saw a sea turtle floating in front of a purple, fan-shaped coral. If we watched video B, which began similarly with fish swimming around multicolored coral but then showed a large shark devouring the fish, we would be less likely later to remember the sea turtle floating next to the purple, fan-shaped coral because the influence of the strong emotion of anxiety interfered with our ability to pay closer attention to some features in the video. Instead, we focused our attention on the features that represented a danger to us.

The PDM-2 describes a rating of 5 as follows: "the individual is appropriately focused, well organized, and able to adapt and learn from experience, even under stress. There is a good ability to express thoughts, affects, and other inner experiences, both verbally and nonverbally. Memory, attention, and executive function are all functioning at a high level, and well-integrated."[34] Concerning Lewis and his capacity for what the PDM-2 refers to as *regulation, attention, and learning*, I think there is ample evidence that when he was in control of his circumstances and not feeling particularly stressed, as when he was organizing and planning for the expedition and learning collaboratively with experts in their fields in Philadelphia, he functioned at a very high level of efficiency. On the other hand, under the stress of interpersonal interactions involving a challenge to his authority, he had trouble both learning and adapting to new styles of behavior that would allow him to more effectively interact with other individuals during his governorship after the years of regimentation he was used to in his military life.

The accuracy of a rating is increased when the clinician's interview with an individual matches the individual's self-reports, records or documents about their life, and the reports of people who know the individual well (e.g., family, friends, employers). Lewis was consistently described in all of these sources as very strong in his ability to focus and be organized but without an equal ability to learn and adapt well under stress, which is when he reverted to a military type of demeanor.

Another important capacity we all possess to varying degrees relates to how well (or not) we are *aware of* our feelings, how deeply (or not) we feel them, and how well (or not) we can read, interpret, and respond to the feelings of other people. Our ability to experience a wide range of emotions (from anger to sadness and grief to happiness) to various *degrees of intensity* is referred to by mental health clinicians as our *affective range*. The *affective range, communication, and understanding* capacity in an individual who is mentally functioning at a high level allows them to respond to a wide range of situations with flexibility and awareness of a wide range of feelings and to be able to accept them and respond to them in empathic and compassionate ways. Anyone can be mildly angry to very angry and mildly happy to very happy. These represent variations in the level of intensity of these emotions, not our response to them. The same is true for other emotions: fear, disappointment, etc.

I believe it is likely that Lewis was able to experience a wide range of emotions and could understand and communicate them in an adequate way most of the time. I think his competency in these capacities is illustrated by how eloquently and descriptively he wrote in the expedition journals and in his letters to his mother, Jefferson, and his friends. I estimate that his abilities fell in the midrange of the scale for this area of functioning. This is based on the difficulty he had in managing specific emotions such as anger, especially when under stress and in situations in which his honor was challenged by other people. Lewis's ability to keep calm even in the face of life-threatening circumstances was a remarkable strength. His response to being charged by a grizzly bear near the Great Falls and his composure and clear directions to Private Windsor on how to extricate himself from a probably fatal fall off a muddy cliff during their exploration of the Marias River on June 6, 1805, are prime examples of Lewis's great ability in this regard.[35] In times of great stress, when confronted with threats from the natural environment, Lewis was as cool, calm, and collected a personality as has ever existed. If Lewis had been a physician, he would be the person I would want taking care of me in an emergency.

We all know that our experiences influence how we view the world. If one or more people early in our lives harmed us, when we grow up we may develop an expectation that all people are motivated by the intention to harm us. If we have had experiences with others that we consider to have been helpful and caring, we are more likely to automatically assume that people we encounter mean to help us. *Mentalization* is a term used to describe the ability to reflect on (or imagine) not only what we think and feel in our own minds but also to imagine that *others might think and feel differently than we do.* This capacity includes imagining what others might think about us. When we can imagine that someone could be different from us, we do not assume that the subjective experience that we have is necessarily the same for another person. We can allow for the possibility that it may not be similar to our own.

We all function along a range of being relatively more or less able to mentalize and reflect on what is in our mind and the minds of others. The capacity for *mentalization and reflective functioning* may be difficult for non-mental health professionals to conceptualize as these processes usually operate outside of our conscious awareness. Mentalizing has been described as the ability to "understand misunderstandings."[36] The more an individual possesses this capacity, the more likely they are to be able to consider many different motivations to understand any particular behavior they observe in others. Individuals who function at a lower level are relatively less able to consider alternative motivations or intentions to explain behaviors they see in others; their outlooks are more rigid, and their conclusions about what they believe is objective reality is significantly narrower.

Lewis's self-descriptions, as well descriptions of him by people who knew him, indicate that he was usually able to reflect on and imagine his own and others' behavior in realistic ways while in a state of calm. However, some of Lewis's most remarkable problems arose when he perceived that others were devaluing or insulting him, in which case his ability to step back and reflect on those behaviors was overtaken by strong, angry feelings. This led Lewis to quickly assign the worst motivations to others' behaviors and thus respond in a manner that was not in his or others' best interests. Multiple examples of this in Lewis's life perfectly illustrate this phenomenon. His interaction with Lieutenant Elliott and with the Nez Perce Indian who threw the puppy in his lap while he was eating his dinner are perhaps two of the most obvious illustrations of his difficulty in understanding that the motivations of others could be different from his own. Instead of interpreting the physically harmless behavior on the part of the Indian as playful teasing or, at worst, a harmless cultural faux pas, Lewis's immediate and automatic reaction was to get up from his seated position, confront the Indian, throw the puppy back at the perpetrator of this insult, strike him, and then pull his tomahawk from his belt and threaten to kill the young man.

Whatever Lieutenant Elliott's interaction was with the young Lewis, Lewis was unable to consider the possibility that Elliott was innocent in the matter. Lewis reacted to Elliott's perceived insults by demanding "satisfaction" and shedding tears. On the return trip on the Columbia, he repeated this type of behavior when he coupled his anger with a physical assault against a native who took a canoe oar mount out of a pile of ashes after Lewis had burned the expedition's canoes to prevent the local tribes from having them. Instead of practicing some "mentalizing" about the dire poverty and need of these Indians, Lewis responded with a threat to burn down a tribal village in response to a perceived insult. Once again, his actions reveal Lewis's relative inability to provide any alternative explanations for others' behaviors in times of great anger. His decisions in these cases also directly disobeyed the prime directive issued by Jefferson, which was to treat tribes with as much kindness as the situation allowed. Clearly, at times, Lewis's ability to think (mentalize) went offline when his anger was triggered by another's insulting behavior.

I sometimes explain this phenomenon to my patients who report some behavior that they feel guilty or ashamed about (e.g., screaming when they did not get something they wanted) by saying, "Your brain was flooded with anger at that moment, and you couldn't think." This reflexive, knee-jerk reaction is a behavioral pattern that is somewhat prominent with Lewis, and the multiple examples within the historical record span a large portion of his lifetime—not just the months in the Columbia River basin, as Nicandri stated.

The fourth of the twelve capacities relevant to mental functioning, *differentiation and integration (identity)*, involves knowing who we are and having confidence in that, even though we may hear other people describe us differently. This ability involves filtering what others think of us and comparing it to how we see ourselves. A realistic view of ourselves means seeing ourselves as human, as possessing certain abilities and skills as well as limitations. Relatively more optimal functioning in this arena involves perceiving ourselves as different from other people as opposed to superior (or inferior) to others. This ability is related to how secure (or insecure) we feel about our identity.

For example, Lewis defined himself as an explorer; he had long wished to lead an exploration party into the American interior. Just before leaving on the expedition, he stated that "the picture which now presented itself to me was a most pleasing one. entertaining [now] as I do, the most confident hope of succeading in a voyage which had formed a da[r]ling project of mine for the last ten years."[37] Given the fact that his very successful completion of this project resulted in his becoming a national hero, we might conclude that Lewis had a high degree of confidence and a sense of security in defining himself as an explorer. On the other hand, given his multiple unsuccessful attempts to find a wife, we might conclude that he felt relatively more insecure when it came to his identity in this area of his life.

A negative result of Lewis's acceptance of others' opinions of him, which contributed to his sense of self-worth, is that negative opinions produced painful feelings that were probably very detrimental to his mental health. The higher Lewis climbed, the harder he could fall. Lewis took very seriously what others thought of him, so he had a very hard fall whenever the ladder was pulled out from under him and he felt disrespected or insulted. Lewis's trip to Washington in 1809 was at least in part his attempt to reconcile his own internal sense of himself as honest in the face of government officials' implied perception of him as dishonest.

The fifth capacity, which is *relationships and intimacy*, is another key to understanding Lewis's life and mental functioning.[38] Lewis did seem to have had many stable, mutually satisfying relationships. He stayed in contact with his mother through letters. Based on some of the teasing comments contained in his letters, it appears that their relationship was a warm one. She supplied nurturing acts to take care of him, and he reciprocated. At the end of his life, while he was living in St. Louis, he was investing in land with the plan of moving her there so that they could be in closer proximity; he was thinking of her welfare. Based on what we know of their exchanges, it appears that he had a positive attachment to his mother.

Meriwether had similarly deep relationships with all of his siblings. In the absence of a biological father, he had uncles who acted as guardians and father figures to him. He also had Jefferson, who was a mentor, friend, and father figure, encouraging Lewis and nurturing his interests and talents to help him achieve his fullest potential. Lewis had a very warm and trusting relationship with William Clark. He also had other good male friends—Mahlon Dickerson in Philadelphia and Amos Stoddard, with whom he exchanged regular correspondence. It appears that he had developed some degree of friendship with William Carr (in St. Louis). Carr was sufficiently familiar with Lewis to be able to comment that Lewis was a "good man, but a very imprudent one" at the time of Lewis's departure from St. Louis in September of 1809.[39] There is a lot of evidence that Lewis's capacity for relationships and intimacy was strong and that he possessed the ability to develop and sustain several very deep, mature, and affectionately positive relationships.

Although some of Meriwether's behaviors could be interpreted to fit a diagnosis of Asperger's syndrome, the friendships he had and their deep and mutual nature weigh heavily against him suffering from an autism spectrum-related illness such as Asperger's syndrome, as proposed by Stephenie Ambrose-Tubbs in *Sacagawea Deserves the Day Off*.[40] Great naturalists require a degree of obsessive-compulsive behavior to be adept at detailed descriptions, such as those Lewis wrote of the several hundred new species of flora and fauna he collected. Having these tendencies in his personality does not necessarily mean that Meriwether was "on the spectrum" as these tendencies are not exclusive to that diagnosis. Writing in 2008, Ambrose-Tubbs suggested that Lewis had a mild version of "Asperger's," the term used in the 1994 edition of the *Diagnostic and Statistical Manual of Mental Disorders*, but the current (2013) DMS-5 has replaced this with the term "autism spectrum disorder." Current diagnostic criteria for autism spectrum disorder include deficits in developing, maintaining, and understanding relationships. There is too much evidence that Lewis was adept in developing and maintaining mutually fulfilling relationships to seriously consider this as the most accurate diagnosis.

The fact that Lewis had difficulty engaging in a long-term romantic relationship is an unresolved conundrum for many Lewis devotees. There seems to have been something in Lewis's personality to account for this, and authors have speculated about the reason. Some factors that resulted in his failure to marry are external to Lewis's personality.

The possible or even probable aversion of some women to live a frontier lifestyle could be one reason he never married. Internal factors also contribute to understanding Lewis's bachelorhood. We know that Lewis's capacity for empathy and caring had its limits when his anger was triggered. If we dissect Lewis's personality as a gentry-class male, with all the accoutrements of such an upbringing, and add to this his extraordinary self-confidence, his military demeanor with a certain inability to tolerate minor errors in others, and his exalted social position as a national hero and explorer, he may have come across to others as arrogant. It is not only possible but highly probable that he was perceived by females who were in the pool of possible life mates as very self-important and therefore a rather unattractive and difficult person to live with. Such a personality could have easily scared off many potential marriage-aged females, particularly young teenaged females, which, based on the historical record, was likely the case with some of Lewis's marital candidates.

It is also important to again highlight that Lewis had many significant losses during his childhood and adolescence; the impact of these losses cannot be dismissed. The death of his father when Lewis was five, the emotional loss of his mother six months later when she married his stepfather, a further emotional and physical loss around age twelve when his mother, stepfather, and most of his siblings moved to Georgia from Virginia, and then the loss of his stepfather, who passed away when Lewis was almost eighteen—all of these experiences at these different stages of his development would result in a lack of security in his sense of himself and would likely cause him to doubt his ability to establish and maintain a long-term intimate relationship with a woman.

In analyzing any male's inability to establish a romantic relationship with a female, the factor of sexual orientation must be considered. Lewis expressed romantic attraction to and interest in several females before his death, and on more than one occasion during the expedition commented in the journals about his appreciation of "handsome" Indian women. Although we will never be able to know for certain what Lewis's sexual orientation was, these writings weigh in favor of Lewis having a heterosexual orientation.

Another important capacity in mental functioning, according to the PDM-2, is *self-esteem regulation and quality of internal experience*.[41] This is related to our level of self-confidence and how positively or negatively we feel about ourselves. Lewis's success in his military career is evidenced by promotions in rank, which provided him with a sense of himself as very competent and capable in his professional life.

Being a member of the gentry likely created a sense in Lewis that he was superior to others in some respects, especially in terms of master-slave relations. This was part of his cultural DNA. His sense of superiority to those he perceived as his social inferiors was most unattractively presented to the public in his scathing review in 1807 of the publication reporting on the events of the expedition authored by Sergeant Patrick Gass and his comments on the advertisement by Private Robert Frazer of his intention to publish his journal. Lewis went so far as to deny his acquaintance with these expedition members by mentioning what he referred to as "several unauthorized and probably some spurious publications now preparing for the press, on the subject of my late tour to the Pacific Ocean by individuals entirely unknown to me." He arrogantly and insultingly described Frazer as "only a private who was entirely unacquainted" with any scientific matters and could provide "merely a limited detail of our daily transactions." Heaping more insults upon Frazer, Lewis added, regarding all unauthorized publications about the expedition, "I presume that they cannot have stronger pretensions to accuracy of information than that of Robert Frazer."[42] His rather ungracious evaluation of the value of Private Frazer's reports on the expedition identified Frazer as perhaps the *least capable* member of the Corps to provide an accurate report.

The publisher of the Gass edition of the expedition journals, which went to press in 1807, took Lewis to task with a public letter to a newspaper that ridiculed Lewis's arrogance and disapproval of the Gass diary, including a scathing comment about Lewis: while "your Excellency was star-gazing, and taking celestial observations, he [Gass] was taking observations in the world below."[43] Such public embarrassment was no doubt a knife to the heart of Lewis's self-perception.

Perhaps the most important two affirmations in Lewis's life occurred when Jefferson selected him to be his personal secretary and later appointed him as the commander of the expedition, which undoubtedly strengthened Lewis's sense of himself as important, competent, and very special. Optimal functioning in this capacity would be identified as holding a realistic view of oneself as a worthy human being who was essentially no better or worse than anyone else—as someone who was "good enough." In other words, Lewis's inner belief that he was valued by others and led a meaningful life was generally strong most of the time, although there were instances when he experienced feelings of inadequacy and vulnerability, his positive self-view was disrupted, and his self-confidence suffered a blow. We can also observe that some of his experiences of rising up the ranks in regard to his accomplishments both in the army and in the Masonic Temple likely contributed to a sense of himself as more special than most people, creating what we might call arrogance or an inflated sense of his self-importance. Bates certainly perceived Lewis in this light. All of the public adulation Lewis encountered after his return in 1806 would have only served to magnify such a personality trait.

Our optimal mental functioning depends in part on our capacity for *impulse control and regulation*, the seventh of the twelve capacities presented in the PDM-2.[44] We can all relate to experiences in which we feel strong and sudden urges or desires to take immediate action. Such impulses may be relatively easy or hard to resist acting upon, depending on the person. For example, individuals diagnosed with attention-deficit/hyperactivity disorder (ADHD) characteristically have significant difficulty taking turns in circumstances requiring patience, and they may often interrupt others who are talking. Individuals struggling with substance use disorders have difficulty refraining from acting on their impulses to drink alcohol or use drugs.

A person is rated highly on this capacity if they can express their impulses in ways that are appropriate for their culture and the situation at hand. On the other hand, a relatively weak capacity to regulate impulses appropriately does not bode well for effective functioning in relationships at home or work. Anger and frustration are normal emotions when we do not get what we want, and how we manage them can mean the difference between our finding a constructive solution to a problem with a coworker and implementing it in a way that satisfies both parties (e.g., by feeling angry yet maintaining a calm demeanor and talking through potential solutions using a calm and respectful tone of voice) and ending up in jail facing an assault charge.

The range of expression of impulses from appropriate to inappropriate depends on the context in which it occurs. A good illustration of this capacity can be found in Lewis's treatment of the Blackfeet man killed at the Two Medicine Fight Site. Lewis perceived and understood the behavior of the would-be thieves as direct threats and insults to him and his men, which, in fact, they most certainly were. But Lewis's interpretation of the Blackfeet's actions led to his emotional response of leaving the Jefferson peace medal hanging around the neck of one of the men they had killed "that they might be informed who we were."[45] It was not sufficient for Lewis to remove himself and his team from the area of conflict and thus escape a profoundly dangerous situation. There were only four of them, and they were about a hundred miles from the nearest help. But in that situation, Lewis's honor was offended, and he interpreted the actions of the Blackfeet as a direct insult. For a man like Lewis, such an insult could not go unanswered—just as both Lieutenant Elliott's insult and Bates's offensive behavior could not be ignored. At the Two Medicine Fight Site, the insult to Lewis's honor resulted in his decision to leave the medal around the neck of the dead warrior as a sign that in some way alleviated the insult in Lewis's mind by metaphorically rubbing this powerful tribe's nose in the dirt. This act, at least in Lewis's mind, allowed him to feel and communicate his sense of superiority to the Blackfeet tribe. While Lewis's response of killing people who were trying to steal his horses and weapons and who he perceived as trying to kill him could be considered appropriate for the context in which he found himself, it could be argued that his action of leaving the peace medal around the neck of the dead Indian was arrogant and ill advised.

How we defend against awareness of our feelings is the subject of the eighth capacity of interest to us in understanding Lewis. This is labeled *defensive functioning*. Defenses are "automatic psychological responses to internal or external stressors and emotional conflicts."[46] They protect us from painful realities, feelings, thoughts, and memories. We all use defense mechanisms to cope with our feelings. The question is, which one(s) are we using? The lower the level of the defense, the greater the degree to which reality is distorted and therefore the greater degree to which it is maladaptive and dysfunctional. As a general rule, individuals who use what is referred to as *higher-level* defenses are considered *neurotic*, while those using *lower-level* defenses are considered *psychotic*. The higher the level of defense, the greater the ability to see reality for what it is—painful though that reality might be. The analysis of this capacity in Lewis is key to my assertion that Lewis functioned at a neurotic level because he could generally view reality accurately.

Defense mechanisms generally operate outside our conscious awareness, and the higher our level of stress, the more likely we are to employ them. In the last months of Lewis's life, the threats of loss of his reputation and financial security were intense. It is my belief, based on what we know about what occurred in the final weeks of his life, that he was experiencing so much anger, hurt, and betrayal that he struggled mightily with processing his strong feelings. The sources of his pain were not targets that he could legitimately deal with by either pulling out his tomahawk or physically assaulting them, as had been his modus operandi along the Columbia River. His choices were to either turn these feelings in against himself or outwardly toward other people. If a relatively mentally healthy person encounters multiple stressors occurring simultaneously that cut deeper than the person's capacity to manage them constructively, such a person could easily decompensate and move from using higher- to lower-level defenses.

In the case of Lewis, I think it is highly likely that he used the defense known as *acting out*. This is a defense mechanism used when a person is unable to cope adequately with conflicted mental content by thinking about it and verbalizing it with words. Instead, they use their actions to express their feelings, without consideration of the negative consequences of their behavior. Such behaviors are usually impulsive and include some form of self-harm, including substance abuse and suicidal behavior. I think the documented reports of Lewis's excessive use of alcohol and his reported suicide attempts on the boat traveling down the Mississippi to Fort Pickering in 1809, where Captain Russell put him under house arrest for two weeks to sober up, are evidence of his acting out. The adverse effect and role played by his alcohol abuse in this scenario are impossible to overestimate. The probability that he relapsed into abuse of alcohol between the time he left the fort and his arrival at Grinder's Stand eleven days later is also documented during this time.

I think it is highly likely that Lewis, in a state of intoxication that greatly magnified his already very high level of anger and frustration (i.e., mental derangement), acted out his despair by turning it all inward and shooting himself in the early morning hours of October 11, 1809. Magnification of existing emotions is a well-recognized effect of alcohol.

If Lewis was suffering from deep depression and despair, adding alcohol abuse to that equation was deadly.

The ninth capacity of mental functioning is referred to as *adaptation, resiliency, and strength*.[47] When we are hit by the storms of life, this capacity speaks to how well (or poorly) we can effectively and constructively weather the resulting turmoil. Whether the storm is the loss of loved ones, financial security, or the endless list of childhood or adult traumas that can befall human beings, anyone can get knocked down in the turbulence. Getting back up depends on how strong we feel inside and our ability to turn hardships into opportunities for growth. Ernest Hemingway, who ironically ended up committing suicide despite all of his fame and fortune, wrote in *Farewell to Arms*, "Life breaks everyone and afterward many are strong at the broken places." This capacity involves "unusual and creative ways of dealing with challenges . . . strengths, such as empathy, sensitivity to others' needs and feelings, ability to recognize alternative viewpoints, and ability to be appropriately assertive."[48]

Throughout his life, Lewis demonstrated tremendous strength and ability to bounce back, both mentally and physically. During his court-martial, he fought back against what he believed to be false accusations threatening to end his budding military career—a situation he experienced as a grave injustice against him. He faced and survived numerous life-and-death situations during the expedition. A lot of evidence exists that Lewis functioned at a high level with regard to overcoming obstacles throughout most of his life. However, his ability to accomplish this while performing a job (for which he was, arguably, poorly suited) deteriorated dramatically in the last year and a half before he died—when the demons Gary Moulton described came calling.[49] For the man who described himself as possessing a "governing passion for rambling,"[50] Lewis the explorer was trying to force himself as a square peg into the round hole of a political administrator, and he felt pressured to interact with others whom he likely viewed as inferior to him. Combining this with the absence of a loving and supportive wife, Lewis began a steady emotional decline that, due to his use of alcohol, did not allow him to activate the more healthy functioning he may have used earlier in his life. His abuse of alcohol in his final months diminished his ability to be adaptive, resilient, and strong.

The final three of the capacities of mental functioning focus on what the PDM-2 describes as issues related to self-awareness and self-direction. I begin my discussion of the tenth capacity of mental functioning by remembering what Socrates said so aptly over 2,500 years ago: "the unexamined life is not worth living." The better we are able to stand outside ourselves and observe our own mental and internal life, the better we can understand ourselves and use this information to help us learn, grow, and develop to our fullest potential. These elements are known as *self-observing capacities (psychological mindedness)*.[51] If we are in the higher range of functioning in this area, we are able to reflect on what has happened in our past, what is happening in the present, and what we anticipate about the future as well as consider how these interact in complex ways. If our ability to observe ourselves diminishes, so does our interest and/or motivation to understand ourselves more deeply. Those who lack self-observing skills, who are not interested in understanding their behavior, are destined to experience the frustrations of life with little or no self-insight and therefore with little ability to alter their behavior. The heavy use of alcohol greatly diminishes any possibility of self-observation.

Stress can also negatively impact this capacity, making it harder for us to be aware of another's subjective experiences and minimizing our appreciation that they might have reacted in a certain way because they are a different person and have different wants and needs than we do. For example, in the absence of major stressors, when someone does not return our phone call or respond to an email, we may be able to reflect on this and be able to take into account various possible explanations—"Maybe they are very busy taking care of something else that is a higher priority at the moment" or "Maybe they never received my email because I mistyped the address—I'll send them another one, just in case that happened." If we are highly psychologically minded, we will be able to consider such alternative possibilities even under stress. Those who operate with little capacity in this area will likely decide that the person in question is purposely ignoring them and will hold on to this opinion without considering alternative explanations. Once again, the heavy use of alcohol, which intensifies any preexisting emotions, would serve as a very negative influence on our ability to exercise healthy, constructive reactions to negative emotions.

It would appear that Lewis's ability to have insight into himself and others was strong when he was not stressed, as evidenced by his expedition journal entry on his thirty-first birthday, upon which I have already commented in relation to Lewis's personality type. However, his capacity for self-insight deteriorated when he was stressed or insulted. There are numerous examples of this in Lewis's life. For example, this decline appears in Bates's description of his encounter with Lewis in the Masonic Lodge ballroom when Lewis sat down at a table with him and Bates got up and left. Lewis "saw red" and quickly lost his ability to be able to stay calm, provide himself with an "internal warning" that his anger had been the source of personal trouble in his past, or come up with any alternative explanation, such as, "Perhaps Bates is upset with me because he does not like the decisions I am making that conflict with his own. It has to be hard for him to work under my authority since he had so much more decision-making power before I arrived to take over the governorship. I will try to have a talk with him when we are back in the office next week and see if we can sort this all out." Instead, Lewis, in his state of marked agitation, felt the need to call for Clark's aid in this fiasco and very likely had to be restrained from demanding a duel or engaging in a physical fight with his secretary.

The next capacity related to self-awareness involves our sense of morality, also known as our superego or conscience. We all have internal standards and beliefs by which we judge ourselves and others, and we learn these starting in childhood. We approve or disapprove of our own behaviors (and even the presence of certain thoughts and feelings) in a way ranging from very harsh to very gentle. Thus, if we have been taught to be honest, when we find ourselves telling a lie we may react with either strong, mild, or even no guilt, depending on how strictly we adhere to our inner moral values and ideals. Known in the PDM-2 as the *capacity to construct and use internal standards and ideals*, this component of mental functioning is relevant to how flexibly (or inflexibly) we interpret the behavior of both ourselves and others.[52] A strongly developed ability in this arena takes into account the possession of well-formulated core beliefs and principles within ourselves but also the recognition of how our choices impact the lives of those around us. A relatively poorly developed capacity results in a more rigid approach to understanding self and others and a strong tendency to what might be referred to as "black-or-white thinking"—i.e., interpreting behavior and people as either "all bad" or "all good."

The capacity to build and use internal standards and ideals requires being mindful that different cultures may hold beliefs and values that vary from our own and takes into account that different people have different capacities. During the expedition, Lewis frequently noted the cultural beliefs of various tribes he encountered, beliefs that significantly differed from Euro-American beliefs. At times, he strayed from the simple recording of beliefs and failed to show any understanding of the tribe's situation, rendering personal judgments on an aspect of a native tribe's cultural values, behaviors, and physical appearance that he did not admire. His inability in this area can be seen in his unflattering descriptions of native women on the Pacific coast and his interpreted comments (based on reports from other tribes) about the powerful Blackfeet as "vicious, lawless and an abandoned set of wretches."[53] Lewis's behavior with several tribes during the return trip up the Columbia showed that he had little patience with and/or understanding of tribal ethics and that he lacked empathy for their state of dire poverty. His behavior during these times, manifested by his burning the canoes that could have been given to needy tribes and thus strengthened the expedition's prestige among the tribes, showed his relative inability to understand a culture other than his own. The examples of his threatening the imprudent man who threw the puppy into his lap and his dealing harshly with Indians who stole items from the expedition not only showed his lack of ability to be sensitive to other's cultural values and needs but also harmed the reputation of the expedition and violated Jefferson's directive to do everything within his power to encourage good relations with the tribes he interacted with. Once again, these are examples of times when Lewis's anger and arrogance got in his way.

In the PDM-2, the highest rating for this capacity is described as follows: "Internal standards support meaningful strivings and feelings of authenticity and self-esteem. Feelings of guilt are balanced with a measure of self-compassion, and so are used as signals for reappraising one's behavior. Others are viewed with a balance of compassion, empathy, and objective criticism."[54] If we look again at Lewis's journal entry on his thirty-first birthday as an illustration of his functioning in this capacity, we can see the presence of his tendency toward what we might call a *harsh superego*—that is, a leaning toward judging himself (and therefore others) through the lens of what a reasonable person would estimate was a rather unrealistic view of himself, given his strengths and talents. He had accomplished so much in his life, yet we see him describing himself as if he had accomplished relatively little. There existed a large gap between his perception of himself as he was and as he thought he should be (his ego ideal).

The twelfth and final capacity required for effective mental functioning according to the PDM-2 is *meaning and purpose*. We all create a story that we tell ourselves (and others) about what we believe to be the meaning and purpose of our life. To construct this, we must be able to reflect on our beliefs, values, actions, and attitudes and on what we consider our philosophy of life and our spirituality (or lack of it), which may or may not include formal religious affiliation. Those who function highly in this capacity "show a clear, unwavering sense of purpose and meaning, along with an intrinsic sense of agency and the ability to look outside the self and transcend immediate situational concerns. . . . New situations and relationships are approached with an open, fresh perspective."[55] Having a sense of agency means having a sense that we have some degree of control over the direction in which we are steering our own ship, despite the winds and waves that may crash against it. The less well developed this ability is, the more likely we are to experience life as meaningless and directionless and ourselves as isolated and alienated from other people. As a result, the doubts we experience about our worth and purpose in life can be profound.

We have every indication from what we know of Lewis that he had a very strong sense of purpose for his life. He always approached his duties with an unshakeable attitude of persistence, determination, hard work, and diligence. His philosophy of life, as he stated in his journal entry on his thirty-first birthday, was to live more for humankind than for himself. He held lofty ideals and set all his strength on fulfilling them. He did so until the base of his supportive structure and foundation began to give way beneath him in the form of the withdrawal of government support for everything he needed to accomplish his tasks. Lewis's patriotism and his desire to see his family succeed were core values and principles that gave meaning to his life. When his financial future was threatened by the U.S. government, this was a direct assault on his identify. His life narrative up until the last few months of his life had led him to expect that this support would always be available—and the shock of discovering that this was not the case, which was far more insulting and devastating to his future than any previous wound caused by any human, caused him to falter and collapse emotionally.

If Lewis had been surrounded by the emotional support of a loving wife and a large extended family, as William Clark was, there might have been a different end to the story of his life. As bad fortune would have it, Lewis had only a very brief and limited safety net in the person of Captain Gilbert Russell, who undoubtedly treated him with kindness, compassion, friendship, and understanding during his convalescence at Fort Pickering in the weeks before his death. Russell and Fort Pickering were a haven of respite for Lewis. But his short stay with Russell was insufficient to put Lewis back on track to lasting mental health. Dr. Benjamin Rush had warned the medical community against the premature discharge of a patient such as Lewis, citing his experience of seeing such unstable patients kill themselves. Russell, however, allowed Lewis to leave for Washington with a vastly insufficient aftercare plan and attended to by a man who was reportedly fond of whiskey. Lewis's travel companion, Neelly, was completely unable to provide proper supervision and support for Lewis as he continued his overland trip to Washington. Neelly engaged in what alcohol rehabilitation counselors refer to as "enabling behavior" by supplying Lewis with additional alcohol. This scenario was reported by Gilbert Russell after Lewis's death. Lewis's relapse resulted in the need to stop and rest en route at the Chickasaw Agency for two days as Lewis was once again reported by Neelly to be "at times, deranged in mind."[56] As noted in chapter 8, it is extremely unlikely that this mental disease was the result of a case of cerebral malaria.

Underlining Neelly's report is the letter from Russell, in which he wrote,

> [B]y much severe depletion during his illness he had been considerably reduced and debilitated, from which he had not entirely recovered when he set off, and the weather in that country being yet excessively hot and the exercise of traveling, too severe for him; in three or four days he was again affected

with the same mental disease. He had no person with him who could manage or controul him in his propensities and he daily grew worse untill he arrived at the house of a Mr. Grinder.[57]

It seems highly probable that Russell was referring to Lewis's propensity to abuse alcohol. The use of the word "propensity" *refers directly to a behavior, not a disease.* Russell's word choice also fits the use of the word "habit" used by Jefferson about the negative effects of Lewis's behavior in his final days. Both men were obviously referring to a behavior manifested by Lewis. Neither "propensity" nor "habit" was referring to malaria (see chapter 8).

If Clark or Jefferson had been with Lewis to provide some emotional support, or if Lewis had not been drinking, his demons would have been greatly diminished and would not have led him to feel such overwhelming despair.

The Subjective Experience (S Axis)

The third and final dimension of the PDM-2 composite relates to the subjective experiences people have of their symptoms.[58] The emphasis in this dimension is on looking at a constellation of symptoms present in any given individual and asking, "What is it like for this person to have the symptoms they have?" In Lewis's case, "What was it like for him to be depressed or experience a substance use disorder?"

Anxiety and depression are symptoms that are present in most psychiatric disorders and may provide some validity to the idea that as human beings we are all more similar than we are different. The opposite side of this coin is that even though these symptoms are very common, every person experiences depression in their own unique way. As a thirty-five-year-old man who had worked very hard to accomplish much professional success in his life, seeing it all come crashing down in a relatively short period of time would have been devastating for Lewis. He probably thought, "I have worked much too hard and for too long for this to be happening to me." When so many external stressors were compounding so quickly during the last months of his life, it is understandable that Lewis would experience the strong feelings of anger, hopelessness, and helplessness typically found in depression.

The wish to self-soothe his painful emotions with alcohol would also be understandable, given its immediate ability to numb painful emotions.

Lewis undoubtedly felt very bad about his situation and, perhaps equally important, due to his Enlightenment worldview, he felt bad about feeling bad. He wanted desperately to trust people and to feel positive about life, but all of the circumstances surrounding him greatly damaged that view, resulting in distrust and anger toward people and an all-encompassing negative attitude toward life. Lewis's depression was produced not only by his external circumstances but also by his internal perception of them. It is far more painful for someone who expects to get a beautiful cake for their birthday to receive a stale loaf of bread than it is for someone who has become accustomed to starving to receive that same loaf of bread.

In sum, my diagnostic impressions are that Lewis had the *type* of personality that was primarily of an *obsessive-compulsive style*, with *depressive and narcissistic tendencies*. My conclusion is that he operated at a *neurotic level* within this style, based on how effectively he functioned overall throughout most of his life. He had many strengths, talents, and abilities that he used to very full potential, and he possessed what mental health professionals might refer to as a lot of *ego strength*. When stressed by negative interpersonal interactions, he seems to have employed defenses against his painful feelings of helplessness and anger by *acting out*. The powerful effect of Lewis's likely excessive alcohol use on his undoing at the end of his life cannot be overestimated. He used it to self-soothe his emotions, but in doing so he decreased his ability to make wise, rational decisions. Without the emotional support he needed to help him maintain his sobriety, it is reasonable to believe he turned his anger inward, bringing about a tragic end to a brave person who in reality had accomplished a great deal in his brief life.

Historical reports by William Clark, William Carr, Mahlon Dickerson, and Thomas Jefferson point out that Meriwether Lewis was an intelligent, honorable, honest, and well-meaning man. Our response to how Lewis coped with the painful circumstances that emerged at the end of his life needs to include not condemnation but sympathy and compassion and the understanding that "there but for the grace of God go I."

Chapter 13

Meriwether Lewis and the Second Man on the Moon

How few there are who have courage enough to own their faults, or resolution enough to mend them.
—Benjamin Franklin

During the bicentennial commemoration of the Lewis and Clark Expedition in 2005, Americans were treated to an excellent thirteen-hour public radio production narrated by Peter Coyote and hosted by Clay Jenkinson, titled *Unfinished Journey: The Lewis and Clark Expedition*, that covered various aspects of the expedition in an informative and entertaining manner. I (David) was privileged to participate in two of these programs, entitled "Traditions of Medicine Meet in the American West" and "The World of Lewis and Clark."

One of the other programs in the series was entitled "The First Space Race."[1] During this episode, Coyote started the program by stating, "The race for the Pacific Ocean and the race for the moon are linked across two hundred years of American history." The episode explored the similarities between the two endeavors and the scientific, administrative, and political factors that enabled their successes. The difficulties in fulfilling each of these massive undertakings and the success of each event were very well dramatized.

At least as interesting as the basic facts of these historically important trips is the life of the second man to step foot on the moon during the Apollo 11 trip in July 1969, Colonel Buzz Aldrin. In many ways, Aldrin's life after returning from the moon parallels the post-expedition life of Meriwether Lewis. Clay Jenkinson, in his book *The Character of Meriwether Lewis*, touches on this same analogy, but, with our emphasis on the medical and psychological aspects of Lewis's life, we believe it is essential that we examine this topic from our point of view.

Edwin Eugene Aldrin Jr., better known to the world as "Buzz," enjoyed a life that was in many ways phenomenally successful. Aldrin's intelligence and his ability to accomplish demanding tasks and function under pressure are the essence of the bravery and abilities of the men and women of the legendary United States space program. Buzz graduated third in the class of 1951 from the U.S. Military Academy with a degree in mechanical engineering. He was then commissioned into the U.S. Air Force and, as many military superstars do, became a fighter pilot, serving in the Korean War. He flew sixty-six missions and shot down two MIG jets in air-to-air combat. With an illustrious military career already behind him in his late twenties, Aldrin went on to earn a doctorate in astronautics at the Massachusetts Institute of Technology and was selected as a member of the NASA Astronaut Corps in the 1960s. His first space flight was on Gemini 12, and he spent five hours in extravehicular activity tethered to the capsule by a cord.[2] One might imagine that floating around outer space, several hundred miles above the earth at the end of a line attached to your command capsule, might rival Lewis's experience at the Great Falls in 1805 that he wrote about so effusively in a journal entry. Buzz was the Meriwether Lewis of the twentieth century in terms of both accomplishment and public recognition. He had everything to live for, had no apparent mental health issues, and by any objective evaluation was the best of the best.

Meriwether Lewis had also achieved much in his remarkable army career by the time he was in his mid-twenties. His rise to stardom did not result from Korea, MIT, or NASA but from a direct invitation from Thomas Jefferson to come to Washington and become his personal secretary in 1801. This quantum leap upward in Lewis's life and the elevated status in American society he enjoyed cannot be overstated. If you can imagine being stationed at a frontier army outpost, performing rather mundane duties, and then one day receiving a letter from the president informing you that you would become a member of his family and work in the president's home, you may be able to tap into the excitement Lewis must have felt upon receiving Jefferson's invitation. As Lewis made his way back to Washington to assume his duties, his heart must have been lighter than air. He no doubt was nearly floating on his horse as he rode along dusty and muddy roads lined with budding green broadleaf trees in a springtime eastern United States forest.

The Soviet Union launched its Sputnik satellite in 1957, threatening America with the possibility of being number two in the space race to the moon. The gauntlet had been thrown down. As my Slovenian physics professor Aleš Strojnik told my physics class at Arizona State University in 1982, "As Sputnik orbited the earth, it sounded off a 'beep, beep, beep' over Moscow, and over Washington it was 'ha, ha, ha'"! Alexander Mackenzie, the intrepid Scottish explorer of Canada, was the English version of Sputnik in late eighteenth-century America. Mackenzie reached the Pacific Ocean on July 20, 1793, after crossing the vast Canadian area of North America, putting the United States in peril of being shut out of the settlement and possession of the western continent.

The presidents in both these eras were justifiably alarmed. President John Kennedy answered the call and entered the United States into a fully committed race against the Soviet Union to become the first country to reach the moon. President Thomas Jefferson realized that it was imperative to beat England, Spain, France, and Russia in the exploration and settlement of the western North American territories. Just as *Unfinished Journey* portrayed, the Corps of Discovery engaged in the first "space race" and Lewis was the man who was expected to make it all happen. To achieve the purposes outlined for the expedition, Lewis, like Buzz Aldrin, was the best of the best.

Both Lewis and Aldrin were born to do great things. From the time he was young, Lewis was familiar with the outdoor life and had many skills that made him the perfect candidate for the job he would ultimately assume. Although he lacked the academic background of Aldrin, who had a doctorate from MIT, Lewis was nevertheless bright, inquisitive, and able to soak up important information. The two men—Lewis the explorer and outdoorsman and Aldrin the pilot and astronaut—were perfect physical specimens. Both were fearless and a bit cocky and self-confident; both were asked by the U.S. president to accomplish great tasks for their country; both were looking for a challenge and found it doing exactly what they loved most.

Aldrin, as he flew through space at 17,500 miles per hour, floated in open space attached to a cord linked to Gemini 12, and then set foot on the moon in 1969, could no doubt echo Lewis's comments 164 years earlier during a fine spring day in present-day North Dakota. As Lewis was leaving Fort Mandan on April 7, 1805, his entry in the journals reveals perhaps more about who he was and what was important to him than anything else he ever wrote during his more than two years on the trail: "I could but esteem this moment of my departure as among the most happy of my life."[3] We believe that moment in Lewis's life was just as he noted; it must have been the very best that he ever experienced.

When Buzz Aldrin returned from the moon, his life's course was comparable to that of Meriwether Lewis after his return from twenty-eight months on the trail across North America. Although the technology surrounding the events of their separate lives was very different, the public viewed these men and their positions in society as equally remarkable. Lewis became the illustrious personage everyone wanted to see, touch, and hear. Endless parties, awards, and ego-flattering conversations with the leaders of the day made his being insulted by Lieutenant Elliott and impertinent Native Americans back on the Columbia River distant memories. Lewis was the toast of every town he entered and was appropriately recognized as a hero. When Aldrin returned, he was celebrated by multi-city ticker-tape parades, dinners, international travel, and the awarding of numerous medals and citations. They were each on top of their respective world.

Both men had gone on life-altering expeditions. How could Aldrin or Lewis ever explain their experiences to another person who had not experienced the thrill of setting foot on the dust of the moon, watching the earth rise over the horizon, or being the first Euro-American to view the Great Falls and the Gates of the Mountains or to face down a charging grizzly bear with an empty rifle and an espontoon? Aldrin was often asked the obvious question of what it was like to be on the moon. He described it as "magnificent desolation."[4] There is no doubt that Lewis, in all of his encounters with the admiring public, was asked similar questions about those vast unsettled lands to the West. We can only wish to have been able to listen to his wonderful stories.

But, within weeks after his return to earth, it dawned on Aldrin that "magnificent desolation" was an appropriate way to describe his post-flight state of mind. By late 1969, after prolonged touring, seemingly endless speeches, and luncheons and hand-shaking with heads of state around the world, Aldrin was physically and mentally exhausted. He became depressed and turned increasingly to his favorite drink, Scotch whiskey, to soothe his depression. One question often asked about the post-expedition depression Lewis may have suffered from might be redirected to Aldrin: What in the world did Buzz Aldrin have to be depressed about? But we need not question this as Aldrin has extensively described his emotional predicament in his own words.

After Lewis's return, he went on a prolonged tour of the eastern United States, met with political and scientific leaders, and attended celebrations held in his honor. Everything seemed to be pointing to an upward path for his life, but there is every indication that he too started down a road to emotional depression. His fall was perhaps not as rapid as that experienced by Aldrin, but nevertheless, the process began. By every report from Jefferson and Clark and the others in the chain of letters that followed his life's path toward his death in 1809, Lewis experienced a set of circumstances that led him to a state of depression. The reasons for this are numerous. For now, we simply note that Lewis's life was following a path analogous to Aldrin's: a strange mixture of public adulation, fame, and personal agony.

Both Lewis and Aldrin were in military careers, and despite the two centuries separating them, both were living and training with hard-drinking men whose habits were both accepted, if not encouraged, by their commanders. This is undeniable. Lewis openly told his mother of "the oceans of whiskey" available to him in 1794 and bragged that he was "able to share it with the heartiest fellow in camp."[5]

Although Lewis was accused of drinking at the time of his incident with Lieutenant Elliott in 1795, four witnesses testified that he was not observably intoxicated. Lieutenant Elliott's party took place inside of his house, and the attendees were drinking brandy. The facts that drinking among the officer corps was ubiquitous in that era and that questions about Lewis's state of intoxication were asked at the court-martial hearing strongly imply that drinking to excess in the army of that time was common.

Surprisingly, Aldrin, although he was a member of a superelite group of pilots and astronauts, experienced similar attitudes and practices. Aldrin writes, "Almost everyone I knew drank alcohol in some measure, astronauts included. The only astronauts who didn't drink while I was a part of NASA were Alan Bean and Bill Anders. For me, drinking was not a problem; it was simply something I did to relax. At least that's what I told myself."[6] This sounds like a comment that may have been made at the party thrown in 1795 by Lieutenant Elliott.

Aldrin's family had a history of mental illness manifested by some type of mood disorder. Both his mother and his grandfather had committed suicide. He likely had a genetic predisposition to mental illness, and when he tried to answer the question of what he should do now that he had gone to the moon, Aldrin became increasingly depressed. He was suffering from the "hypochondriac affections" and "melancholia" of the twentieth century. As many people would do, Aldrin sought out comfort from a source that his reason told him would offer some relief to his depression: alcohol. Emotional pain is accepted by professional alcohol rehabilitation specialists as a predisposing factor for alcohol use disorder.

In their attempt to discredit the idea that Lewis suffered from post-expedition depression and alcohol abuse, several Lewis biographers have asked questions about Lewis's mental state and alcohol use in a way that implies that it was improbable that he was either depressed or abused alcohol. If you simply replace Aldrin's name with Lewis's, you can see the futility of such arguments. Just as previous Lewis authors have noted, Lewis was a fighter, not a quitter—as was Aldrin. Aldrin was immensely successful and enjoyed phenomenal public adulation—yet, by his own admission, he was depressed.

In an attempt to discredit the notion of Lewis's alcohol use, the question is often posed concerning Jefferson's decision to give command of the Corps of Discovery to an "alcoholic"—to Lewis. These questions can be asked about Aldrin with even more negative implications. If NASA knew, in the relatively enlightened times of the 1960s, that Buzz Aldrin was an alcoholic, why would they have chosen him to be a Gemini/Apollo astronaut and sent him to the moon? If Aldrin was an alcohol abuser, why wouldn't the NASA medical staff have known about it, and why didn't his fellow astronauts report him? Surely such a problem in one of their elite astronauts would have been noticed by such a sophisticated group as NASA. The Gemini and Apollo missions took place in a time when such problems were much more in the consciousness of both medical science and the public than during the time of Lewis, when America was locked in a culturally accepted, whiskey-soaked period of alcohol abuse. If we apply the questions designed to show the improbability of alcohol abuse by Lewis to Aldrin and consider the reality of Aldrin's life, we are left with the conclusion that the belief that Lewis could not have been a heavy drinker is naive.

Aldrin tried in various ways to both deny and address his depression. Unlike Lewis, who apparently never had a successful and loving relationship with a woman, Aldrin had more than one. Aldrin's multiple love interests only supplied a momentary relief from his increasing disillusionment, however, and, since the alcohol's effect was at least temporarily helpful, he decided to increase his drinking.

In July 1971, Aldrin hoped to start a new position as commandant of the test pilot school at Edwards Air Force Base in California. Things seemed to be looking up. But the novelty of that command was quickly tarnished, and he finally sought medical help—not for his depression or alcohol use but for his back and neck pain.[7] Aldrin, with all of his intelligence and his living in an era with relatively good awareness of alcohol abuse, was still unable to face his drinking problems and was instead complaining of back and neck pain. He visited his Air Force flight surgeon and was referred to Brooks Medical Center in San Antonio, Texas, where the severity of his problems started to be identified.

When Lewis returned from the expedition, like Buzz Aldrin, he was courted by the intelligentsia, heads of government, and the adoring public. But, given that Lewis was a man whose "darling project" was to head an expedition into the unknown, use his skills as a naturalist to describe plants and animals, and write glowing prose about the many adventures he lived through, what type of satisfaction could he possibly find in attending never-ending parties with politicians slapping him on the back, being offered another drink, or being told how wonderful he was? If Lewis became so tired of the Shoshone "national hug"[8] upon meeting that tribe in August of 1805, one must wonder how much he would have enjoyed all the praise heaped upon him by politicians and dignitaries month after month? It was no doubt a welcome novelty for several weeks, but in all probability Lewis, just like Aldrin, may have found all the public adoration tedious after a while—and perhaps even irritating.

When Aldrin finally received medical attention at Brooks Hospital, he took the opportunity, with the help of modern medicine, to explore the problems behind his aimlessness and depression. He explored his family history of mental illness and his strained relationship with his father in his psychotherapy, and his mother's and grandfather's suicides were recognized as significant factors in his own depression. Aldrin had the best physicians of his day addressing his issues. The medications they had in the pharmacopeia were not as effective as many we use today for Aldrin's types of problems, but nevertheless, his treatment was vastly superior to anything that Lewis ever received.

When Lewis became ill, he had no Brooks Medical Center to turn to for help. He had no physicians who understood the psychological issues he faced that were contributing to his problems. All Lewis had, in any realistic assessment, was a physician who was ill prepared to treat almost any physical or mental problem and who practiced in a culture that accepted and even encouraged alcohol abuse.

So, let us revisit and expand some of the common questions asked by Lewis and Clark authors and apply them to Aldrin's situation. If NASA knew that there was mental illness in Aldrin's family, why would they have let him become an astronaut? If Aldrin was an alcoholic or even a hard drinker, why would NASA have allowed him to go to the moon? These are entirely legitimate questions and are just as easy and reasonable to answer for Aldrin as they are for Lewis.

NASA saw nothing in Aldrin, given his brilliant career at West Point and in the Air Force, that would have suggested any mental illness at the time he began his career as an astronaut. Even though he admitted to drinking, nearly all the other NASA trainees drank as well. There was nothing unusual about it. Aldrin was obviously not consistently drinking to excess during his years as an astronaut. Aldrin's drinking took place in an America that was substantially more aware of the problem of alcohol abuse than was the world of Meriwether Lewis. Although there was likely some significant drinking during Lewis's years with

Jefferson, just as with Aldrin, this was accepted, expected, and given a pass by everyone (see chapter 4). Having a problem with alcohol was vastly more common and expected among men (and women) in Lewis's day than in Aldrin's. Since NASA looked the other way when astronaut trainees abused alcohol in the 1960s, why would anyone in Washington in 1801–03, or Frederick Bates in the rough-and-tumble frontier town of St. Louis, have been concerned about Lewis's alcohol intake? Comparing these two scenarios makes any thought that Lewis's behavior would have raised a red flag seem ludicrous. Clearly, Lewis's and Aldrin's behavior did not and would not have rung any alarm bells with their colleagues because it was common, accepted behavior.

Despite the medical interventions Aldrin obtained, by 1973 Aldrin's marriage had failed and his drinking had also spiraled out of control. These two sad occurrences were, without a doubt, related. He attended a twenty-eight-day rehabilitation program and remarried, but within two years he and his second wife had divorced and he had fallen off the wagon again. He acknowledged that he suffered from depression, yet he failed to acknowledge his abuse of alcohol. This is strikingly common with those who suffer from alcohol use disorder. Even an astronaut failed to recognize that alcohol was not a soothing and benign medication to help him cope with depression but was actually fueling his increasing depression and dependence on alcohol.

Social and career disappointments were factors in the lives of both Lewis and Aldrin. After landing on the moon, Aldrin wanted to be named the commandant of the Air Force Academy but was passed over and assigned to work in the Air Force Test Pilot program. Although Lewis was not passed over for any expected promotion, he was assigned to a position that he was capable of performing but that was not a good fit for his personality and talents.

Lewis was faced with Aldrin's problem of finding purpose in activities that he was more than capable of performing but was not well suited to and did not particularly enjoy. What do you do after training for years to fulfill your passionate desire to become an astronaut and then fly to and walk on the moon? What could Lewis do after becoming the president's personal secretary at twenty-six, rubbing elbows with famous and powerful people who helped to prepare him for his upcoming expedition (his "darling project"), traveling by land and water across an uncharted continent, doing scientific research, and then coming home to fame and a promising future? Instead of realizing his opportunities for happiness, he was thrust into a world filled with political intrigue. The result? Lewis, like Aldrin, became depressed.

Psychologist Tom Horvath notes that Lewis in 1804 "knows where he starts, where he's going, and the route is roughly known. Day-to-day challenges were met with ingenuity and persistence. This is a different kind of adversity than having to walk into a room and convince people that you are a worthwhile person."[9] The latter scenario represented the personal set of challenges faced by the conquering explorer turned governor. This type of situation, where one attempts to fit a square peg into a round hole, is experienced by most people. This is neither a novel nor a contentious concept.

Given the fact that Jefferson wanted Lewis to complete the journals as soon as possible, Lewis's assignment to such a demanding position should have been postponed until after the journals were completed. This conflict only added to Lewis's troubles in St. Louis. This was all unnecessary. Jefferson had the power to avoid such a mistake but failed to realize the trap he had created for Lewis.

We think it impossible that walking on the moon and leading the Corps of Discovery did not significantly affect the egos of Aldrin and Lewis. They both were fully aware of their spectacular success. Both Lewis and Aldrin then experienced a succession of emotional blows that, quite predictably, had a terrible effect on their elevated sense of themselves.

Buzz Aldrin, as a commander of the Test Pilot School at Edwards Air Force Base in California, was responsible for training both test pilots in the Air Force as well as funneling some of these men into astronaut training. In a series of crashes in which two expensive planes were lost and three pilots were almost killed, the blame was placed on Aldrin. As a result, he was not promoted from colonel to brigadier general as he had hoped. He was informed by a four-star general that his school would no longer be supplying future astronauts to NASA. Astronaut training was what Aldrin knew, and that was taken away from him. The same general personally insulted him by saying, "Well, let me get this straight, Colonel Aldrin. Why do you call this place the Aerospace Research Pilot School? Don't you think a better name would be the

Air Force Test Pilot School?" Aldrin attempted to defend himself by replying, "We're trying to run a top-notch test pilot school and astronaut training facility here, sir." Aldrin recalled that the general "cut me off short" and added, "Colonel Aldrin, that's the problem. Why do you have that course here? . . . Oh, you came from NASA and you think you're hot stuff around here because you were an astronaut? Well, I don't."[10] It should be noted that this discussion took place in front of all of the junior officers involved in the program. This was a severe personal and public humiliation for Aldrin. Shortly after this episode, Aldrin moved on from his life as a retired astronaut, second man on the moon, international celebrity, etc., and began selling lawnmowers, Cadillacs, and VWs.

For Lewis, the publicly insulting letter from Gass's publisher that referred to him as "your Excellency," coupled with other degrading remarks in 1807, was similar to Aldrin's wounding by his superior officer. When Lewis received a letter from the War Department with more insulting comments about his alleged inappropriate use of government funds and the refusal to honor his expenditures, the heady days of his post-expedition glory must have seemed far in the past.

When victims of depression are down, it is a cardinal rule of mental health that their ability to respond to emotional assaults is more compromised than it would be if they were not in a depressed state of mind. After Aldrin produced his television ad for VW, he received a letter accusing him of being "un-American" because he had endorsed a German automaker. Aldrin observed, "Ordinarily I would have cast off such worthless drivel as the rumination of somebody-with-too-much-time-on-his-or-her-hands. But in my unsteady frame of mind, the letter had a devastating effect that fed into the familiar blue funk."[11] He made several more observations about his mental state during these times of emotional turmoil and reported on his "recurring apprehension about the future." He added, "As a man, a strong man, a let's-get-it-done-and-here's-how-to-do-it man, I was not entitled to fail; when I could not control the situation, feelings of inadequacy and frustration flooded over me." Aldrin's answer? "More and more, I turned to alcohol to ease my mind and see me through the rough times. Because I could handle my drinking—or so I thought—and could consume a lot of alcohol without becoming uncontrollably inebriated, I refused to see it as a problem. As far as I could see, there was nothing wrong. It was a time when almost everyone I knew was drinking heavily, so why not me?"[12] During Lewis's lifetime, when this exact set of behaviors was also rampant, it is easy to believe that he too could have written such a statement.

Buzz Aldrin's honor was grossly insulted, but Lewis's honor was arguably more front and center for him than it would later be for the second man on the moon. Aldrin was never court-martialed as the result of his reaction to a perceived slight of his honor, as was Lewis. At any slight to his honor, Lewis on repeated occasions displayed his verbal and sometimes physical wrath toward the offenders. Just like the boy who had hacked the goose to death in colonial America and the young Ensign Lewis who had cried and demanded "satisfaction" from Lieutenant Elliott in 1795, Governor Lewis would soon suffer insults to his honor that he could not ignore, understand, or accept. Once he assumed his duties as governor, the people insulting his honor were not relatively powerless Native Americans throwing puppies in his lap and stealing remnants of burned canoes out of a fire but malignant and clever politicians who were making his life miserable.

The roots of Lewis's personality issues may be found in the comments of Thomas Jefferson in his introduction to the 1814 edition of the expedition's journals. Jefferson, as someone who knew Lewis and his family personally and had spent significant time with Lewis himself, provides primary evidence of Lewis's underlying personal and familial tendency to depression or anxiety. Jefferson's linking Lewis's mental state with that of members of his family is both important and consistent with the modern medical understanding of the genetic predisposition to depression often found in families.

Lewis biographer Richard Dillon, as well as other Lewis scholars who are not well acquainted with the science of mental health, in their efforts to discredit Jefferson's observation of Lewis's "hypochondriac affections," grossly misstate Jefferson's position. Dillon writes that Jefferson "tended to damn Lewis as an insane suicidist."[13] We do not see Jefferson implying any such charge of insanity but instead understand him to be referring to Lewis as a person who had some degree of neurotic behavior. Neurotic people have a firm grasp on reality. Insane people lose that sense of reality. This is not just an esoteric point. This is important, and Dillon and others who support his line of reasoning, unaware of these distinctions, misstate the clinical situation and significantly err in their psychological interpretations of Lewis.

Dillon attempts to nullify the insightful comments of Jefferson by stating, "It was up to Jefferson to set things right, to make amends for his country's shabby treatment of its greatest explorer. . . . But he failed. . . . Jefferson later became convinced of a strain of insanity existing in the Lewis lineage—a strain no historian before or since has ever turned up."[14] In this strange line of reasoning, Dillon is arguing that we cannot believe Jefferson's statements, even though he was in a position to know them to be true, because no historian has been able to confirm them. Jefferson knew Lewis and his family personally. Just because we do not have documentation from other family members, this does not negate the truth of Jefferson's statements. This is a convoluted, straw-man argument. Jefferson's comment about Lewis's "hypochondriac affections" did not have the same meaning as Dillon's term "insanity," which he uses in a rather cavalier manner. The two are vastly different.

Other documentation related to Lewis's mental health include William Clark's specific and reliable statement in a letter to his brother on the day he learned that Lewis had died: "I fear O! I fear the waight of his mind has over come him."[15] This powerful statement makes the efforts by murder theorists to deny or minimize Lewis's mental health issues an exercise in futility. These same theorists challenge the assertion of Jefferson that he observed Lewis from time to time showing "hypochondriac affections." That term, as used by Jefferson, referred to anxiety, fear of disease, and possibly depression (see chapter 8).[16]

Most importantly, Lewis was not emotionally stable at this point in his life and was not enjoying success in his career. He was trying to make the best of his situation in St. Louis and was involved in both governmental and personal pursuits. Lewis's sense of honor would not allow him to knowingly perform at a low level. But all of the personality traits and behaviors that Lewis had developed prior to this time came right along with him on his departure from the public adulation in the East to the outskirts of civilization in St. Louis. He still had the tendency to lash out at others whose behaviors seemed insulting or incompetent, was short-tempered with the perceived stupidity of others (as displayed to Drouillard and Shields when they met the first Shoshone and scared him off in August 1805 near Lemhi Pass), and had a military commander type of personality, which would not suit him well in a political position where he lacked the complete authority he and Clark had shared during 1803–06. In addition, as his friend William Carr of St. Louis wrote, Lewis left St. Louis in September 1809 with his personal affairs in a state of derangement.

Lewis's many responsibilities, coupled with his drinking and depression, did not permit him to progress with either finishing the expedition's journals or even keep in contact with his close ally and friend Thomas Jefferson. As a result, Jefferson's emotional support and approval of Lewis, which no doubt had a substantially positive influence on Lewis's emotional health, started to erode. Secretary of War Henry Dearborn wrote to Lewis, "No communication except some Drafts for Money, has, for many Months, been received from the Executive of Louisiana." As Ambrose writes, "A worse rebuke quickly followed." Instead of a personal greeting at the start of fatherly correspondence to the explorer of the Missouri River and its tributaries, Jefferson's letter "opened with a complaint: 'Since I parted with you in Albemarle in Sept. last I have never had a line from you.'"[17]

This was Lewis's moment similar to when Buzz Aldrin's commanding general laid waste to Aldrin's ego. When the general addressed Aldrin's command-related failures and noted that he was not a big deal just because he was an astronaut, the effect on Aldrin, by his own admission was devastating. This letter from Jefferson likely had a similar effect on Lewis.

It is well documented by mental health professionals that turmoil in interpersonal relationships is a chief contributing factor in the development and/or worsening of a psychological mood disorder. Do people become depressed because they are unable to get along with others? Or, are people unable to get along with others because they are depressed? Well, the answer to both of those questions is "yes." (This same principle is true for alcohol use and depression). Psychologist Kay Redfield Jamison notes that depressed people "not only are influenced by the events in their lives, they also have a strong reciprocal influence on the world and people around them: they often alienate others with their anger, withdrawal, or violence."[18] Over and over again, Jamison notes, "intense interpersonal discord" is a key contributing factor in depression and suicide.[19]

The frightful relationship between Lewis and his secretary, Frederick Bates, was due to the close working relationship of these two people who were both prone to highly inflated self-honor, selfishness, self-confidence, and narcissism. Bates apparently hoped that once Lewis assumed the governorship, they would enjoy a collegial relationship. But, despite his stated intentions, Bates seems to us to be the ultimate personification of a self-absorbed bureaucrat—precisely the kind who might make another person's life miserable just because he could. Bates, who was the acting territorial governor of Louisiana during the months prior to Lewis's arrival, was undoubtedly insulted when Lewis fired a number of his appointees and took over command of the ship of state, relegating Bates, the governor, to a subordinate position. He did not like his demotion. Although the two men were Masonic Lodge brothers, there is no indication that they ever liked each other personally and every indication that they disliked each other intensely. This change in the command of Louisiana started a feud that would only escalate in future months.

Lewis's military mentality, thoroughly entrenched by his status as commander in chief of the Corps of Discovery and his sense of his own honor and importance resulting from the public attention he had received for the previous two years, did not sit well in a work situation that required multiple interactions with others, a team effort, and an ability to see and understand others' ideas and desires. Bates, by many reports, had a temper at least as short as Lewis's. When a Pennsylvanian addressed Bates's "barbarous conduct" toward Lewis, Bates responded with the following:

> I told you this morning that it was false—and I repeat that it is an impudent stupidity in you to persist the assertion. In return for the personal allusions with which you have honored me, I tender to you my most hearty contempt.... I pledge my word of honour that if you ever again bark at my heels, I will spurn you like a puppy from my path.[20]

The malignant character of Bates was brought forward by William Clark, who in July 1810 wrote that Bates was a "little animale whome I had mistaken as my friend," adding that he had "neither love nor respect for" the man.[21] Historian Jim Holmberg, notes that Clark made these accusations of Bates's honor during times when such comments could easily result in a duel; they were therefore not made without serious consideration.[22]

Bates went on to undercut Lewis's leadership in his letters to Washington politicians and members of the new Madison administration. This prompted the horrible, honor-destroying accusations from Secretary of War William Eustis, described by both Henry Clay and Albert Gallatin as utterly incompetent in any field. Eustis's derogatory comments as he refused federal payment of IOUs signed by Lewis carried the authority of the American government, condemning Lewis for failing to ask permission to spend money for various government assignments in Louisiana. With the federal government refusing to honor Lewis's financial commitments on behalf of the Upper Louisiana Territory, Lewis became anxious about his personal finances and the real possibility of financial ruin. As Clark wrote, "[H]is Crediters all flocking in near the time of his Setting out distressed him much."[23]

All this emotional distress was born from Lewis's sense of personal embarrassment and loss of honor. Lewis wrote,

> This occurrence has given me infinite concern as from it the fate of other bills, drawn for similar purposes, to a considerable amount cannot be mistaken. This rejection cannot fail to impress the public mind unfavourable with respec to me, nor is this consideration more painful than the censure which must arise in the mind of the Executive from my having drawn public monies without authority. A third, and not less, embarrassing circumstance attending the transaction is that my private funds are entirely incompetent to meet these bills, if protested.[24]

This anxious letter by Lewis harkens back to an earlier time in 1795 when, as a younger man, he addressed similar issues regarding his honor and its importance to his life. Responding to the accusations of Lieutenant Elliott during his court-martial trial, Lewis stated, "[I]t is very disaggreable to hobble through life with a broken reputation, I conceive the duty of every man to connect intimally [intimately], their life and reputation by all possible ties, to the end. That when the one makes its exit the other may also."[25]

The cumulative assault on Lewis's ego by the harshness of his friend and mentor Jefferson, the implications of the actions of the federal government under new and unfriendly leadership, and the interpersonal strife with Bates was far more challenging than anything that Lewis had ever encountered previously. Even the insult by Lieutenant Elliott in 1795 that caused Lewis "to be very much hurt" and to shed tears as a result of his loss of honor could not compare with the current situation. It is apparent from all reports that he was becoming despondent. This was not the result of some unspecified personal weakness, as proposed by some past Lewis authors, but the culmination of a storm of personality-assaulting circumstances imposed on a man with narcissistic tendencies who characteristically escalated any criticism to the level of interpersonal war. Lewis was depressed, and he was drinking to the point that he purchased over three hundred gallons of whiskey sometime in 1809.

Lewis and Buzz Aldrin had both led lives of great accomplishment and service, both were honest, and both ended up in positions that insulted their honor at the hands of lesser men. Both were far removed from the happiest days of their lives—Lewis leaving Fort Mandan in command of his "darling project" and Aldrin stepping off a ladder onto the gray, dusty surface of the moon.

Were Aldrin and Lewis just emotionally weak individuals? No. Lewis and Aldrin were men whose remarkable accomplishments were disappearing in the rearview mirror of their lives. The future was looking desolate for each of them, Aldrin due to his inability to ever match his experience of being the second man on the moon and Lewis due to the emotional fallout of a lack of intimate love, assaults on his character from individuals with the power to ruin his life and devastate his finances, and, most profoundly, his depression caused by these difficulties and his increasing use of alcohol to numb all his emotional pain.

Of all these factors, by far the most personally devastating for Lewis was his alcohol abuse. Alcohol abuse, in all cases, makes everything worse. This is a tragic and common scenario. Without honor and respect, Lewis said that his life was not worth living. For both Aldrin and Lewis, the immediate answer to their depression seemed to be found in a whiskey bottle. This scenario is so compelling and complete that the only thing missing is a video to confirm it.

We think it would be naive to believe that Lewis was not drinking heavily after his return to society. Are we to believe that, at all those parties staged in Lewis's honor after his return, during a time in America when hard liquor flowed like lemonade at a modern Fourth of July party, Lewis did not drink a significant amount of whiskey? And then, of course, the IOU signed by Lewis for eight barrels of whiskey certainly represents a problem for those who choose to deny he had such a habit.

Jefferson wrote after Lewis's death that Lewis's affliction "was probably increased by the habit into which he had fallen & the painful reflections that would necessarily produce in a mind like his."[26] The meaning of the term "habit" here is obviously, in the context of Jefferson's knowledge of the incidents leading to Lewis's death, referring to a state of alcohol abuse. In order to limit the implications of this, one biographer takes the position that "habit" is a reference to malaria, which we have shown is incorrect (see chapter 8).[27]

Clay Jenkinson allows for a wider interpretation of Jefferson's "habit" comment, including such possibilities as "whoring, masturbation, addiction to laudanum, sleeping through the day, or for that matter keeping to himself and avoiding the company of others."[28] Jenkinson also notes that there is no evidence in the journals of Lewis having a drinking problem.[29] We do not dispute this. But the journals only cover the time frame involved in the expedition, and for over a year of the expedition, the men had no access to whiskey. In addition, Lewis was happily engaged in his "darling project" during this period.

We agree with Jenkinson's assessment that Buzz Aldrin was able, due to expert substance abuse guidance, a loving and patient family, and other emotional supports, to conquer his problems. As of 2021, Aldrin is still living the life of the person who was the second man on the moon. Jenkinson also accurately noted that all of the emotional supports of a loving family and modern pharmaceutical treatment for depression that aided Aldrin in his recovery were totally absent for Lewis.[30] Lewis's inability or ultimate disinterest in finding a loving wife, total lack of effective medical treatment for his depression, and alcohol abuse were far more than he was able to handle. This does not in any way mean that Lewis emotionally weak. Given no effective intervention, very few people could emerge from this catastrophic combination of factors unscathed.

It is noteworthy that Lewis was without a doubt a very honest man. His friend Mahlon Dickerson, writing in his diary, paid tribute to his late friend as "the most sincere friend I ever had."[31] William Clark noted his sincere feelings for his friend and co-commander when he wrote, "I do not beleve there was ever an honest er man in Louisiana nor one who had pureor motives than Govr. Lewis."[32] Lewis's honesty and his resulting trust in benevolent human nature, as evidenced by his participation in the Freemasons (who encouraged their members to lead virtuous lives), and his belief in Jeffersonian Enlightenment thinking, did not work well for him once he became encumbered by the political world of self-serving and back-stabbing bureaucrats.

Buzz Aldrin was also an honest man. In what must be one of the most painful ironies in human history, the honesty of this U.S. Air Force fighter pilot, NASA astronaut who had earned a Ph.D., and the second man on the moon led to his failure at a Beverly Hills auto dealership. He was reportedly too honest to be a convincing car salesman.[33]

Both Meriwether Lewis and Buzz Aldrin led spectacularly successful lives in service to America. Their lives exhibit startling similarities in personality and achievement but not in outcome. Aldrin received the help and support he needed, and he survived and thrived—Lewis, sadly, did not.

Chapter 14
Murder or Suicide?

Be careful how you think; your life is shaped by your thoughts.
—*Proverbs 4:23 (Good News Translation)*

The essence of our research for this book has been interesting to us, and we hope the topics we cover have been enlightening for our readers. We have addressed a number of the issues that have been cited by various individuals as either the cause of or contributing factors to the tragic death of Meriwether Lewis. We have endeavored to honestly and fairly address the many opinions about these issues and have come to the inescapable conclusion that many of the previously published opinions, particularly when they involve issues of medicine or psychology regarding Lewis's life and death, are unsupportable and erroneous. Rather than the suicide arguments being "readily countered," as asserted by the late historian John Guice,[1] it seems to us, as a physician and clinical psychologist, that the exact opposite is true. Guice provided extensive testimony during the mock coroner's jury held in 1996, much of which reflected either a misunderstanding or a misrepresentation of the issues he addressed.[2] Clay Jenkinson provides a synopsis of Guice's forty arguments against Lewis's suicide in *The Character of Meriwether Lewis*.[3] In reading through Guice's list, the only medically related opinions that we agree with are that Dr. Ravenholt's theory of syphilis is implausible and that a forensic exam of Lewis's remains should be performed. His other medically and psychologically based opinions are either factually incorrect or do not reflect an accurate understanding of the issues involved.

Various Lewis authors and historians other than Guice have expressed their opinions through the years that Lewis did not commit suicide and that the case in favor of his suicide is so weak as to be nearly impossible. Olin Wheeler was one of the first of these modern writers to offer his opinion of the improbability of Lewis committing suicide. He expressed his doubts "that a young man of 35, the Governor of the vast Territory of Louisiana, then on his way from his capital to that of the nation, where he knew he would be received with all the distinction and consideration due his office and reputation, should take his own life."[4]

Lewis biographer Richard Dillon took on the mantle of clearing Lewis's name of the "crime" of suicide by writing, "Is it likely that the cause of Lewis's death was self-murder? Not at all. If there is such a person as the anti-suicide type, it was Meriwether Lewis. By temperament, he was a fighter, not a quitter. . . . Sensitive he was; neurotic he was not. Lewis was one of the most positive personalities in American history."[5] Dr. Eldon Chuinard attacked Thomas Jefferson's acceptance of Lewis's suicide with the accusation that Jefferson impugned the character of Lewis "It seems to me that Jefferson's ready acceptance of Lewis's death by suicide was a disgraceful way to treat a man."[6] More recently, Patricia Stroud in *Bitterroot: The Life and Death of Meriwether Lewis*, takes up the fight against Lewis's suicide and comes down on the side of murder.

Tony Turnbow, an excellent historical researcher, also believes Lewis was the victim of murder. Turnbow seems to take a more pro-murder than anti-suicide approach. He comes to his conclusions based on his analysis of the dangers of the Natchez Trace around Grinder's Stand in 1809.[7] Thomas Danisi takes an alternative route in his treatment of the debate by denying any role of mental illness or alcohol abuse in Lewis's death. He simply states that he was trying to end his suffering from malaria by killing himself.[8]

Another case in point is Vardis Fisher, whose occasionally humorous book (*Suicide or Murder?*) completely ignores Gilbert Russell's critically important report that Lewis's mental problems at Fort Pickering resulted from his imprudent use of liquor. This inconvenient truth is also conveniently ignored by several other supporters of the murder theory. In a recent episode of the radio program *The Thomas Jefferson Hour*, host Clay Jenkinson and his guest, Idaho state historian HannaLore Hein, discussed Fisher's book.[9] They noted that one of Fisher's arguments attacking the suicide theory was that because Jefferson had an affair with a married woman when he was in France, his comments about Lewis's death could not be believed. The logical connection between these two facts escapes us. Additional convoluted logic in his book, as noted by Jenkinson and Hein, does not speak well of his arguments.

We must note that the only physician or mental health professional who supports the murder theory is Eldon Chuinard, M.D., an orthopedic surgeon. His opinions on the nature and results of Lewis's wounds have been criticized as incorrect by multiple medical experts in trauma surgery, emergency medicine, and forensic pathology (see chapter 9). Not one medical expert I consulted with regarding this issue supported Chuinard's claims concerning Lewis's wounds. And yet, Guice listed Chuinard's opinion as his *premier* piece of evidence against the suicide theory.[10] If Guice believed Chuinard's opinion was his blue-ribbon piece of evidence, then the rest of the evidence in favor of the murder theory had to be weak indeed.

In our careers, we have seen some segments of the public express distrust of both medicine and psychology. The public's nonacceptance of these professions occurs perhaps more frequently within the arena of mental health. A significant percentage of the public will never seek treatment for mental health-related issues, for a variety of reasons. More often than we would care to admit, those in the most need of such treatment are the least likely to seek it. Buzz Aldrin's reflections on his problems are a living and breathing case in point. Personal shame, denial, religious convictions, and fear are but a few of the reasons people don't seek help. Human beings are imperfect; we are frequently wrong. Errors in judgment often come from people we might expect to be wiser. Some armchair psychologists/psychiatrists believe they know the patient better than the patient's physician or psychologist and decide on their own, based on nothing but their faulty human reason, that medication and/or psychotherapy is not needed or would be unhelpful. But denial is not restricted to mental health-related issues. Many people today are taking inadequate precautions during the height of the Covid-19 pandemic, believing that the virus causes nothing more than a common cold for everyone it infects. All these poorly considered actions regarding both physical and mental health leave us speechless and have consequences that are all too often tragic.

One of the hallmarks of mental illness is that the suffering victim has very little or even no insight into the condition from which they suffer. If that is true in this modern time of relative enlightenment, it was even more true in 1809, when many mental/medical problems were unrecognized by the medical community. As a physician dealing primarily with a patient's physical health, if I (David) see a patient complaining of chest pain and shortness of breath (a physical problem), and, after ordering various tests and labs, diagnose that patient with a heart attack and both show and explain to the patient their abnormal EKG and lab tests along with a dire warning that if they ignore their problem they may die, chances are at least good that they will follow their treatment plan of being admitted to the hospital and treated by a cardiologist. But with numerous psychological disorders, ailments that many have suffered from throughout their life that have led to their personal and professional lives being left in shambles, some people will miss and cancel follow-up appointments, discontinue taking their medications without physician consultation, and revert to their own fallacious opinions about their mental conditions. This has been our occasional but not uncommon clinical experience for many years.

Psychologist Dr. Kay Redfield Jamison has done years of research into suicide, and her findings cannot be dismissed as "psychobabble." Her research provides exactly the type of evidence and clinical experience in dealing with mental illness and suicide that directly apply to Lewis's life and cannot be readily countered. Jamison's authoritative and data-driven analysis reveals that the comments of the anti-suicide authors regarding the unlikeliness of Lewis's suicide are, at best, uninformed. Just as a patient can accept or reject a clear medical diagnosis, the reader can accept or reject the convincing evidence that links Meriwether Lewis's death to a mental health-related issue.

The motivation to commit suicide results from an extremely complex web of neurobiology, behavioral medicine, sex of the individual, genetics, and compounding factors such as alcoholism and drug addiction. Mental illness affects a significant percentage of the population.

As Marti covered in chapter 10, mental illness comes in a dizzying array of varieties and severities. Neurotic mental illnesses may be subtle and may allow the sufferer to go through life with a minimum of difficulty. The problems the person encounters during their life, although they cause some personal difficulty, are often easily hidden. People who are neurotic (which Richard Dillon, in his biography of Lewis, denied was a problem with Lewis)[11] are among the most functional of those who suffer from mental illness, despite the fact that they can be in significant emotional pain. Neurotics are in touch with reality, but their personalities have developed so that they may be particularly sensitive to environmental stress, are overly sensitive, and may be particularly susceptible to additional problems such as alcohol and drug abuse. The evidence that Lewis was neurotic is, without question, compelling.

Some authors have either diagnosed Lewis with bipolar disorder or referenced others who support such a diagnosis in their criticisms of the suicide theory. Marti has covered why she does not believe that the evidence suggests that Lewis suffered from bipolar disorder (manifested by alternating manic and depressive states). Based on multiple reports from Lewis's closest friends, it is rather apparent that he did occasionally suffer from unipolar depression, a type of mood disorder that does not include manic episodes. Depressed people generally report feeling sad, a lack of interest in activities that bring them pleasure, being very sensitive to failure or rejection, low self-esteem, feelings of inadequacy, guilt, loss of interest in sex, relationship problems, trouble sleeping or sleeping too much, changes in appetite, trouble concentrating, irritability, hostility, or aggression. Many people who are depressed are successfully treated today with medication and/or psychological therapy. But many of these patients, in an attempt that may be either unconscious or conscious, try to treat their feelings of depression by numbing them with alcohol and/or illicit drugs. Why would an otherwise intelligent person take this path? Because, as Tom Horvath, a specialist in alcohol abuse treatment, states, "Alcohol can be easily purchased, its use is socially acceptable, its use can be easily hidden, and it always works."[12] But every coin has two sides. One side is "it always works," but the other side of the alcohol coin always represents destructive consequences—just ask someone like Buzz Aldrin.

Many have noted that Meriwether Lewis was undergoing a good deal of personal turmoil in the months before his death. His conflict with Frederick Bates, failure to find a wife, personal embarrassment over his financial situation, and the actions of federal government bureaucrats pushing him toward financial and personal ruin were very real threats to Lewis and are mentioned in the historical record. Mental health professionals note that the difficulties in life such as those experienced by Lewis in 1809 do not cause suicide but can precipitate it. We do not believe that Lewis's depression was solely responsible for his death, but it played a large role.

It is well known that loss of financial means, loss of love, divorce, and personal disaster are experienced by many people. Yet not all of those who experience such trauma commit suicide. Given Lewis's intelligence, his accomplishments in both exploration and government service, and his plans for the future, don't these factors eliminate suicide from the list of potential causes of his death? As Lewis biographer Richard Dillon declared, "[I]f there is such a person as the anti-suicide type, it was Meriwether Lewis."[13] Lewis was a shining star in America in 1809. As one Lewis author noted, in denial of Lewis's mental problems, "Lewis was an extraordinarily able, well directed person, why did he commit suicide?"[14]

A similar case is made that others had to deal with virulent politicians, so why would that contribute to Lewis's emotional trauma? Are we to believe that, because numerous others had experienced the pain of dealing with governmental bureaucrats, the threat of personal financial ruin as a result of that mistreatment would not be a profoundly depressing event for Lewis? That type of reasoning is not sound.

Some scholars have noted that particular life difficulties in and of themselves are not the cause of suicide. Al Álvarez, according to Dr. Jamison, "describes better than anyone the highly personal interpretation given to events by those who are suicidal." Álvarez notes:

> A suicide's excuses are mostly casual. At best they assuage the guilt of the survivors, soothe the tidy-minded and encourage the sociologists in their endless search for convincing categories and theories. They are like a trivial border incident which triggers off a major war. The real motives which impel a man to take his own life are elsewhere; they belong to the internal world, devious, contradictory, labyrinthine, and mostly out of sight.[15]

Guice, in his attempt to discredit the suicide theory, also attacks those who suggest that Lewis's preparation of a last will and testament after leaving St. Louis for Washington was a sign of his mental derangement. Guice wrote, "So the fact that he writes a Will on the way down the river enhances him in my view. It doesn't show he's getting ready to blow his brains out."[16] In addressing this issue, it was most informative to discuss this with Dan Sturdevant, J.D., past president of the Lewis and Clark Trail Heritage Foundation. Sturdevant spent his legal career in the field of estate planning. He has had extensive experience with people making wills and trusts. He believes that Lewis's lack of making a will in St. Louis and then doing so during his final weeks is highly indicative of a state of great mental stress and of Lewis's belief that he might not ever make it to Washington. He does not believe that this is simply a matter of a prudent man covering his bases, as Guice suggested. So, once again, we have two opinions, one from a man with no experience in dealing with the motivations of those making final wills and another from a man who has extensive professional experience with people doing that same task. We will let the reader decide whose opinion holds more validity. In order to accept Guice's reasoning, one would need to accept that Lewis decided to make a last will during this time based on clear thinking and a lucid mind. However, if one accepts the statements by numerous people who had firsthand knowledge of Lewis's depressed and unsound mental state during those last weeks (Clark, Carr, Russell), which resulted in his confinement and medical treatment at Fort Pickering, Guice's reasoning is without merit.

Two of the most convincing pieces of historical testimony we encountered in our research on Lewis are the observations made by Thomas Jefferson and William Clark concerning the mental state of Lewis, which they had witnessed firsthand. Although many of those who support the murder theory criticize these two pieces of evidence, they usually do so by either minimizing or twisting the evidence. Jefferson reported on Lewis's "hypochondriac affections," which was a reference to a form of mental illness (anxiety, fear of disease, and possibly depression) that was present in multiple people within Lewis's family lineage (see chapter 8).

Vardis Fisher notes that Jefferson's comment has been refuted by contemporary Lewis family members.[17] His reasoning is convoluted. If his claim is true, we must conclude that these reported family members cited by Fisher lived in more modern times and were therefore significantly separated in time from both Meriwether and his ancestors as well as from Jefferson. How could they possibly know Jefferson's comments were invalid? We know from historical documents that Meriwether's half brother Dr. John Marks was confined to a mental hospital for a time. If that is true, then Fisher's point is false. There is significant statistical and research evidence supporting the idea that some types of mental illness have a genetic component. This fact is beyond question and weighs on the side of such a predisposition existing in Meriwether Lewis if it was present in other family members.[18] Those who minimize Jefferson's comments about Lewis's mental state either criticize Jefferson for improperly disclosing this information about Lewis ("throwing Lewis under the bus") or simply discount it as unreliable.

Those who think along these lines appear to do so for a couple of reasons. Jefferson's evidence is clear that some obvious issues developed with Lewis that were also seen in the past with other members of the family. If this were not so, then Jefferson's very public pronouncement of these facts, if they were knowingly false, would put Jefferson in the position of publicly lying about Lewis and his family and thus inviting public disapproval and scorn. Jefferson, a man who has been accused by some of occasionally acting solely in his own interest, would not have risked his reputation by giving such personal information on Lewis if he did not believe it to be true. For Jefferson, knowingly spreading lies about Lewis would be acting against his own interest. Jefferson would have had no motive to act in such a way.

Many suicide critics cite Jefferson's comments and ask, Why would Jefferson have given the command of the Corps of Discovery to Lewis if he knew of his alcohol or personality problems? The answer is simple and consistent with our clinical experience. If Jefferson witnessed any symptoms in Lewis prior to the expedition, they were so subtle that he either failed to appreciate the importance of such observations or thought nothing of them. The profound effect of Lewis's post-expedition mental derangement and death only occurred when the "demons" Moulton described came calling and Lewis answered the door. What Jefferson observed in Lewis and wrote about in his letter of April 18, 1810, was a postmortem observation that took into account Jefferson's early observations of Lewis's personality in relation to the reports of

Lewis's death. To phrase this a bit differently, Jefferson's observations of the young Lewis (pre-expedition) became significant only in light of what ultimately happened to Lewis. History is filled with such events. Our own lives are replete with similar occasions. Who has not said to themselves, "If I had only known about that bit of evidence before I acted, I would have decided on a different course of action" or "I should have seen that bad thing coming my way"?

A favorite target of the anti-suicide group is Lewis's reported problems with alcohol. They either outright deny his drinking or justify his abuse because many other men during those times also drank excessively. Guice, in contrast to other murder theorists who deny that Lewis used alcohol, noted, "Yes, he at times did drink. It is safe to say that at times he got drunk, and one of those times may have been on his arrival at Fort Pickering." Guice also adds that, during Lewis's stop-overs in Philadelphia and the parties there with his friend Mahlon Dickerson and their "cavorting with the girls," alcohol may have been a part of his life. Then, in a sudden apparent minimization of alcohol abuse that we find incredible, Guice adds, "But drinking in the young republic, and especially on the frontier, was par at a time when par was pretty high. The amount of whiskey drunk on the southern frontier seems astronomical by modern standards."[19]

In trying to interpret Guice's statement, we feel he is attempting to provide some justification of the probably excessive amount of drinking that Lewis, Dickerson, and their bachelor friends engaged in while making the rounds of the parties held in Lewis's honor in Philadelphia after his return. Guice's line of reasoning may be that Lewis might have been drinking excessive amounts of alcohol at some points in his life, but so was nearly everybody else in the United States, so we shouldn't think it excessive or give those reports much weight. Maybe we are misinterpreting Guice's statement, but his use of "but" as the first word in a sentence following his admission that Lewis probably drank too much seems to be an attempt to justify Lewis's frequent and probable alcohol abuse. Our knowledge of both the social and U.S. military culture of this time makes it all the more obvious that these social occasions in Philadelphia were likely lubricated with copious amounts of alcohol. Guice, although he is an advocate for the murder theory, unintentionally helps us make our case that Lewis, at least on occasion, used excessive amounts of alcohol. Guice subsequently asks, "Where is the hard evidence that Meriwether Lewis was an alcoholic? Many writers echo the charge of alcoholism, but none point to creditable evidence."[20] In our minds, the question of Lewis's alcohol abuse has been answered by some very strong circumstantial evidence in addition to the already existing historical record.

The coroner's jury of 1996 is often touted as an authoritative and comprehensive exercise in evaluating the evidence surrounding Lewis's death. Although there are a number of individuals whose testimony we are in no position to question as they are the experts in their fields and we are not, there was some medical testimony given regarding Lewis's alcohol use and the historical record on which we are qualified to comment. The coroner's jury was a great publicity project designed to increase the public's knowledge and interest in the upcoming Lewis and Clark bicentennial commemoration from 2003–06, but it promised much more than it produced in valuable testimony, particularly when it came to medical and psychological issues that applied to Lewis.

On Lewis's final trip, when he arrived at Fort Pickering, it was reported by the commanding officer, Gilbert Russell, that Lewis had been intoxicated when he arrived and that he was put on a treatment of "claret and a little white wine" to help him sober up.[21] Two of the experts on the coroner's jury, Guice and Dr. Thomas Streed, a criminal psychologist, criticized this aspect of the historical record and used it to imply that Russell's letter lacked credibility and therefore that the position that Lewis had an alcohol problem was weak. Guice flatly states in his book *By His Own Hand?*, "It is safe to say that at times he got drunk, and one of those times may have been on his arrival at Fort Pickering."[22] We would fully agree with some of Guice's statement but would question why he limited Lewis's drunkenness to Fort Pickering. It seems that he was attempting to avoid identifying Lewis's alcohol abuse as a chronic problem that had existed prior to that date. The IOU for eight barrels of whiskey makes Lewis's previous and significant use of whiskey credible, however, and as we fill in more of the jigsaw pieces of Lewis's personal situation, Guice's acknowledgment of Lewis's drinking takes on more weight.

Streed testified on alcohol and drug use in individuals who commit suicide. Streed stated, "Twenty-five percent of all suicide victims are alcohol dependent and that's the operative word. It doesn't mean that they drink a lot, they are dependent upon alcohol."[23] His opinion seems to miss the point entirely. The amount of alcohol an alcohol-dependent person is drinking is subjective and meaningless. The point is that the alcohol they are drinking, whatever the amount, is causing them a significant problem.

Streed follows up with, "Lewis drank frequently but there's no evidence of dependency in the sense that he had to have a drink and then once he started it was impossible or difficult for him to stop. Are there indications of—let's call it ruckus behavior. Yes, there are but is this alcohol dependence? There is no evidence of that."[24] We are at a loss to explain how Streed would be able to determine this as well as how Lewis's purchase of eight barrels of whiskey would not be evidence of such a dependence. When a person is frequently drinking and their drinking is by all reports causing them problems in their life, it is clinically pointless and impossible to effectively argue that such a person is not "alcohol dependent."

Streed then adds:

Lewis is endorsed by President Jefferson as commander for Discovery. This again flies in the face of an individual entrusting a very important mission upon someone they might have had a lack of confidence in because of alcohol abuse. There is no evidence of alcohol abuse during the expedition. Lewis' harsh enemy, the biggest enemy that he probably had, Frederick Bates, never criticized Lewis concerning his drinking habits.[25]

Guice augments Streed's point by stating the following during the coroner's jury regarding Jefferson's decision to give Lewis command of the expedition: "I suggest to you it is not likely he would put the expedition in charge of a person if he knew that that person had a history of alcoholism and mental problems and instability."[26]

This argument seems to be a popular line of reasoning among supporters of the murder theory, but it is easily countered by the point that during the time when Lewis was preparing for the expedition in 1801–03, he did not have an apparent alcohol problem. As we extensively covered earlier in this chapter, alcohol abuse was often not even a recognized problem in the early years of America. Intoxication was a common and accepted part of life for many years in America. Jefferson, without a doubt, drank significant amounts of wine, at least as often as every evening with dinner. We note yet once again that members of the U.S. Army were routinely given sufficient daily quantities of hard liquor to put them into a state of mild intoxication. Given these parameters, it would require a significantly large amount of alcohol intake by anyone in this scenario to be labeled as having an alcohol problem in 1803. Just getting drunk with your daily gill (four ounces) ration in the army would not have been considered a problem by anyone. If there is no recognized problem, there is no problem to report.

Further testimony from Streed regarding Lewis's reported treatment at Fort Pickering by Captain Gilbert Russell for his "free use of liquor" is not accurate. Streed, again trying to criticize Russell's account of Lewis's state and thus cast doubt on the credibility of Russell's entire report, writes that "an astounding aspect of this, after writing or making these observations Russell also remarks that he deprived him several days of alcohol except for claret and some white wine. Again if an individual has a drinking problem, these aren't the sorts of things that one would normally prescribe even in medicinal quantities."[27]

There is no merit to this comment. The untreated withdrawal of an alcohol-dependent person who has been drinking heavily may be a life-threatening medical problem. It is not a simple case of discontinuing the alcohol and drying out. The neurological system of alcohol abusers who have been drinking heavily has adjusted to the chronic presence of the depressing effects of alcohol. When the alcohol is removed abruptly, they may experience life-threatening symptoms as a result of a neurological rebound, including anxiety, headache, vomiting, sweating, confusion, high blood pressure, seizures, nightmares, restlessness, tachycardia (racing heart), and hallucinations. This severe rebound reaction is not the same thing as the DTs (delirium tremens), which may start forty-eight to seventy-two hours after the discontinuation of heavy alcohol drinking and include hallucinations and delusional thinking. That is a completely separate problem.

So, how would modern medicine treat this problem? What would Dr. Rush have done? Did Russell do the correct thing by giving Lewis some wine over a period of days to help wean him off of the hard liquor?

Is there really anything that is "astounding," to quote Streed, in terms of Russell's observations or his treatment of Lewis?

In today's medicine, a withdrawing alcohol abuser would be administered medication to sedate their hyperactive nervous system (these medications would include some members of the benzodiazepine class of sedative-hypnotic medications). Some of these medicines have become quite familiar to the American public by their trade names: Valium, Librium, Ativan, and Librium.

Since Rush did not have any benzodiazepines back in the early 1800s, what would he have done to help Lewis in such a state as Russell reported? Rush wrote specifically in his 1794 pamphlet regarding the use and abuse of "spirituous liquors" (hard distilled liquor) that "[f]ew men ever become habitual drunkards upon wine" and that its effects "upon the temper are likewise in most cases directly opposite to those . . . of spirituous liquors." Since Rush believed hard liquor to be a stimulant, in order to prevent "any inconveniences from the sudden loss of their stimulus upon his stomach," Rush's treatment was to drink "plentifully of camomile or any other bitter tea, or a few glasses of sound old wine every day." He observed that switching whiskey or rum to beer and wine could cure their addiction. He wrote, "I have great pleasure in adding, that I have seen a number of people who have been effectually restored to health, character, and to usefulness to their families and to society by following this advice."[28] Alcoholics Anonymous and other twenty-first-century alcohol treatment organizations would likely disagree with Rush's methods of 1794, but these quotations document that providing wine is exactly how he and other physicians treated a hard liquor addiction withdrawal in those days.

What is easily understood is that, rather than giving a questionable and harmful treatment to Lewis, Russell, by the standards of 1809, provided *exactly* the correct medical treatment that was available to him. Lewis responded very well to this entirely appropriate treatment and at least temporarily improved. Rather than casting doubt on the credibility of the Russell report, in this case we should give him a gold star for his treatment of Lewis. This adds to the validity and credibility of his written report on Lewis's condition.

What are the symptoms of delirium tremens, and could Lewis have been exhibiting this problem? If we bet with the odds, we would have to bet against this situation as only 3 to 5 percent of chronic alcohol abusers become victims of the DTs. However, if we simply consider the symptoms of this most severe form of alcohol withdrawal, it might be a convincing picture of Lewis's situation. People with the DTs most definitely show signs of "mental derangement" with the usual symptoms of profound confusion and autonomic nervous system hyperactivity, which includes agitation, tremors (shaking), high blood pressure, and a high heart rate, certainly all very profound signs of an "indisposition." Since it is reported that Lewis was successfully withdrawn from his alcohol intoxication over about ten days at Fort Pickering, and given the reports of his mental condition, this must be a consideration even though the odds are against it. Once the derangement recurred near or at Grinder's Stand, reports are that Lewis had started drinking once again and thus would not have been in a state of alcohol withdrawal with its possible profound mental side effects.

Dr. Rush, based on his copious astute observations in the early nineteenth century that have earned him the title of father of American psychiatry, described the danger of discharging a person in Lewis's condition too soon and without further observation of their mental condition. Lewis's departure from Fort Pickering provides a good example of such a case. With strangely prophetic accuracy, Rush stated,

> We should be careful to distinguish between a return of reason and a certain cunning, which enable mad people to talk and behave correctly for a short time, and thereby to deceive their attendants, so as to obtain a premature discharge from their place of confinement. To prevent the evils that might arise from a mistake of this kind, they should be narrowly watched during their convalescence, nor should they be discharged, until their recovery had been confirmed by weeks of correct conversation and conduct. Three instances of suicide have occurred in patients soon after they left the Pennsylvania Hospital, and while they were receiving the congratulations of their friends upon their recovery.[29]

The problem in directly applying this comment to Lewis is that we really have no idea what type of mental illness Rush is referring to in his statement.

Another error expressed by Streed is his comments regarding the possible use of opium by Lewis during his final days. He states, regarding Lewis,

> Yes he used opium for malaria, but there is again, no evidence of any kind of an abusive relationship or a dependency. So it's highlighted in the sense that there are researchers over the years that would say yes, the individual was using alcohol. There may be a bifurcated problem in the use of alcohol and drugs in the sense that the combination of these things may result in some kind of synergistic relation, in other words, heightened reaction. But again, there is no evidence of this having occurred before.[30]

Opium and laudanum are narcotics that are potent central nervous system depressants, just as alcohol is a central nervous system depressant. There is no question that there would be a "synergistic relation," which Streed notes as only a possibility. The mixing of significant amounts of alcohol and opium is a deadly combination, and given the reported symptoms of Lewis's "mental derangement," his alcohol abuse, and the successful treatment of wine in getting him through the withdrawal period, any concurrent use of opium was indeed a serious problem. In addition, the laudanum and/or opium pills alone that Lewis may have been taking in the final weeks could have been sufficient to put him into a mental state of derangement. Opium and its other pharmacologically active ingredients such as codeine and morphine, which were present in the raw opium pills Lewis was likely taking, are by themselves very potent neurologic depressants.

If you have ever had surgery or had a painful medical procedure performed, then you likely have experienced some of the potent neurological side effects and pain relief provided by opium derivatives. After several days of intense post-operative ankle pain, the result of a painful ankle injury and surgical repair, I (David) was given intramuscular Demerol, a potent derivative of opium. I took that medication every three to four hours, and after a few days I was fearful that my mind had left me, never to return. On another occasion, after cervical spine fusion surgery, I awoke from a morphine-induced hallucination (mental derangement) that Elvis Presley had just been in my room singing

Silent Night. I was convinced that Elvis had just given me a personal performance, and I asked my amused wife, Marti, if she too had heard him. This story still gets laughs in our household.

Imagine what happens when a potent drug like ethanol (in excess) is mixed with opium. The effects of this mixture on a person's thinking ability are impossible to overstate. The combination, if both drugs were in a sufficiently high amount in the bloodstream, could have killed Lewis. When present in lesser quantities, they would have altered his presence of mind and his hold on reality to that point that he could be considered "deranged." Even if neither of these drugs was in his body during the time he was at Fort Pickering, if he had been drinking excessively and using opium in the recent past, the withdrawal from these drugs could have put him into a state of "derangement."

Are we to believe that the fact that many people had an alcohol use disorder in 1809 somehow made Lewis's alcohol abuse less dangerous? That type of argument is truly a bridge too far. We have noted that Jefferson's report of the "habit" into which Lewis had fallen should be considered alcohol abuse syndrome and that, given his difficulties in St. Louis, he had a recurrence of his mental health-related "hypochondriac affections" and drank some of those several hundred gallons of whiskey that he purchased in 1809 from Isaac Miller in a futile effort to rid himself of his emotional torture. Given all of the other evidence we have explored of the alcohol-abusing American culture of that era, the firsthand reports of Gilbert Russell of Lewis's admission of his free use of liquor, and the potentially poisonous nature of the various medications Lewis may have been taking, this scenario of Lewis's final days becomes intuitively obvious. What does not make any sense and cannot be justified is the argument that Jefferson's reference to Lewis's "habit" referred to a return of malaria.

Firsthand reports of Lewis's mental state during his final days come not only from Jefferson but also from his dear friend William Clark. Historian James Holmberg, editor of *Dear Brother: Letters of William Clark to Jonathan Clark*, provides historically profound and convincing evidence in the now published letters of William Clark concerning his close friend Meriwether Lewis. These include eight letters from William Clark written between late August 1809 and early March 1810. As Holmberg notes, "[F]our of the letters are particularly significant because they chronicle Clark's reaction to Lewis's death and pass on information he received about his friend's suicide."[31] Clark's first reference to the emotional distress he witnessed in Lewis was in his initial letter of August 26, 1809. Clark noted that "his Crediters all flocking in near the time of his Setting out distressed him much. which he expressed to me in Such terms as to Cause a Cempothy which is not yet off," adding that "if his [Lewis's] mind had been at ease I Should have parted Cherefully."[32] Holmberg hits the nail on the head with his evaluation of the significance of these statements: "This is a very important passage concerning Lewis's state of mind at this time. For Clark to be so obviously concerned about his friend's distress and relay it to Jonathan indicates the extent of his worry for him and the degree to which Lewis's mind was unsettled."[33] We could not agree more. Those who believe Lewis was murdered must perform philosophical backflips to either deny or minimize such information.

Clark's observations of Lewis's emotional state are an 1809 version of a clear description of significant depression and anxiety. No one who reads them can come to any other conclusion. Anyone asking what Lewis had to be depressed about need wonder about that no longer. The Clark letters provide direct evidence that Lewis was significantly emotionally affected by his problems during 1809. Lewis's problems were so great that they even affected his empathic friend's emotions. The references Clark makes to Lewis being distressed "much" and to Clark's own empathic reaction to the situation strongly imply that Lewis's emotional reaction was more than just a fit of slight anger or disappointment at the actions of his creditors or something that amounted to a slight insult or just being "sad."

Lewis's shedding of tears at the slight he perceived that led to his court-martial trial, his anger, and his behavior in several incidents analyzed in chapter 10 are evidence of his strong reactions to the profound insults he suffered at the hands of Elliott, several unnamed Native Americans, Bates, Eustis, and Madison and to the disapproval of his lack of producing the journals by his father figure, Thomas Jefferson. By multiple reports, particularly those of Clark, who referenced Lewis's mental state during their last visit, the evidence of Lewis's significant clinical anxiety and depression is overwhelming. This does not require any new interpretation.

In *River of Promise*, historian David Nicandri traces the onset of Lewis's emotional deterioration back to the hardships and dangers he encountered during the 1805–06 era in the Columbia River Valley. As Marti has previously noted, Lewis's behaviors during this time period were not confined to this time; they had been present during his entire adult life. Lewis's tendency toward imprudent actions and overconfidence was noted by a member of Jefferson's cabinet. Attorney General Levi Lincoln commented that Lewis would be much more likely, "in case of difficulty, to push too far, than to recede too soon."[34]

Lewis had noted in his court-martial testimony that without his honor his life was not worth living. His personality traits of honesty and his strong or even extreme sense of honor, coupled with the reprehensible actions of the U.S. government and Lewis's own highly personalized interpretation of those actions, which is typical of someone in the midst of depression, set Lewis into a further emotional tailspin. None of this evidence needs to be tortured, fabricated, ignored, or contorted to fit this picture, as is necessary for nearly all of the evidence cited by supporters of the murder theory.

On numerous occasions, Lewis reacted to slights to his honor and reputation with a grown-up version of the little Southern boy, a member of the gentry, who was bitten by a goose and then hacked the bird to death with his toy sword. When the offending "goose" is not a bird but high-ranking officials in the U.S. government, getting rid of the offending entity is not quite as easy.

Clark's report of Lewis's depression prior to his departure from St. Louis is magnified by his comments regarding Lewis after his death. When Clark was informed of the death of Lewis on October 28, 1809, he wrote to his brother Jonathan the same day with a profoundly insightful description of his belief that Lewis had committed suicide:

> [T]o day I Saw in a Frankfort paper caller the Arguss a report published which givs me much Concern, it Says that Govr. Lewis killed himself by Cutting his Throat with a knife, on his way between the Chickaw Saw Bluffs and nashville, I fear this report has too much truth, tho' hope it may have no foundation. . . . I fear O! I fear the waight of his mind has over come him, what will be the Consequence?[35]

This report from Lewis's most trusted and dear friend is an immense problem for those who attempt to discredit Lewis's reported suicide. When this letter from Clark burst on the historical scene in 1998 and Holmberg published *Dear Brother* in 2002, another seemingly insurmountable piece of evidence was laid in the path of the murder theorists. Of course, in order to attack the suicide theory, something must be done to discredit Clark's observations on Lewis's emotional turmoil. If true, they represent a piece of very insightful evidence that can only be interpreted in one way—Lewis was emotionally distraught.

The latest published response and challenge to Clark's report comes in Patricia Stroud's *Bitterroot*, published in 2018. Stroud writes that the original letter is "lost" and

> exists only in typescript at the Filson Historical Club in Kentucky. And the letter that Clark refers to as having been received at Jonathan's house, which Lewis wrote from New Madrid, has never been located. That one of these letters should not be known in the original, and the other nonexistent, is curious. Why have these two crucial missives disappeared when so many others of Clark's to Jonathan still exist? Clark's phrase from his "lost" original letter, "I fear this report has too much truth," is suspiciously similar to the statement of the so-called James Howe, who wrote Bates from Nashville, "I fear there is too much truth in it." All unknown to Clark, was there foul play, even a carefully planned conspiracy behind these missing, or possibly recreated, letters?[36]

Stroud's point is clear. She believes there is no original Clark letter and that therefore the typescript letter attributed to Clark may be, or is, a fake—fabricated by some unknown individual to support their nefarious intentions. Therefore, these comments did not originate from William Clark and are not to be believed.

As human beings, we are all capable of error. Stroud's comment on Clark's letter is a case in point. Her assertion that the original Clark letter is "lost" is simply not true. The original letter according to James Holmberg, "survives and is in the Filson Historical Society's collection."[37] Since the original letter does exist, this line of attack against Lewis's emotional state by way of an argument against the credibility of Clark's reported comments joins a growing list of murder/anti-suicide theories that are unequivocally false.

Lewis's depression should not be thought of as a sign of any emotional character weakness. Nor is it a fictitious label placed on him, as biographer Stroud asserted when she wrote in the introduction to her biography of Lewis that she could not find "any indication of the pathologically depressive, alcoholic, or suicidal behavior that has been attributed to him."[38] Lewis was not weak. He was the victim of virulent politicians who emaciated him, violated his great sense of honor, insulted his honesty, and promised to ruin all of the valuable work and rewards that he had accomplished and obtained both during and after the expedition. Our picture of Lewis is not that of a pathetically weak-kneed personality. Anyone whose inner core values are violated to the extent that these politicians violated those of Meriwether Lewis, promising personal ruin to his life, would be depressed. Everyone has their breaking point. There is a chink in everyone's armor.

This is not a clinical scenario that requires a great deal of hand-wringing to reach an insightful diagnosis. We have seen situations very similar to this in our professional practices hundreds of times. Anyone who has been involved with either physical or mental health would readily accept such a diagnosis and be able to cite hundreds of examples of similar experiences in their own practices. The current medical and psychological understanding is that people will often self-medicate with a substance that relieves their depressive symptoms of anxiety and loss of pleasure in life. In the case of Meriwether Lewis, such relief probably came via his use of alcohol, which was easy to obtain, socially acceptable, and always worked.

Was Lewis, at least in part, drinking because he was depressed? Or was he depressed because he was drinking? The two scenarios are equally likely. For those who are depressed and are treating their depression with alcohol, it always works both ways.

To accurately view Lewis and his final days through the lens of 1809, we must view his behavior in relation to the widespread abuse of alcohol in American culture. Although Lewis was not actively drinking to the point that it caused him to have a mental health issue during his time with Jefferson, there can be no doubt—no doubt whatsoever—that during his years with Jefferson there was probably, at a minimum, daily wine drinking going on in the president's house. Jefferson is not believed to have been a heavy drinker, but it would be impossible to deny his frequent drinking given the fact that during his years as president his wine collection "swelled to more than 20,000 bottles."[39] In fact, as we have noted previously in this book, an Italian dinner guest at Monticello was out of luck when he requested a simple glass of water to enjoy with his dinner. There was no water to drink that evening at Monticello—only alcohol. This is not to suggest that Jefferson had an alcohol abuse problem. But, alcohol was readily available and frequently consumed in his home.

At the time that Lewis was in Washington in 1801 until he left for the West, he was at the top of his game. His life was rewarding, challenging, and fulfilling. He was being academically prepared by the leading minds in the country to go on the 1803 equivalent of the 1969 moon shot. He was a grown-up version of the contented little Virginian who went out into the night to hunt with his dogs. Things could not get much better for Lewis than they were in 1803. He was thriving in this milieu of respect, encouragement, the furthering of his scientific education, and rubbing elbows with the political and societal elite of his era. He was the golden boy of America in 1803—just like Buzz Aldrin was a hotshot of the 1960s U.S. space program. But when Aldrin failed as a Cadillac and VW salesman and Lewis's financial future and personal honor were on their way to disaster in 1809, both faced a 180-degree departure from their earlier life trajectories. They reached their mental breaking points and sought some relief in the form of alcohol. The key difference in the outcomes of the two men was that Aldrin had a loving support system and modern medical treatment available to him. Lewis had neither.

To effectively build the case that Lewis was murdered, murder theorists must attack the credibility of the reports that reference alcohol as a chief factor in Lewis's death. This seems a nearly impossible task. In addition to all the reports of Lewis's alcohol use during his earlier life, we still have the IOU for three hundred and twenty gallons of whiskey (eight barrels) dated August 1809 and other whiskey purchases made earlier that same year documented in his personal financial log and signed documents. These 1809 purchases make all the reports of Lewis's alcohol abuse from Gilbert Russell, Thomas Jefferson, James Neelly, and

Pricilla Grinder fit like a glove. There is a documentable trail of alcohol use throughout Lewis's adult life, from the culture in which he lived to his partaking of "oceans of whiskey" when in the militia (1794), to his comment that "to my great comfort I have this Day been so fortunate as for the price of one dollar to procure a quart of Rum for a christmas dram"[40] (1795), to his probable use of alcohol as a contributing factor to the event that led to his court-martial during the fall of 1795, and to the culture of alcohol drinking of the U.S. military in that era. We have covered in some detail the erroneous opinions relating to this issue, ranging from the testimony of some in the coroner's jury hearing in 1996 to numerous others who attempt to deny that Lewis used and abused alcohol. The combination of these multiple reports from unrelated sources makes his alcohol abuse a virtual certainty.

Some have argued that Captain Gilbert Russell's report to Thomas Jefferson citing Lewis's alcohol abuse was actually written by someone other than Russell, implying a mysterious conspiracy to murder Lewis. Neelly's testimony of Lewis's suicide, alcohol use, and state of mental derangement has also been attacked as not credible. Even if Tony Turnbow is correct that Neelly was not with Lewis on the night he died but was instead seventy miles north in Franklin, Tennessee, where he was involved in a lawsuit, and that Neelly was not an honorable fellow and, as Russell indicated, was an alcohol abuser himself, it does not make any difference to our argument. Neelly never claimed in his letter to have been an eyewitness to the death. Neelly was motivated to cover his failure to accompany and protect Lewis from his use of whiskey, and he states in his letter to Jefferson that he was not present at the time of Lewis's death. He was simply reporting the facts to Jefferson as he had been told them by Pernier and Pricilla Grinder.

Neelly's report could have been followed up and investigated by both Jefferson and Clark, but neither ever did so. Even if we ignore the Neelly report, it makes very little difference to the probability of Lewis's state of mental derangement brought about by alcohol abuse. There are multiple other sources of the same information, including his friend William Carr, who noted at the time of Lewis's departure from St. Louis for Washington, "Our Governor left us a few days since with his private affairs altogether deranged. He is a good man, but a very imprudent one—I apprehend he will not return."[41]

We then have Pricilla Grinder's description of the "deranged" Meriwether Lewis's last hours. If one attacks Grinder's testimony, as many have, she then joins the long list of supposed frauds who somehow participated in a coordinated deception to unjustly portray Lewis as a depressed alcohol abuser and as someone who was, at least occasionally, mentally deranged (Carr, the boatmen, Clark, Russell, Neelly, Grinder, Pernier, Jefferson, etc.). What would have been her motivation to be untruthful in describing Lewis's final hours? When consistent testimony is received regarding Lewis's state of health from multiple sources, most of whom did not know each other, the trustworthiness of such testimony become extremely difficult to ignore.

One of the possible participants in the proposed fraud, Captain Russell, reported on an event that would have been witnessed by other soldiers at Fort Pickering. His well-documented treatment of Lewis's alcohol withdrawal was not only medically correct for that day but also confirms Lewis's drinking problem. That medical treatment took over a week to accomplish. The somewhat public setting of Fort Pickering would not be a good choice of a venue for lying about Lewis's condition. In addition, Russell did not need to concoct such a story about Lewis's admission of alcohol abuse and his public mental derangement to protect himself and account for a death that had occurred miles away from his command. In addition, there are multiple reports by Russell in the historical record that document his observations of Lewis's troubles. Amazingly, some Lewis authors have completely ignored these reports in the formulation of their theories that Lewis did not commit suicide.

Another obvious question is that if Pernier, Lewis's servant who was with him at Grinder's Stand, was in any way involved in Lewis's death, why would Pernier bother to travel back to Charlottesville to report to Lucy Marks, Lewis's mother? Pernier could have simply gotten "lost" on the way; he could have never showed up at Locust Hill and gone on with his life in some other location, probably without anyone even caring.

The main target of the murder theorists is the credibility of each of these people and their reports about Lewis. The reliable reports from Jefferson, Clark, the boatmen who transported Lewis down the Mississippi, Russell, Neelly, Carr, Stoddard, Grinder, and Pernier all point to Lewis's state of mental derangement. If all their reports are erroneous, they all become either mistaken (Jefferson and Clark), participants in an assassination, or knowing participants in a negative story about Lewis, thus becoming either people of poor character or outright liars. It is also worthy of note that the reports of Lewis's alcohol abuse come from multiple people who lived miles apart and did not even know each other. Did some master conspirator contact all these people and give them instructions about what to say about Lewis and his drinking? Did the same conspirator also visit William Clark and Thomas Jefferson with instructions about what they should write in their postmortem comments? Was Clark sorely mistaken in his eyewitness account of Lewis's depression? If someone ordered an assassination, why didn't the assassins simply wait behind a tree on the Natchez Trace and shoot Lewis in the back as he passed by rather than attack him at an inn? That scenario would have made some sense. The murder theorists who attack the credibility of these witnesses usually are convinced that there is no credible evidence that Lewis was either depressed or abusing alcohol. This theory is the quintessential house of cards.

A common objection has been made through the years by critics of the suicide theory, from Vardis Fisher's book (originally published in 1962) to Patricia Stroud's recent book (2018). Stroud writes that since Lewis "had proven himself a crack shot on many occasions . . . it is inconceivable that he would have missed on his first attempt."[42] Such assertions do not stand up to the findings of forensic pathologists who are experienced in determining the source of a death by gunshot. It is not uncommon for a suicide victim to hesitate just before pulling the trigger, given their mental anguish and confusion.[43] If Lewis were in a state of mental derangement as a result of alcohol intoxication, his usual skill as a marksman would have been drastically diminished. If his first shot were a superficial head wound, the force of the bullet would have undoubtedly caused a concussion that would have added to the confusion of Lewis's mind. One must realize that Lewis did not have a clear head while pointing the pistol that ended his life. He would probably have been in a state of tremendous anxiety and confusion. Arguments against Lewis shooting himself that are based on his previously excellent marksmanship ring completely hollow. I note that Dr. Glenn Wagner, former San Diego County coroner and chief medical officer, had no concerns about the veracity of Lewis's wounds as described in the historical documents. Showing excellent marksmanship when shooting a weapon with a clear mind while hunting or for self-defense is an entirely different situation than suffering from severe depression and alcohol intoxication and pointing a pistol at your head or chest with the intent of killing yourself. The murder theorists' objection on this point displays a fundamental misunderstanding of the situation.

Various Lewis scholars, in their efforts to reject Lewis's possible suicide, note that his failure to find a wife was not unusual and that other men he knew were single too. Is one to believe that the loneliness and unhappiness of other men who wanted to marry but had not found a wife would make Lewis feel better about his own unwanted bachelorhood? Such logic borders on absurdity, yet that is the line of thinking. Guice went so far during the 1996 coroner's jury to state, "You know, most people say that the reason he committed suicide was because he didn't find a girlfriend or a wife."[44] Guice's statement is a misrepresentation of the truth. We are not aware of any suicide theorist who argues that Lewis's failure in romance was "the cause" of his suicide. It was a factor, but it was not the cause.

It might be considered common knowledge, and thus not in need of scientific study, that having close, emotionally satisfying relationships with people is beneficial for good mental health. Although many people live wonderful and satisfying single lives by choice, filled with friends, family, career, and activities, most people seek out a mate for life, get married, and raise children and consider these to be some of the joys of life. Lewis publicly stated his desire to marry on many occasions, so the disappointment he felt in being single appeared to be significant, based on his own reports to his friends.

The absence of those joys of life, particularly for those who want them, can be significant. Mental health professionals have firmly established many risks for depression and suicide. One of the obvious factors is a lack of emotional connection to others. Lewis lacked emotional connection to a female (a wife) that, according to his writings, he was so desperately seeking. This does not suggest that there is anything wrong with such a desire. It is a positive thing and is what has made the world go around for millennia. Such a loving and supportive relationship forms a necessary part of life for many, and its absence when it is desired, particularly in the face of extreme personal adversity, can add significantly to the challenge of life's devastating moments. It is not our intention to insult the memory of Lewis but simply to allow his own words and his social situation in 1806–09 to speak in his absence.

The exalted status in society that Lewis attained in 1806–09 made him, at least on paper, the most eligible bachelor in the United States. Many have speculated on why he did not or could not find a wife. If there had been one failed courtship, it would be an easy matter to conclude that some reason other than Lewis's own personality or behavior had been at fault. Perhaps the woman in question had another love interest. Or, maybe she did not want to live in St. Louis after becoming used to the relatively refined culture of the East. The latter explanation has been proposed regarding Lewis's failed pursuit of Letitia Breckinridge. Maybe the prospective bride was not interested at that point in her life in tying the knot, although Breckinridge did marry shortly after her contact with Lewis.

There were multiple potential candidates to become Mrs. Lewis, and Lewis either struck out with or rejected all of them. This points to the possibility that perhaps there was something within the personality of Lewis—his demeanor, attitude, or habits—that discouraged his multiple romantic prospects, leading to his comment that he was "now a perfect widower with rispect to love."[45] Lewis's failure in this arena of life can either be explained by a remarkable amount of discrimination on his part, so that no woman could measure up to his standards, or to some very unattractive personality traits that he exhibited toward potential wives—or it could be a combination of both of these factors.

His repeated reference to various females in his letters provides some insight into his thinking. Lewis wrote, "My little affair with Miss A--N R--h has had neither beginning nor end on her part."[46] This statement points directly to the possibility that Lewis was not an appealing prospect to many women. Miss A. R. apparently never did, nor ever would, have any interest in Lewis. His disappointment is seen in his November 3, 1807, letter to his friend Mahlon Dickerson:

> I feel all that restlessness, that inquietude, that certain indiscribable something common to old bachelors, which I cannot avoid thinking my dear fellow, proceeds from that void in our hearts, which might, or ought to be better filled. Whence it comes I know not, but certain it is that I never felt less like a heroe than

at the present moment. What may be my next adventure god know, but on this I am determined, to get a wife.⁴⁷

These are not the personal writings of a man who is poking fun at himself or his bachelorhood. He is anxious and is feeling depressed about it. Unfamiliar with twenty-first-century psychological jargon, he describes his feelings as "restlessness, inquietude," a "void" in his heart.

Lewis doesn't stop there but proceeds to address questions to Dickerson about other "bewitching gipsies" with whom they had interacted in Philadelphia in the preceding months. He asks about Miss E. B., "whose memory will remain provokingly important in spite of all my philosophy. Have you heard from her? How you seen her? How is she? Is she well, sick, dead or married?"[48] In an 1808 letter to his longtime friend Major William Preston, Lewis rehashes his frustrations with some of his romantic interests, describing them with notes of humor: [Y]ou have gained that which I have yet to obtain, a wif," adding his observations of his failed courtship:

> [S]he is off, passed—off the hooks, I mean in a matrimonial point of view; be it so, the die is cast, may god be with her and her's, and the favored angels of heaven guard her bliss both here and/ and hereafter, is the sincere prayer of her very sincere friend, to whom she has left the noble consolation of scratching his head and biting his nails, with ample leasure to ruminate on the chapter of accedents in matters of love and the folly of castle-building.[49]

On his way to St. Louis in 1807, Lewis made a stop in Fincastle, Virginia, at the home of William Clark's future father-in-law. It was here that he soon identified, with the help of his brother, an apparently attractive candidate to become Mrs. Lewis, Letitia Breckinridge, whom his brother Reuben reported was "one of the most beautiful women I have ever seen."[50] Apparently, Lewis had previously been interested in Letitia's sister Elizabeth, but after meeting Letitia, he wrote that "my soul revolts at the idea of attempting to make her my wife."[51] This comment indicates that Lewis was not going to accept just anybody but was rather selective. He was probably not as desperate as some of his writings suggest. One might also wonder whether there was any woman who would have been good enough for Meriwether Lewis, conqueror of the West, presidential secretary, and the 1806 version of the second man on the moon.

His romantic failures obviously caused Lewis some "intrapsychic conflict" (to use a contemporary term from the mental health field) as a result of the immense sadness felt by nearly all humans when their romantic intentions are frustrated or thwarted. These personal mental reactions to unrequited love would create a negative self-image, sadness, frustration, disappointment, and ultimately anger. Lewis had no outlet for these negative feelings except to share them with his closest friends, Dickerson and Clark, and/or try to numb his feelings with alcohol. Any attempt to deny his feelings and follow the advice of the modern American cartoon "psychologist" Homer Simpson to push our feelings deep down inside where they will never bother us again would be a blueprint for personal emotional misery. But, that seems to be exactly what Lewis did with such feelings.

Paul Russell Cutright, in an excellent article published in *We Proceeded On*, argued that Lewis may have begun to numb his feelings of discontent about his bachelor status by increasing his intake of alcohol during the days prior to arriving in St. Louis on March 8, 1808.[52] Although such an explanation is totally possible and even probable, there is no direct evidence that this was the case. Written records indicate that Lewis was drinking porter and other types of beer in Philadelphia, but again, this does not make his alcohol use into a vice during that time in his life. The personally written and signed IOU for eight barrels of whiskey in August of 1809 presents a much greater problem for those who attempt to minimize or outright deny Lewis's eventual alcohol abuse. Some may try to minimize Lewis's drinking this vast amount of alcohol by noting that much of it must have been destined for other than personal use. My question to those who pose that question would be, "How many of those several hundred gallons of whiskey, if procured for his own use, would not represent a real problem?" Let's theorize that Lewis only intended fifty of those gallons for himself. Does that somehow make the situation any better? We think not. There is no escaping this conclusion, given the historical record of this period in his life. The idea that Lewis was not a drinker, as proposed by Patricia Stroud, John Guice, and other Lewis biographers (see chapter 4), is simply not credible.

The most important thing to note concerning Lewis's romantic history is that he reportedly wanted a wife yet did not have one. The potential ramifications of his undesired state of bachelorhood are multitude. Since Lewis did not have a wife, despite his stated desire, what are we to conclude?

1. The possibility that Lewis and Clark were both gay has been presented in articles printed in *We Proceeded On* in 2015,[53] but we think there is no credible evidence to support this idea. We consider the articles that explore this theory, although they provide the Lewis and Clark community with yet another novel historical interpretation, an exercise that started with a conclusion and selectively misrepresented situations reported in the journals to suit an already decided outcome.

2. It is not recorded anywhere, to our knowledge, that Lewis had any serious relationships with women in his post-expedition life. This lack of a historical trail for Lewis's romantic life means very little to us. If his love life was nonexistent and he was a lonely bachelor. as he described himself to Clark, are we to assume that he was celibate for the thirty-seven months after the expedition? Given our experience in our careers and with people in our own lives, in our judgment it is a stretch to believe this. If Lewis had no willing female companions (an almost ridiculous thought), prostitution was certainly available to him. We believe it is possible that he hired prostitutes.

3. Lewis did not share his mother Lucy's Methodist faith, which would have harshly condemned sexual behavior outside of marriage. He did belong to a Masonic Lodge, which, although it may not have approved of prostitution, would not have had a strong voice to address such issues in the private sex life of an advanced Mason, particularly if such a practice were carried on in secret. This was not the sort of behavior that most men normally publicly advertised, particularly if that man was the head of the local Masonic Temple and governor of the territory. We doubt Lewis would have ever shared about his visits to prostitutes with fellow Masons. If he did, it most certainly would have been kept a secret by a brother Mason—perhaps with the exception of Frederick Bates.

4. Although many of the reported end-of-life symptoms exhibited by Lewis may align with a diagnosis of neurosyphilis, we must remember that the odds against such a scenario are remarkably high—even if Lewis had contracted the disease in his post-expedition life and it was untreated. Neurosyphilis would have to be included in the differential diagnosis of his end-of-life illness. But, if we consider the odds, neurosyphilis is not the probable cause of Lewis's death. Remember that many other psychiatric and medical illnesses share some of the same mental symptoms as neurosyphilis. That is why syphilis is called "the great imitator."
5. If Lewis was not drinking on a daily basis, we suspect that he was binge drinking relatively frequently. We claim this due to our knowledge of drinking habits in the United States during the last three years of Lewis's life, his behavior during the last days of his life, and his purchase of eight barrels of whiskey with a handwritten IOU signed by him on August 22, 1809. Binge drinking is a known risk factor for engaging in high-risk behaviors such as having sex with a prostitute and the resulting high probability of contracting a sexually transmitted disease. It is possible that Lewis may have been infected with a venereal disease in his post-expedition life. Did he seek treatment for it? We believe that he would have, given his personality. There is no evidence for such a scenario. But, the treatment would, at best, have been unreliable. Mercury treatment was not nearly as effective as the modern antibiotic penicillin G.
6. Could Lewis's probable drinking to excess have interacted with malaria, syphilis, or any of the other common infectious diseases present at that time? Or, could some of the medications he was using have adversely affected him?

   Alcohol abuse is known to cause suppression of the normal immune system. If Lewis's drinking was fairly consistent and prolonged, rather than occasional binge drinking, his immune response to either a potential malarial or syphilitic infection (or any other infectious disease) could have been blunted. There is little doubt that any malarial parasites present in Lewis and any possible recurrence of the disease would have been made worse by his alcohol abuse, but the malaria picture leading to Lewis's death as presented by Danisi and Jackson is not accurate (see chapter 8).

It is unlikely that Lewis's reported mental derangement was the result of mercury poisoning. The ionic salt of calomel present in Dr. Rush's pills would not have passed into his brain to any significant degree and therefore would not have produced neurological symptoms associated with mercury poisoning. Mercury in its elemental form may have affected his neurological system, but *he would not have recovered from such a problem in just over a week at Fort Pickering on a diet of reduced alcohol.*

There is no doubt that most of the medications available to Lewis were not very effective in treating any of his medical issues. Any mercury he took, either calomel or otherwise, would have damaged his kidneys, intestines, and other protein-containing structures in his body (see chapter 5). He had no effective medical care for any of his "indispositions." But neither did anyone else in 1809.

The only physician who ever examined Lewis's body (Samuel B. Moore, M.D.) did so in 1848. His mission, from the Tennessee State Commission, was to locate the grave for the purpose of erecting a monument. The commission's report concluded that "it seems to be more probable that he died by the hands of an assassin," thus disputing the decades-old narrative of Lewis's reported suicide.[54] This type of exam, over forty years after Lewis's death, would not have approached the competence of a modern-day forensic exam, nor did it even pretend to. A physician in 1848 would have provided very little authoritative insight into Lewis's manner of death.

Another interesting reference from the past regarding wounds on Lewis's body comes from a National Park Service employee when the Lewis burial site monument was refurbished in 1928. The employee, Delong Rice, reportedly saw a wound in the skull when the body was "accidentally" exposed. He commented, "Isn't it interesting that a man who killed himself had a bullet hole in the back of the head?"[55] This type of report is exactly why a forensic exam should occur on the remains of the body in this gravesite. This sole report from a nonprofessional on a body that was not embalmed and not appropriately housed in an adequate casket is problematic because it suggests that a hole in the skull was the result of a bullet wound. According to Anthony Leo, M.D., this type of irregularity could have a host of causes and is not necessarily caused by a bullet wound.[56]

If a hole in the back of the skull existed—and Lewis was the shooter—the skull wound would have to be the result of the second shot as such a wound would have been instantaneously deadly, preventing any self-inflicted second shot to the torso. If Lewis's remains were exhumed, a team of modern forensic pathologists would be able to investigate such a wound and determine if it was consistent with a self-inflicted gunshot. But it is not certain that Lewis did have such a wound, and there is no proof that the body exhumed in 1848 or viewed in 1928 "accidentally" was even that of Lewis. The presence of a physician on the team in the nineteenth century provides little of value for any forensic-related conclusions in 2021. To put much credibility in the findings of that group would be similar to showing faith in the treatments performed by physicians of that day.

The coroner's jury of 1996 contains what we believe is valuable and relevant information on various aspects of the imagined exhumation, but some of the medically and psychologically based testimony was not accurate. Multiple questions should have been asked in follow-up examination of some of the "witnesses"—questions that were never asked until we have asked them in this book. In our work, we have attempted to address the questions that should have been answered by the medical and psychological experts of the coroner's jury. The coroner's jury was an excellent promotional activity for the upcoming bicentennial commemoration of the expedition of Lewis and Clark, but it promised much more than it produced related to medical and psychological issues surrounding Lewis's death.

Another inaccuracy of Guice's testimony in the coroner's jury is illustrated in his opinion on suicide. He stated,

> We have more tolerance toward it, better understanding of it now, but the easiest thing to do for Jefferson was to accept it as a suicide and I think with all due respect to any local officials who may be listening to me now, we even see evidence of this today, that officials, if they're able to declare a homicide a suicide, it's a

much cleaner operation. You don't have to do an investigation, you don't have to have trials.[57]

This statement is incorrect in almost every parameter. The modern determination of a suicide must meet certain criteria. Deaths are categorized by the "manner" of death, which can be homicide, natural, accidental, suicide, or undetermined. A homicide occurs when a death is caused directly by the actions of another person; this does not necessarily refer to a criminal act. An accidental death may occur from such actions as a fall off a cliff or a drug overdose. A natural death occurs as the result of some disease process. An undetermined manner of death means that the death was not deemed natural, accidental, a suicide, or a homicide. Lewis's death was almost certainly neither an accident nor natural. If he died as the result of two gunshot wounds, an accidental scenario is not believable. Suicide is not a wastebasket designation for deaths with an undetermined cause assigned by medical examiners who are too lazy to thoroughly investigate the manner of death.[58] No qualified medical examiner should default to the designation of suicide when the manner of death is actually undetermined.[59]

In our careers as a physician and a psychologist, as we have described in detail in this book, the issues regarding the proposed suicide of Lewis are issues that we have studied, treated, and understand. At the risk of sounding grandiose, which is not our intention in any way, we must in all honesty note that, except for Drs. Chuinard and Ravenholt, the community of scholars who believe that the suicide theory can be dismissed, to our knowledge, does not contain a single individual who has any training, expertise, or experience in any of the issues that were likely to have contributed to Lewis's death. Some physicians provided testimony during the 1996 coroner's jury whose opinions supported the suicide theory (e.g., Dr. Francisco), but his supporting comments were not highlighted or followed up on by the people asking the questions.

We have not commented much on the historical theories and challenges related to the various individual reports of Lewis's death by suicide. The historical evaluation of such texts does not fall within our area of expertise. Although we are not experts in the academic evaluation of historical texts, it is painfully apparent, based on the interpretations published by several previous authors, that a good deal of the historical evaluation of Lewis's death is erroneous and, at best, not logical. One does not need to have an advanced degree in history to determine the improbability of many of the historical interpretations offered by various Lewis authors. The theoretical puzzle depicted by the various murder theories is missing so many pieces as to be nearly unrecognizable. Many others who are more skilled and qualified than the Drs. Peck to evaluate historical documents have addressed the historical weaknesses of the murder theory, including the nonexistent conspiratorial letters from General Wilkinson, the identification of the letters from Neelly and Russell as forgeries, and the inconsistencies in Grinder's story over the years of her life.

Some who argue that Lewis was murdered believe that various letters from Neelly and Russell are forgeries because handwriting experts have stated that the original letters were written by someone other than the reported author. Of course, that assertion is readily countered by the idea that a secretary wrote the letters for these men, who then signed them. But even if you reject the Neelly and Russell letters as evidence, the other reports from William Carr, William Clark, and Thomas Jefferson still must be dealt with. For our conclusions to be correct, there is no need to manipulate various diseases like syphilis and malaria and propose highly unlikely scenarios. There is no need to deny direct testimony by multiple people about Lewis's depressed mental state near his end or to propose conspiracy theories based on nonexistent evidence to reach a logical conclusion. The suicide scenario withstands the probable truth that Neelly was a bad guy who abandoned Lewis on the Natchez Trace, drank too much, and was actually in Franklin, Tennessee, instead of being with Lewis as he should have been. Many murder theorists use this as evidence for their theory, but it makes no difference in our professional judgment concerning Lewis's personal situation during the final weeks of his life. That someone other than Gilbert Russell may have written the damning letter about Lewis's condition at Fort Pickering, thus making the letter attributed to Russell a forgery, is of little consequence. The "Russell letter" reporting Lewis's admission of alcohol abuse does not present a picture that is an outlier view of Lewis's alcohol abuse. Rather, this and other reports by Russell support all of the other evidence in favor of the theory of suicide.

The best review available of the murder/suicide debate is found in an article by Clay Jenkinson. In his summary of the murder theorists' beliefs, he lists forty different ideas commonly presented by those supporting the theory that Lewis was murdered. Many of these ideas display a serious misunderstanding of mental health and medical issues. Many follow a line of reasoning that is mystifying to us as well as to many other scholars. Some of them border on the ridiculous, or, as Jenkinson appropriately states, are "essentially incoherent."[60] All of them ignore or disagree with the overwhelming evidence that we have presented. If detractors of the suicide theory disagree with our opinions, we would welcome, and in fact request, any correction showing us the errors in our thinking. Guice's statement that the suicide arguments are all "readily countered" is just wrong. It is not a little wrong; it is completely wrong.

The suicide theory exists largely because of the testimony of three of Lewis's closest friends, Clark, Jefferson, and Dickerson. In addition to those three, his friend William Carr, the one to whom Lewis gave the responsibility of tending to his financial affairs in St. Louis, described Lewis as a "good but imprudent man," noting that he was leaving for Washington with his personal affairs "altogether deranged."[61] All these men agreed. They were in a position to know. Their knowledge was firsthand knowledge—not filtered through anyone. Their observations are in our estimation both credible and accurate. All the parameters of their reports fit together like a tailor-made suit.

As we noted in our introduction, we were not at Grinder's Stand on the night of October 10 and the predawn hours of October 11, 1809. We did not see who pulled the triggers of the guns that killed Meriwether Lewis. It is possible that all we have researched and presented here is entirely true but a very bad person came along that night and shot Lewis. Of course, if that were true, then Pricilla Grinder's story and all the other reports of Lewis's situation once again become a problem for the believers of such a scenario.

We consider ourselves to be fortunate to have had our lives touched by the story of Meriwether Lewis and the other members of the Corps of Discovery. In our association with many people within the world of Lewis and Clark, we have found that this story of adventure has given many of us added meaning and enjoyment. It is a difficult task for many to accept that our heroes may disappoint us. For some people, the idea that Lewis might have ended his own life due to depression and alcohol abuse is not something they choose to believe. For reasons of their own, they are unable to accept such a conclusion. As for his mother Lucy, it was just too painful. Suicide, even in our relatively enlightened culture, is still judged negatively due to a lack of empathy and understanding of the causal factors. But, in our professional experience, this tragic scenario has collided with our lives on too many occasions to believe that Lewis would somehow escape these all too easily documented circumstances and the resulting human behaviors that resulted in his personal tragedy.

We have had many magical moments along the trail of Lewis and Clark. The wilderness of western Montana, undoubtedly quite similar to what it was two hundred-plus years ago, often transports us back to 1805, such as when we visit the Gates of the Mountains outside of Helena or the Missouri River at the confluence of the Dearborn River, which I (David) painted for the cover of this book and through which the Corps of Discovery paddled their canoes upstream in July of 1805. To sit atop Lemhi Pass and gaze westward as Lewis did in August 1805 and read his thoughts on that day so long ago is an experience that every fan of this story should experience. The story of Lewis and Clark and the Corps of Discovery has something of value and interest for everyone. As Steve Ambrose philosophized at our cabin in 2000, "If the story of Lewis and Clark had been written for a Hollywood production, it might appear too spectacular and contrived to be considered an actual historical event."

Perhaps new and novel theories concerning Lewis's death will be proposed by people without an in-depth understanding of all the issues we have covered who desire to present yet another interpretation of history. If we wanted to make up our own novel theories, all we would need would be a good textbook of human pathology. We could start on page one and, by the end of the book, come up with several hundred new medical theories to explain the death of Lewis. Each one would contain a shred of truth that might justify it as a possibility. But, to do so, all of the existing evidence that points directly at suicide would need to be ignored or countered. That evidence may be ignored or disbelieved *but never factually countered.*

Although much of what we have presented is the result of our evaluations and judgments, some of what we have done in this work agrees with work already done by others. We have attempted to give credit where it is due when the ideas we have presented have been, at least in part, covered by other scholars. We are not the first authors on Lewis to believe that he committed suicide. Others have come to the same conclusion through evaluating the data based on their own backgrounds. We trust that our medical and psychological insights will help those readers who lack a background in these fields and will perhaps in some way help to illuminate not only the fate of our shared hero Meriwether Lewis but their own paths through life.

The emotional and alcohol-related problems experienced by Lewis live on in our world today. They are thriving and in many ways are more complex and rampant than they were for those alive in 1809. People continue to treat others in grossly unfair and harmful ways, just as certain people treated Lewis. Victims of this behavior often react in predictable ways and experience emotional despair. Every reader knows people who are suffering from some of the problems we have covered. Millions are depressed and are self-medicating with alcohol *because it always works*. But this is a very sharp two-edged knife that we guarantee will cut very deeply. We encourage readers to be friends to the depressed and suffering, and if you need professional help, we hope that you will seek it.

We finish our work in this book with a thought that I (David) wrote toward the end of *Or Perish in the Attempt* that expresses our ongoing historical fantasy. I reflected that

> in my occasionally romantic imagination and admitted fascination with the story of Lewis and Clark, I fantasize that someday, on one of my outings in western Montana, I will come around a corner on a forest trail or over the top of some windswept ridge and discover the Corps of Discovery sitting around their campfire. I will be hailed by a friendly shout from William Clark and be invited to sit down with them and hear some of their stories and enjoy a bite of the white pudding. As the fire snaps and sparks, I ask the men what it was like to be trapped on the Great Falls plains while being pelted with giant hailstones or how they endured their weeks of grueling labors on the Missouri and crossing the Bitterroots.[62]

These are the kinds of thoughts that are predominant for us regarding the life of Meriwether Lewis. Lewis was a man of vast talents. He was a committed American patriot. He accomplished much of honor to both himself and his country. As is true of all of us, his feet were made of clay. He lived in a culture that was not altogether good for a man of his psychological constitution. His culture both produced and aggravated some of the personality issues that led to his death. What Lewis has left behind for us to enjoy and relive is not the tragic aspects of many of the topics of this book but the adventure, excitement, and wonder of the deeds that he and the Corps of Discovery both experienced and accomplished. Lewis's memory is justly held sacred by many Americans. To some he is a hero, and to many Native Americans he represents the beginning of the end of their way of life—but to everyone, he is a legend. The spectacular popularity of the Lewis and Clark story in the American psyche will live on for future generations of Americans as well as future physicians and psychologists who will likely add to, or perhaps challenge, our interpretations. We look forward to that.

We think that the exhumation of Lewis's remains should take place. As forensic pathologist Glenn Wagner said to us, America has spent enormous amounts of money and time to repatriate the bodies of our fallen military heroes from abroad. This has occurred even when just a few bones of an individual have been found. Our military heroes are sacred to the memory of all Americans. This country wants to know the unknown questions surrounding the deaths of fellow Americans and, as much as possible, bring their stories to a truthful close. For Lewis, the end of his life's story has not yet been told. The U.S. Department of the Interior granted approval for an exhumation to the Lewis Family on January 11, 2008, and subsequently reversed the decision on April 2, 2010. There is no legitimate reason, particularly since the Lewis family has requested it and a previous administration granted permission for an exhumation, for that exam not to occur.[63] It is somewhat mystifying to us that the U.S. government can assume control over the remains of Meriwether Lewis and deny permission to over 200 members of the Lewis family who have petitioned for decades for a forensic exam to occur. Perhaps the study of Lewis's remains will not resolve all the questions, but it would at least ensure that everything has been done that can be to solve the riddle of Lewis's death. Lewis was a patriot who deserves the best that can be provided to his memory by his beloved America. As long as there are unanswered questions about his fate, and as long as his surviving family desires it, we should do whatever is within our power as a nation to provide those answers.

Now that we have spent well over eighteen months researching and writing this book, we have asked ourselves what we would change in Lewis's life story if it were in our power to travel back in time and influence his life.

We wish, as Steve Ambrose proposed in *Undaunted Courage*, that Lewis had been provided a supportive environment after his return in 1806 in the War Department and aid from those who could have helped him to finish the journals. Lewis had an exceptionally large amount of self-confidence that was not always be guided by wisdom. The lure of a governorship was probably very enticing to such a high achiever as Lewis. The appointment of the Louisiana governor was up to Jefferson, and in our opinion he erred greatly in appointing Lewis to that position. Without the fallout that Lewis experienced from holding that position, many of the terrible assaults on Lewis's personality and emotional health would have been eliminated. If he had been able to focus all his attention on completing the journals, the demons that visited him in St. Louis would have never knocked on his door. The government bureaucrats who helped to kill him would have bitten some other victim. But Jefferson, the idealist, despite his great human abilities in political theory, was also capable of great error. His human reason, which he so admired and which supported and guided his way through life, did not lead him to the best decision in this instance.

If we could, we would have encouraged Lewis to consider staying in the U.S. Army and pursuing his further career there. By all reports, he loved the life of a soldier, and his emotional makeup was compatible with such a job. We also wish we could have introduced him to a supportive and loving woman to be his wife. Away from the frontier of St. Louis and working on the journals in Philadelphia, he would have been able to meet more potential life partners. The political intrigue and emotional distress he experienced in St. Louis could have been replaced with the emotional fulfillment of completing the journals and enjoying life with his wife. We wish that there were no nasty, vindictive, self-interested, and duplicitous people in the world—in short, no narcissists. But that problem of human nature will never vanish; perhaps it is only getting worse.

But all of our hopes and wishes for the past are simply not available. History cannot be relived. Our limited influence as friends might not have been sufficient to change the course of Lewis's life.

We believe in the veracity of our analysis of the issues as presented in this work, and we will continue to believe that Meriwether Lewis was a talented, brave, honest, conscientious, and patriotic yet tarnished individual. We are all tarnished in some ways. Like Lewis and Jefferson, we too have made and will make mistakes in life. Lewis was broken in some ways, just as we all are.

We wish we could have been friends with Meriwether Lewis. We are certain, as both William Clark and Mahlon Dickerson noted, that he was a sincere and good friend. His firsthand accounts of many of the events of his life and the people he knew would be some of the best stories anyone in history could possibly tell.

Appendix

A Conversation with Dr. Glenn Wagner

Glenn Wagner, D.O., is a forensic pathologist and former chief medical officer for the County of San Diego, California. In his nearly fifty years of professional experience, Dr. Wagner has performed over fourteen thousand postmortem exams. His reflections on various questions I (David) posed on October 5, 2019, regarding a possible postmortem exam on the remains of Meriwether Lewis are fascinating.

Dr. David Peck: What fields of study are included in the specialty of forensic pathology?

Dr. Glenn Wagner: Forensic pathology, at least in the United States, is actually a multidisciplinary specialty, obviously, looking at pathology issues tied to medical-legal investigations. But there is also anthropology, odontology (dentistry), criminalistic forensic psychiatry and psychology. All those disciplines come together. In general, there are seven basic questions that always need to be asked and answered: Who? What? When? Where? How? By whom? and Why? Generally, it takes specialized training in all those areas to address those seven questions. Even after all of that, the one question that is least likely to be satisfactorily answered is why. Why does a person do what they do under those circumstances? But they do it. It is so critical to understanding all the others. Forensic pathology is a subspecialty of pathology, and pathology is the study of altered anatomy and physiology as a result of trauma, infection, congenital defects, anatomic variants, and environmental conditions.

Peck: If Lewis's body were not embalmed, what effect would this have on his remains?

Wagner: Lewis died in 1809, so we are talking over 231 years ago. His state of preservation is going to be dependent largely on where he and how he was buried—whether the casket emplacements have held up over the time . . . a high water table, acid ground, a lot of plant activity will all degrade any remains. Obviously, a body that is embalmed, particularly arterial embalming, is most of the time good for a little bit longer. But "from thus we come and thus we go," and so the question becomes, If we were to exhume Lewis's remains today, what would we find? We may find dust, we may find a skeleton, we may find partial or complete mummification or a relatively intact body—based on the continuity of the casket and his burial spot. Given the expectation and the knowledge that he is on National Park land and that the water table is not an issue, nor the acidity, I think there is a really good chance that his remains will not only be skeletal but with connective soft tissue.

Clothing should still be quite intact, which would provide a great deal of information that remains unanswered at this point in 2020. We are constantly uncovering Native American remains from the same area that are considerably older than Lewis, and [we] are able, through DNA studies with forensic anthropology studies and imaging, to extract considerable information. A person of Lewis's stature should be no different.

Assuming that we have material to work with, the question becomes, What might you find in the forensic examination? The information that we have is that he sustained two gunshot wounds, one to the head that appears to be a "graze" wound and one to the body, which presumably was the more lethal. If the gun was held close, regardless of whether he held it or someone else did, there would likely still be powder burns and lead residue on the skull itself. Now, if there is tissue on the skull, powder burns might be present there, but identification of its presence might require scanning electron microscopy or some more specific means of analysis. But the demonstration of a gunshot wound, the entrance wound, the character of that entrance wound, that give you information, on caliber, distance, proximity, and trajectory, are all fair game. The additional findings that we might be able to determine, and would be interesting to know, [is] if Lewis were right- or left-handed—I don't know. But there are generally changes in the skeletal structure to support an anthropologist working with a pathologist to be reasonably certain as to whether a person is right- or left-handed. And since we are talking about holding a gun to your head, which way it's pointed is kind of important in terms of right- or left-handedness.

Depending on how much of the body is left, we may have organs. It's highly unlikely, because the decomposition process for those organs are stimulated by the internal environment, the amount of bacteria and the enzymes. But there still may be enough material that you not only could predict the trajectory but the organs hit and where they are hit and the level of bleeding over time, which is of interest.

My understanding is that when his death was reported to the army, it was reported as a suicide. But in further review, some folks felt that a two-hour survival time, which is what he reportedly had, would suggest that it was not a suicide. I'd have to disagree with that position. Gunshot wounds kill by exsanguination [bleeding], and depending on what the bullet hits will determine how quickly you are going to bleed. Loss of about 30 percent (of blood volume) will put you into shock. Loss of 40 percent will likely kill you if you are not treated medically. The question becomes, here, If it were a suicide and the first gunshot wound is a head wound, a graze wound, would he likely have a concussion or a subdural hematoma? We are talking about a 50-caliber ball fired out of a flintlock. Probably a brace of pistols; he had two of them. My guess is that he would probably have great difficulty if he had a concussion, reloading. So, I'm pretty certain that he had two pistols available when this event occurred, if it's self-inflicted. The second [wound] was somewhere over the chest, exiting in the lower left back area, which would suggest a right to left and downward direction. So, he may or may not have gotten part of his heart. He may or may not have gotten his lungs. But he most certainly got a portion of his liver, stomach, and small intestine, and the descending colon, and probably the left kidney. Well, of all of those, the ones that are going to bleed the most aggressively are the liver and the kidney. So, he could have very well survived two hours, if in fact that report could be validated.

Peck: What infectious diseases, as well as the presence of alcohol or opiates of some combination, might still be detectable within the remains?

Wagner: The hair is generally long surviving and is a very useful study. Bone and nails, if they were to survive, would certainly reflect heavy metal poisoning. Soft tissues subjected to DNA and RNA [analyses] are likely able to indicate if a person has been exposed to malaria, typhoid, or any number of infectious diseases. I'm reminded, for example, of a recent study in England involving mass graves from the black plague where they actually picked up DNA from *Yersinia pestis* [the causative organism of the plague] in the teeth of those remains. They are significantly older than Lewis's remains. So, I'm comfortable, if we have something to work with and we use the right techniques and the right specialties, we can answer, reasonably definitively, what risk factors Lewis may have had from infection/malaria, chronic alcohol use, and, if reported correctly, opioid abuse.

One of the questions that comes up is, What is the significance of the presence or absence of soot, or stippling? And it is related to the assessment of distance. In pathology, we usually describe distance as associated with gunshot wounds as *contact, loose contact, intermediate,* or *distant.* In contact and loose contact, soot is deposited on the skin and oftentimes into the wound, including the bone. Loose contact, you get the same, but it is in a lesser "dosage," if you will. Intermediate, you won't get any soot at all deposited on the wound because a fired gun is like a controlled explosion. The powder is gone, but the unburned powder will be deposited on the skin, giving it a freckling or stippling effect. And anything that is a gunshot wound that does not have stippling is a distant gunshot wound by definition. Which can be relatively close . . . usually not closer than a foot. So, a foot to infinity for distance. So, going back to the question, if the soot were found on him, on the skull or chest plate, it would certainly be consistent with a suicide, but it does not exclude that injury being cause by another [person]. It just indicates the distance between his body and the barrel of the gun was small.

In a comprehensive forensic evaluation, particularly where an anthropologist, maybe a dentist, a chemist, as well as a pathologist are all engaged, there is a lot of data that may come in from all the material relative to pre-existing disease, infectious process, trauma, as well as any anatomic variants that may be a function of age, gender, or ethnicity, and we've got plenty of studies based on forensic archaeology, if you will, based on mummies and skeletal remains, that suggest that given the right tools that most if not all of the conditions—alcoholism, malaria, heavy metal poisoning, opiates—could be addressed. Let me take them point by point.

Malaria would be the most challenging because it circulates in the blood. If the liver or the spleen were still present, even if they were desiccated [all the moisture removed; dried out] DNA and RNA studies should be able to identify the *Plasmodium* [the causative organism of malaria]. In the absence of those, the question of, since he reportedly died of trauma, whether a blood clot somewhere could remain for that study to be done, I don't know how clear identifying malaria on marrow or bone might be. But if they can pick up *Yersinia pestis* in teeth of medieval people dying of the black plague, I would think that malaria, which is worldwide, would be equally easy to detect with the right techniques.

The same thing is true with heavy metals. Arsenic, mercury . . . They tend to be deposited in bone and hair and nails. These structure oftentimes do survive. Opiates are a little bit different story. I would guess that morphine, codeine, or variations of those drugs would most likely show up in hair than anyplace else.

So, the only other question becomes, What about alcohol? We know he was an alcoholic. Can we prove that? If we had a liver, it would be easy. We'd look for cirrhosis, and we'd look for microscopic changes that would come from that. Long-term alcoholics tend to have enlarged hearts. If he had a heart and it was imaged, or sectioned, and there wasn't that bad of coronary disease present, and it was a large heart, that would be in support of, but not exclusive for, alcohol-related cardiomyopathy. The brain is unlikely to survive, but even the brain will show signs of long-term alcohol use, mostly focused on the mammary bodies. Unless he was significantly malnourished, I don't know that we could take it much further than that. I think that the historical record shows that he was a pretty well-established alcoholic, so I think it is less an issue in terms of its presence rather than what would be the contributing factor of alcohol being a risk factor for suicide.

Peck: What would you expect to find if Lewis had committed suicide? What are the key things you would look at?

Wagner: The question of suicide, from a manner of death, which is how we certify cases for purposes of death certificates, is very different from natural, accidental, homicide, or undetermined. *With suicides, you have to show intent.* Contrary to what many believe, only about 25–30 percent of suicides leave notes. So, we are looking at the circumstance in which that person dies—shooting themselves, hanging themselves, jumping off a building or a height—and then looking at risk factors that would indicate intent rather than an accident or death at the hands of another that would make it a homicide. The risk factors for Meriwether, from my perspective, is a young guy who got fame, just by his escapade with Clark and doing some eight thousand miles in the expedition. But during that period of time, he drank. And in fact, before that ever started, there was a drinking issue that might had led to his court-martial and other reports of his use of alcohol. That suggests to me that alcohol abuse was a life-long companion for him.

At the time that he was exposed to the medical treatment of the time and he studied under Dr. Rush in Philadelphia, for a period of time, he would have been introduced to tincture of belladonna and opiates. And I would anticipate that he would have probably used those as he needed to as well. More critically, the reports of his being depressed and trying to kill himself in the past take on more important positions because it indicates that this idea of death and the ideation of suicide wasn't new. There is pretty good evidence that he did try to hurt himself or kill himself in the past, and right before his death in Tennessee he had been the governor of Louisiana and, contrary to the success of his exploration, his governorship was not well received. And I suspect that combination would put him into a "funk" that could have very easily set the stage for him to, either under the influence of alcohol or drugs or both, to shoot himself and to end it. Particularly in middle age. One thing I find with today's suicide folks, there is no ethnicity, no gender, but it [middle age] is a time when people take what turns out to be a long-term fix for what may be a short-term problem. But finances, relationships gone bad, an unhappiness with their condition, those people are most at risk as compared to a younger or older person, where there are slightly different risk factors.

Peck: Do you think that exhuming Lewis's body for a forensic evaluation would solve the riddle of how he died?

Wagner: It's more likely to than not because it would be based on more than speculation, witness reports, or past testimony. Having said that, it's likely to raise other questions relative as to why he did what he did. Such a forensic exam may raise questions which have not even been asked in the past two hundred years. But, if I'm given an opportunity of having something to work with versus nothing, I'll always take something. The value to that, aside from the historical, is that [a] medical legal investigation of death itself is really a story of a person, of how they lived as well as how they died. The vast majority of cases, it's like a jigsaw puzzle. There are parts missing. And you kind of arrange what you have and, based on your knowledge of anatomy, pharmacology, physiology, toxicology, you kind of fill in the blanks. It is very clear that every person has a story to tell and that the story is worth hearing. The dead do have an opportunity to speak to the living, and we have an obligation to listen and learn.

The question of the value of a forensic evaluation, particularly of historical material, we are always interested in getting more information than we've had before, whether that's George Washington or King Tut. Meriwether is no different than that. Assuming that there are remains left, given the relative protectedness of his current interment area, an exhumation and a multiple team approach would answer plenty of questions that have been posed in the past relative to malaria, heavy metal, opiates. But it would also answer the question as to right- or left-handedness, relative condition at the time of death, in terms of just bone structure, and probably raise, with the DNA capabilities we have today, questions I can't imagine until I see what we have. And then, try to fill in the blanks. That's part of that jigsaw puzzle that makes it so fascinating. And well worth it! I'm really impressed with what the Italians and Austrians have been able to do with the iceman—Ötzi. He's over three thousand years old. Not only did they determine that he didn't die from environmental exposure, . . . [they determined that he died] from a homicide. And through an analysis of his DNA, they claim to have traced and identified some nineteen living people! That's a three-thousand-year-old story. . . . That's pretty impressive! So, if that can happen, can you just imagine what Meriwether has to say, given the opportunity?

Peck: Would you characterize alcoholism as a disease that frequently affects socially and professionally high-functioning adults?

Wagner: That is a good question. Alcoholism or alcohol abuse is prevalent in all groups. And there are plenty of socially and politically functioning adults who are alcoholic. The question I guess becomes, and it's one you can't answer, is, if they weren't drinking, would they be even better in their social and professional functioning? Or, has alcohol provided a cloak by which they can carry out those activities in a better position? I think there is not a straight answer to that. Alcohol or any kind of addiction is a liability. Some people are able to take liabilities and turn them into strengths. And you'd have to profile Meriwether not just physically but psychologically in order to come to a position on that. Will they [alcoholics] die earlier? Probably. On the other hand, some people say that [drinking alcohol] adds to your longevity . . . just don't abuse it.

Peck: Do socially and politically functional people sometimes abuse opioids?

Wagner: I'm not so sure it's an either/or situation. Individuals who are inclined to have an addictive personality are inclined to have several addictions. The alcohol, certainly, can lessen your state of awareness or in some cases increase it. The same thing is true of opiates. They both have been around for a very long time. You can trace the use of both back thousands of years, and I don't know [that] they are necessarily exclusive. At least in the population that I see today, the vast majority of people have both on board at the time of their death.

Peck: How many deaths have you investigated that you ultimately determined to be suicides?

Wagner: I've been involved in medical-legal investigations close to fifty years and have in excess of fourteen thousand autopsies that I have done as well as countless others where I have been present while monitoring pathology residents and fellows in their post-graduate medical training. In general, in a medical-legal population, 25–30 percent of your caseloads are going to be suicides. And a significant number, probably about 10 percent, are going to be by gunshot wounds. And it's that experience over time that translates into hundreds, sometimes thousands of cases that you can compare and contrast and draw conclusions from based on the parameters that each case presents.

Peck: Please tell us about a suicide postmortem.

Wagner: A medical-legal examination exists from a public health or public safety perspective for the purpose of certifying a death certificate. There are a lot of questions on a death certificate, but the questions that must be addressed or answered is, who they are, what killed them (cause of death), and an opinion on the manner of death. Most interest in the case is not the identification (that is expected) or the cause of death but the manner of death. There are five or six categories as defined at CDC [Centers for Disease Control] level and each of the states. Homicide, which is death at the hands of another, natural, an accident (an act of God), undetermined, or suicide. The undetermined stands out in that after a really extensive effort to get the parameters, you just don't have enough to be able to answer it. So, it is kind of a "dump term," for lack of a better word.

Suicide on the other hand, presents more issues for the forensic pathologist and his team because families don't want to hear that their loved one has died from a suicide. There are plenty of cultural issues that are tied to that, let alone family values. What all suicides must be able to show is intent. That is what becomes critical with Meriwether. Does he have a history of suicidal ideation? Attempts? What other risks factors were present with Lewis? Do the injuries, if present, support a self-inflicted wound or not? In the absence of a suicide note, is this going to be enough? It has to be brought to a level of reasonable proof. That varies from court to court. You want to call a death a suicide only with a great deal of investigation and probably soul-searching. And [more than] all the other manners of death, I think suicide requires a behavioral analysis if at all possible because that is where you are going to get the clues for their inclination to hurt themselves or kill themselves.

So, the question becomes for me, Why are you here and why are you talking [to me about this]? Well, I had an interest in this case and whether or not there was adequate evidence, or could be adequate evidence, to address the circumstances of Meriwether's death. In doing that, I found that reading about the Lewis and Clark Expedition, in a number of different parameters with descriptions of day-to-day activity, gives me an insight into the behavioral aspects that I think strengthen my position that Meriwether was an alcoholic, a long-term alcoholic, may very well have had an opium dependency, let alone anything he might have been exposed to in terms of infectious diseases from malaria to syphilis, for that matter. It's a very interesting question. What we have is a very prominent American who happens to die in 1809, been buried for 231-plus years, and there is some interest in either exhuming him for possible burial at Arlington because he was an army captain or at least answering questions that remain unanswered to both his family's and the general public's satisfaction at this time. So, a forensic inquiry, especially one that is multidisciplinary, would provide the objective data and the technical results that would enable one to answer many of the questions that have been raised. In doing so, is it likely that we may get more questions? You bet! That's the excitement of forensic pathology and medicine. Because for every question you answer, another set of questions come up that need to be answered. All within that who, what, when, where, how, why, and by whom.

Peck: In speaking with Meriwether Lewis's four-times-great-grand-niece, who lives in Virginia, she told us that many Lewis family members have been petitioning the government to have Meriwether's body exhumed. The [National] Park Service has denied their request. What would be your argument for why the Park Service should allow the exhumation of Lewis's body?

Wagner: The question, I guess, is what are the expectations and needs of existing family members to repatriate their own and to control that burial versus accepting war dead where they fall. We go to great lengths to find our war dead, recover them if at all possible, and repatriate them. So, I think the Park Service's argument [that it will disturb the site, is unnecessary, and will set a bad precedent] doesn't hold water. Nonetheless, it's been a barrier so far. It seems to me that is something that could be easily taken to Congress or the Executive Branch who give the marching orders to the Park Service and the Department of Interior. It is a mountain to climb, but it is a mountain that can be climbed. The question then is, What do you know about what's there and the negatives of going to whatever expense? I would argue that you probably could evaluate the burial site without disturbing it. That's an argument that could be taken to the courts.

Peck: Lewis's burial monument is near Hohenwald, Tennessee, a few hundred feet from Grinder's Stand. What studies could be done above ground to study the grave site?

Wagner: The most useful today in terms of determining what you have of forensic value is ground-penetrating radar. And that is readily available. Having spent many years in the military and on federal investigations, there may be others—spectrographic and satellite analysis—that would add to that, and probably a combination of those would answer what you have to work with as well as the locations and set the stage for any further discussions. It's probably worth doing that. The flip side of that [is] those who say, "Let a dead man lie where they are . . . that's their place." I can't argue with that either. It gets into the cultural values of the community you are dealing with and whether or not today's capabilities allow for greater flexibility or greater liability in making those decisions.

Peck: Would you be able to tell with aboveground techniques if there was a body present in the grave?

Wagner: In all probability, yes. But every case is different. If he was in a lead coffin or is buried deeper or there is more debris on top of it, it may be more difficult. But the capabilities we have today enable us to identify remains that are buried. So, the level of intactness allows for that possibility to be very real. So, the answer today is yes. The question as to a suicide or a homicide is really the most pressing situation here and in most cases would go to the court, with all of the arguments being presented by both sides. There is no question in my mind that you could make an argument for this not being self-inflicted or inflicted by another. But in the absence of a confession, the risk factors remain the same. In the same light, the question is, What makes it a self-inflicted injury? Well, that is where we are starting from, and we are making a set of questions that asks, Is there anything that excludes a suicide? Given the belief that the risk factors are there for a suicide, and if the answer is no, there is nothing contradictory, you have at least equal standing if not more than another scenario that has it as a homicide. There is nothing unique about a wound, most of the time, or a postmortem interval, most of the time, that throw it one way or the other. It's all the parameters. So, a person who wants to make another argument, I value that argument, I say, go for it, and let's see what you have and compare and contrast. Ultimately, it will be the public and the family that will be the jury on this case.

Peck: Is there likely any neurologic tissue left in Lewis's body (spinal cord/brain) that might shed any light on various issues such as heavy metal toxicity or syphilitic infection that Lewis might have had?

Wagner: Generally, central nervous system tissue would not survive because it is mostly water. Having said that, I have recovered skeletal remains where the brain is the size of a thimble but is still there. Given the current DNA/RNA testing capabilities, I think you could consider addressing something like a neurosyphilis case. I think it would depend on much of what we've been defining as the operating parameters for a forensic investigation. That is, What do you have? and What is the condition of what you have? and What does it lend itself to being studied [with] in terms of technique? I'm intrigued with the fact that I think there is a possibility. I'd be surprised if there is anything left. But the world is full of surprises, and that is the whole reason [for] pursuing this investigation from a forensic perspective.

Bibliography

Adhikari, Bipin, et al. "Perceptions of Asymptomatic Malaria Infection and Their Implications for Malaria Control and Elimination in Laos." *PLoS ONE* 13, no. 12: article e0208912.

Ahsan, Shagufta, and Joseph Burrascano. "Neurosyphilis: An Unresolved Case of Meningitis." *Case Reports in Infectious Diseases* (2015): article 634259. doi:10.1155/2015/634259.

Aldrin, Buzz. *Magnificent Desolation: The Long Journey Home from the Moon.* London: Bloomsbury, 2009.

Allen, Jon G., Peter Fonagy, and Anthony W. Bateman. *Mentalizing in Clinical Practice.* Washington, DC: American Psychiatric Publishing, 2008.

Ambrose, Stephen E. *Undaunted Courage: Meriwether Lewis, Thomas Jefferson and the Opening of the American West.* 1st ed., 15th printing. New York: Simon & Schuster, 1996.

Ambrose-Tubbs, Stephenie. *Why Sacagawea Deserves the Day Off and Other Lessons from the Lewis & Clark Trail.* Lincoln: Bison Books, University of Nebraska Press, 2008.

American Psychiatric Association. *Diagnostic and Statistical Manual of Mental Disorders.* 5th ed. Washington, DC: Author, 2013.

Anderson, Sarah Travers Lewis Scott. *Lewises, Meriwethers and Their Kin.* Baltimore, MD: Genealogical Publishing Co., 2008

Armitage, David. "In Defense of Presentism." https://scholar.harvard.edu/files/armitage/files/in_defence_of_presentism.pdf.

Azevedo, Bruna Fernandes, et al. "Toxic Effects of Mercury on the Cardiovascular and Central Nervous Systems." *Journal of Biomedicine and Biotechnology* (July 2012): Article 949048. doi:10:1155/2012/949048.

Bakeless, John. *Lewis and Clark: Partners in Discovery.* New York: William Morrow & Co., 1947.

Benemann, William. "My Friend and Companion: The Intimate Journey of Lewis and Clark" [part 1]. *We Proceeded On* 41, no. 1 (February 2015): 5–16.

———. "My Friend and Companion: The Intimate Journey of Lewis and Clark" [part 2]. *We Proceeded On* 41, no. 2 (May 2015): 27–34. lewisandclark.org/wpo/.

Bentley, James R., ed. "Two Letters of Meriwether Lewis to Major William Preston." *Filson Club History Quarterly* 44 (1970): 170–75.

Bergh, Albert Ellery, ed. *The Writings of Thomas Jefferson.* Vol. 13. Washington, DC: The Thomas Jefferson Memorial Association, 1907.

Berrettini, Wade. "Genetics of Major Mood Disorders." *Psychiatry (Edgmont)* 1, no. 2 (2004): 34–48.

Betts, Edwin Morris, and James Adam Bear Jr., eds. *The Family Letters of Thomas Jefferson.* Charlottesville: University Press of Virginia, 1986.

Blum, Deborah. *The Poisoner's Handbook: Murder and the Birth of Forensic Medicine in Jazz Age New York.* New York: Penguin Books, 2010.

Brown, David, and Thane Harpole. *Warner Hall: Story of a Great Plantation.* Gloucester, VA: Data Investigations, 2004.

Cairns, Earl E. *Christianity through the Centuries: A History of the Christian Church.* Grand Rapids, MI: Zondervan, 1981.

Chan, Thomas Y. K. "Inorganic Mercury Poisoning Associated with Skin-Lightening Cosmetic Products." *Clinical Toxicology* 49, no. 10 (2011): 886–91.

Chang, Helen Y. "A Brief History of Anglo-Western Suicide: From Legal Wrong to Civil Right." *Southern University Law Review* 46, no. 1 (Fall 2018): 150–94.

Cherrington, E. H. *The Evolution of Prohibition.* Westerville, OH: American Issue Press, 1920.

Chuinard, E. G. "How Did Meriwether Lewis Die? It Was Murder" [part 2]. *We Proceeded On* 17, no. 4 (November 1991): 4–10. lewisandclark.org/wpo/.

———. "How Did Meriwether Lewis Die? It Was Murder" [part 3]. *We Proceeded On* 18, no. 1 (January 1992): 4–10. lewisandclark.org/wpo/.

Colarusso, Calvin A. *Child and Adult Development: A Psychoanalytic Introduction for Clinicians.* New York: Plenum Press, 1992.

Cottret, Bernard. *John Calvin: A Biography.* Grand Rapids, MI: William B. Eerdmans, 2000.

Crosby, Michael. "Hypochondriac Affections." *We Proceeded On* 39, no. 3 (August 2013): 8–15. lewisandclark.org/wpo/.

Crozatti, Lucas Lonardoni, et al. "Atypical Behavioral and Psychiatric Symptoms: Neurosyphilis Should Always Be Considered," *Autopsy Case Reports* 5, no. 3 (July–September 2015): 43–47.

Cutright, Paul Russell. "'Rest, Rest, Perturbed Spirit.'" *We Proceeded On* 12, no. 1 (March 1986): 7–16. lewisandclark.org/wpo/.

Danisi, John, and Thomas C. Danisi, "Uncovering Jefferson's Account of Lewis's Mysterious Death," *We Proceeded On* 38, no. 4 (November 2012): 18–27. lewisandclark.org/wpo/.

Danisi, Thomas C. *Uncovering the Truth about Meriwether Lewis.* Amherst, NY: Prometheus Books, 2012.

Danisi, Thomas C., and John C. Jackson. *Meriwether Lewis.* Amherst, NY: Prometheus Books, 2009.

Dart, Richard C. *Medical Toxicology.* 3rd ed. Philadelphia: Lippincott Williams & Wilkins, 2004.

Davis, Larry E. "Unregulated Potions Still Cause Mercury Poisoning." *Western Journal of Medicine* 173, no. 1 (2000): 19.

Di Maio, Vincent J. M. *Gunshot Wounds: Practical Aspects of Firearms, Ballistics, and Forensic Techniques.* 2nd ed. Boca Raton, FL: CRC Press, 1998.

Dillon, Richard. *Meriwether Lewis: Personal Secretary to President Jefferson, Continental Pathfinder, Governor of Upper Louisiana.* Santa Cruz, CA: Western Tanager Press, 1988.

Finney, Charles G. *The Character, Claims, and Practical Workings of Freemasonry.* Cincinnati: Western Tract and Book Society, 1869.

Fisher, Vardis. *Suicide or Murder? The Strange Death of Governor Meriwether Lewis.* Athens, OH: Swallow Press, 1993.

Flick, Arend. "The Gilmer Daybook and the 'Constitutional Disposition' of William Lewis." *We Proceeded On* 47, no. 2 (May 2021): 14–21. lewisandclark.org/wpo/.

———. "William Diven, the Jay Treaty, and the Court-Martial of Meriwether Lewis." *We Proceeded On* 45, no. 4 (November 2019): 11–18. lewisandclark.org/wpo/.

Fried, Stephen. *Rush: Revolution, Madness, and the Visionary Doctor Who Became a Founding Father*. New York: Crown, 2018.

Ganguly, Swagata, et al. "High Prevalence of Asymptomatic Malaria in a Tribal Population in Eastern India." *Journal of Clinical Microbiology* 51, no. 5 (May 2013): 1439–44.

Garrett, Michael. *Psychotherapy for Psychosis: Integrating Cognitive-Behavioral and Psychodynamic Treatment*. New York: Guilford Publications, 2019.

Guice, John D. W. "'It Seems to Be More Probable . . .': Why Not Homicide?" In *By His Own Hand? The Mysterious Death of Meriwether Lewis*. Edited by John D. W. Guice (pp. 73–105). Norman: Oklahoma University Press, 2006.

Guice, John D. W., ed. *By His Own Hand? The Mysterious Death of Meriweather Lewis*. Norman: University of Oklahoma Press, 2006.

Hacker, J. David. "Decennial Life Tables for the White Population of the United States, 1790–1900." *Historical Methods* 43, no. 2 (2010): 45–79.

Hamilton, David. *The Healers: A History of Medicine in Scotland*. Edinburgh: Canongate, 1981.

Hendrix, James P., Jr., and Guy M. Benson, "Did Meriwether Lewis Ever Live in Georgia?" *We Proceeded On* 44, no. 3 (August 2018): 12–14. lewisandclark.org/wpo/.

Holmberg, James J., ed., *Dear Brother: Letters of William Clark to Jonathan Clark*. New Haven, CT: Yale University Press, 2002.

Holmberg, James J. "'I Fear the Waight of His Mind Has Over Come Him': The Case for Suicide." In *By His Own Hand? The Mysterious Death of Meriwether Lewis*. Edited by John D. W. Guice (pp. 17–72). Norman: Oklahoma University Press, 2006.

Idro, Richard, et al. "Cerebral Malaria: Mechanism of Brain Injury and Strategies for Improved Neuro-Cognitive Outcome." *Pediatric Research* 68, no. 4 (October 2010): 267–74.

Jackson, Donald. *Letters of the Lewis and Clark Expedition*. Vol. 2. Urbana: University of Illinois Press, 1978.

Jamison, Kay Redfield. *Night Falls Fast: Understanding Suicide*. New York: Vintage Books, 2000.

Jenkinson, Clay. *The Character of Meriwether Lewis: "Completely Metamorphosed" in the American West*. Reno, NV: Marmarth Press, 2000.

———. *The Character of Meriwether Lewis: Explorer in the Wilderness*. Bismarck, ND: Dakota Institute, 2011.

———. "Meriwether Lewis's Mysterious Death on the Natchez Trace." In *By His Own Hand? The Mysterious Death of Meriwether Lewis*. Edited by John D. W. Guice (pp. 3–16). Norman: Oklahoma University Press, 2006.

Johnson, Paul. *A History of the American People*. New York: Harper Perennial, 1997.

Kenny, Anthony. *The Rise of Modern Philosophy*. Oxford: Oxford University Press, 2006.

Klausner, Jeffrey D. "The Great Imitator Revealed: Syphilis." *Topics in Antiviral Medicine* 27, no. 2 (May 2019): 71–74. https://www.ncbi.nlm.nih.gov/pmc/articles/PMC6550356/.

Komlos, John. "On the Biological Standard of Living of Eighteenth-Century Americans: Taller, Richer, Healthier." *Research in Economic History* 20 (2001): 223–48.

Kumar, Vinay, Abul Abbas, and Jon Aster. *Robbins and Cotran Pathologic Basis of Disease*. 9th ed. Philadelphia: Elsevier Saunders, 2014.

Kushner, Howard I. *American Suicide*. New Brunswick: Rutgers, the State University of New Jersey, 1991.

Lender, Mark Edward, and James Kirby Martin. *Drinking in America: A History*. New York: Free Press, 1987.

Lepore, Jill. "The Sharpened Quill." *The New Yorker*, October 16, 2006. https://www.newyorker.com/ magazine/2006/10/16/the-sharpened-quill.

Lingiardi, Vittorio, and Nancy McWilliams, eds. *Psychodynamic Diagnostic Manual*. 2nd ed. New York: Guilford Press, 2017.

Long, Stephen Meriwether. "British Lieutenant Colonel Banastre Tarleton and the American Revolution: Drama on the Plantations of Charlottesville." *Meriwether Connections* 24, no. 1 (January–March 2005) and no. 2 (April–June 2005).

Luther, Martin. *Basic Luther: The Ninety-Five Theses, Address to the Nobility, Concerning Christian Liberty, A Small Catechism*. Springfield, IL: Templegate Publishers, 1994.

MacGregor, Carol Lynn. *The Journals of Patrick Gass, Member of the Lewis and Clark Expedition*. Missoula, MT: Mountain Press, 1997.

McCleskey, Clayton. "Methodists: Drinking Still a Touchy Topic." *The Christian Century*, March 21, 2011. https://www.christiancentury.org/article/2011-03/methodists-shun-bottle-no-one-wants-talk-about.

McFerrin, John B. *History of Methodism in Tennessee*. Vol. 1, *From the Year 1763 to the Year 1804*. Nashville: 1869.

McWilliams, Nancy. *Psychoanalytic Diagnosis: Understanding Personality Structure in the Clinical Process*. 2nd ed. New York: Guilford Press, 2011.

Meacham, Jon. *Thomas Jefferson: The Art of Power*. New York: Random House, 2012.

Meacham, Sarah Hand. *Every Home a Distillery*. Baltimore: Johns Hopkins University Press, 2009.

"Meriwether Lewis's Court-Martial Proceedings, November 6–11, 1795." In *Uncovering the Truth about Meriwether Lewis*, edited by Thomas C. Danisi (appendix B). Amherst, NY: Prometheus Books, 2012.

Millon, Theodore. *Masters of the Mind: Exploring the Story of Mental Illness from Ancient Times to the New Millennium*. Hoboken, NJ: Wiley, 2004.

Mitsis, Philip. *The Oxford Handbook of Epicurus and Epicureanism*. Oxford: Oxford University Press, 2020.

Moulton, Gary E. *The Lewis and Clark Expedition Day by Day*. Lincoln: University of Nebraska Press, 2018.

Moulton, Gary E., ed. *The Journals of the Lewis and Clark Expedition*. 13 vols. Lincoln: University of Nebraska Press, 1983–2001.

———. *The Lewis and Clark Journals: An American Epic of Discovery*. Lincoln: University of Nebraska, 2003.

Nicandri, David L. *River of Promise: Lewis and Clark on the Columbia*. Bismarck, ND: Dakota Institute Press, 2009).

———. "The Study of Lewis and Clark: Where We Are Now and Where We Ought to Go Next." *We Proceeded On* 44, no. 3 (August 2018): 5–9. lewisandclark.org/wpo/.

Noll, Mark A. *America's God: From Jonathan Edwards to Abraham Lincoln*. New York: Oxford University Press, 2002.
Oregon Public Broadcasting. *Unfinished Journey: The Lewis and Clark Expedition*, Oregon Public Broadcasting, Public Radio International, Lewis & Clark College, 2005.
Pascal, Blaise. *Pensées*. Translated by A. J. Krailsheimer. New York: Penguin, 1966.
Peck, David. *Or Perish in the Attempt: The Hardship and Medicine of the Lewis and Clark Expedition*. Lincoln, NE: Bison Books, 2011.
Pelton, Robert. *Historical Christmas Cookery*. West Conshohocken, PA: Infinity Publishing, 2002.
Pollard, Joseph P., Donald W. MacCorquodale, and Reimert Thorolf Ravenholt. "Editorial: Meriwether Lewis' Cause of Death." *Epidemiology* 6, no. 1 (January 1995): 97.
Principe, Lawrence M. *The Scientific Revolution: A Very Short Introduction*. Oxford: Oxford University Press, 2011.
Pybus, Cassandra. "Jefferson's Faulty Math: The Question of Slave Defections in the American Revolution," *William and Mary Quarterly* 62, no. 2 (April 2005): 243–64.
Randolph, Thomas Jefferson, ed. *Memoirs, Correspondence and Private Papers of Thomas Jefferson, Late President of the United States*. Vol. 3. London: Henry Colburn and Richard Bentley, 1829.
Ravenholt, Reimert Thorolf. "Triumph Then Despair: The Tragic Death of Meriwether Lewis." *Epidemiology* 5, no. 3 (May 1994): 366–79.
Ronda, James P. *Lewis and Clark among the Indians*. Lincoln: University of Nebraska Press, 1984.
Rorabaugh, W. J. *The Alcoholic Republic: An American Tradition*. Oxford: Oxford University Press, 1987.
Rowland, Lewis P. *Merritt's Textbook of Neurology*. 8th ed. Philadelphia: Lea & Febiger, 1989.
Rush, Benjamin. *Medical Inquiries and Observations*. 4 volumes. Philadelphia: Arno Press, 1972.
Schouls, Peter. "Descartes and the Idea of Progress." *History of Philosophy Quarterly* 4, no. 4 (October 1987): 423–33.
Smith, Daniel, and Michael Hindus. "Premarital Pregnancy in America 1640–1971: An Overview and Interpretation." *Journal of Interdisciplinary History* 4 (Spring 1975): 537–70.

Staloff, Darren. "Lecture 13: Women and the Family." *The History of the United States*. Springfield, VA: Teaching Company, 1998.

Starrs, James E., and Kira Gale. *The Death of Meriwether Lewis: A Historic Crime Scene Investigation*. Omaha, NE: River Junction Press, 2012.

Taylor, Dale. *The Writer's Guide to Everyday Life in Colonial America: From 1607–1783*. Cincinnati: Writer's Digest Books, 1997.

Tramont, E. C. "*Treponema pallidum* (Syphilis)." In *Mandell, Douglas, and Bennett's Principles and Practice of Infectious Diseases*. Edited by Gerald L. Mandell, John E. Bennett, and Raphael Dolin. Vol. 2. 5th ed. (pp. 2474–90). Philadelphia: Churchill Livingstone, 2000.

Turnbow, Tony L. "The Man Who Abandoned Meriwether Lewis." *We Proceeded On* 38, no. 2 (May 2012): 20–31. lewisandclark.org/wpo/.

Weigley, Russell F., ed. *Philadelphia—A 300 Year History*. New York: W. W. Norton & Co., 1982.

Wheeler, O. D. *The Trial of Lewis and Clark 1804–1904*. New York: G. P. Putnam's Sons, 1904.

Wright, Louis B. *The Cultural Life of the American Colonies*. Mineola, NY: Dover Publications, 2002.

About the Authors

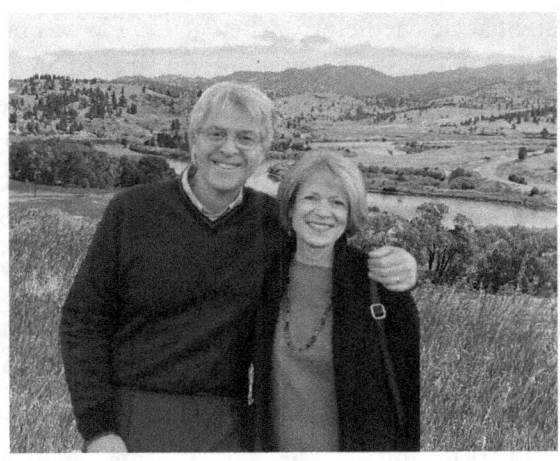

Dr. Marti Peck, grew up in Malvern, Pennsylvania. She earned her B.A. in Psychology at West Chester University (Pennsylvania), where she was a member of the Psi Chi International Honor Society for Psychology, and was recognized as the Social Science Student of the Year during her senior year. She obtained her master's degree in counseling psychology at Arizona State University in 1981 and subsequently earned her Ph.D. in clinical psychology from the California School of Professional Psychology, San Diego in 1989. She completed eight years of postdoctoral study in adult psychoanalysis and is certified by the American Psychoanalytic Association in this specialty. She is a senior faculty member at the San Diego Psychoanalytic Center and also instructed first-year medical students in psychological aspects of medical practice from 2013–16 at the University of California, San Diego, as an adjunct professor in the Department of Psychiatry. She has been in private practice in San Diego for over thirty years.

Dr. David Peck is a native of Santa Barbara, California. He has roots in Montana; his mother Ann was born and raised in Helena.

Dave earned a B.A. and M.Ed. in biology/secondary education from Arizona State University. After teaching high school biology in Tempe, Arizona, for four years (McClintock High), Dave's native interest in science and medicine led him to switch careers. He earned his medical degree (D.O.) in 1987 from Western University of Health Sciences, College of Osteopathic Medicine of the Pacific. He was board certified in family medicine and was a shareholding member of Sharp Rees-Stealy Medical Group in San Diego, where he practiced in the Department of Urgent Care for twenty-one years. Dave is the author of *Or Perish in the Attempt: The Hardship and Medicine of the Lewis and Clark Expedition* (Bison Books, University of Nebraska Press, 2011). He co-produced a Montana PBS documentary based on *Or Perish in the Attempt* in 2016. He is a nationally recognized speaker and has presented to numerous medical societies and historical meetings as well as teaching courses on Lewis and Clark at various venues, including the Chautauqua Institute in western New York.

Marti and Dave live in San Diego, California. They enjoy cycling, hiking, cooking, playing the piano, traveling, spending time at the beach or their cabin in Montana, and visiting and making new friends.

The authors can be contacted through their website: lewisandclarkmedicine.com and via email at lewisclarkmed@gmail.com.

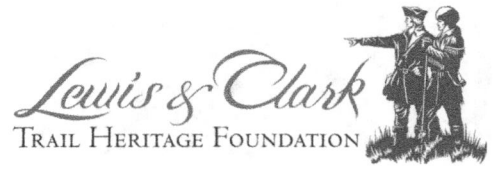

A Special Note to Our Readers

It has been our privilege to belong to a great organization called the Lewis and Clark Trail Heritage Foundation (LCTHF) for a number of years. This organization is dedicated to educating the public about the many facets and adventures of the Lewis and Clark Expedition.

The LCTHF acts as the keeper of the story and steward of the trail in promoting education and scholarship as well as in preserving and protecting the landscape through which the Lewis and Clark Expedition passed. The LCTHF is a charitable, nonprofit, 501(c)3 organization that works in partnership with the Lewis and Clark National Historic Trail, a unit of the National Park Service, in interpreting the Lewis and Clark story and stewarding the trail. The LCTHF holds meetings, activities, and events around the country for its members and the general public, publishes a quarterly journal of scholarly articles (*We Proceeded On*) as well as a newsletter and events calendar, and works to ensure that accurate information about the expedition is available to all.

Please join us and a growing group of interesting people and further your knowledge and enjoyment of what we consider the greatest adventure in American history. For more information, visit lewisandclark.org and lewis-clark.org.

Proceed on!

Endnotes

Introduction
1. Nicandri, "The Study of Lewis and Clark," 8.
2. Guice, *By His Own Hand?*, xiv.
3. Moulton, *The Lewis and Clark Expedition Day by Day*, 646.
4. Holmberg, "'I Fear the Waight of His Mind," 67.
5. Jenkinson, "Meriwether Lewis's Mysterious Death," 14.
6. Pascal, *Pensées*, 85 (aphorism 188).
7. Ambrose, *Undaunted Courage*, 465.

Chapter 1. Life in Early America
1. Meacham, *Every Home a Distillery*, 24–26.
2. Taylor, *The Writer's Guide to Everyday Life in Colonial America*, 121–22.
3. David Peck's six-times-great-grandmother, Jane Hall, was also born in Philadelphia in 1745, the same year as Benjamin Rush. Benjamin Rush's mother was Suzanna Hall. As of the date of the publication of this book, we are still attempting to connect the two Hall families through our genealogical research.
4. Staloff, "Lecture 13: Women and the Family."
5. Pelton, *Historical Christmas Cookery*, viii–ix.
6. Pelton, *Historical Christmas Cookery*, 96–97, 90–91.
7. Pelton, *Historical Christmas Cookery*, 171.
8. Smith and Hindus, "Premarital Pregnancy in America," 537.
9. Meacham, *Thomas Jefferson*, 25–26.
10. Max Roser, "Mortality in the Past—Around Half Died as Children," Our World in Data, June 11, 2019, ourworldindata.org/child-mortality.
11. Hamilton, *The Healers*, 121.
12. Hamilton, *The Healers*, 92.

13 Weigley, *Philadelphia—A 300 Year History*, 232–33.
14 Weigley, *Philadelphia—A 300 Year History*, 220.
15 Mary D. McConaghy, Michael Silberman, and Irina Kalashnikova, "Penn in the 18th Century: School of Medicine," Penn University Archives & Records Center, 2004, https://archives.upenn.edu/exhibits/penn-history/18th-century/medical-school.
16 Wright, *The Cultural Life of the American Colonies*, 182.
17 Charles Blake, *An Historical Account of the Providence State* (Providence, 1868), 19, as cited in Wright, *The Cultural Life of the American Colonies*, 184.
18 Ambrose, *Undaunted Courage*, 52.
19 Traders and explorers venturing into the western region brought back tales of ample land and economic opportunity. My (David's) six-times-great-grandparents Patrick and Jane (Hall) Magee participated in this westward movement. After marrying in Christ's Church, Philadelphia, on Christmas Eve 1765, they moved west to south-central Pennsylvania.
20 "Montana's Indian Country," Discovering Lewis & Clark, www.Lewis-Clark.org/article/2975.
21 Ronda, *Lewis and Clark among the Indians*, chaps. 2–3.
22 Joann Loviglio, "Cause of Mozart's Death Revealed—218 Years Late," *Chron*, August 18, 2009, https://www.chron.com/news/bizarre/article/Cause-of-Mozart-s-death-revealed-218-years-1735278.php.
23 Wikipedia, s.v. "Demographic history of the United States," https://en.wikipedia.org/wiki/Demographic_history_of_the_United_States; Hacker, "Decennial Life Tables"; Komlos, "On the Biological Standard of Living."
24 "Reign of Terror," *Encyclopedia Britannica*, https://www.britannica.com/event/Reign-of-Terror.
25 Johnson, *A History of the American People*, 255–56.
26 As cited in Johnson, *A History of the American People*, 256.
27 Irving Brandt, *James Madison: Secretary of State, 1800–1809*, James Madison, Vol. 4 (1953), 306, as cited in Johnson, *A History of the American People*, 257.
28 Jenkinson, *The Character of Meriwether Lewis* (2000), 107.
29 Ambrose, *Undaunted Courage*, 407.
30 Johnson, *A History of the American People*, 258.
31 *Encyclopedia Britannica*, s.v. "Haitian Revolution," https://www.britannica.com/topic/Haitian-Revolution.

32 Ambrose, *Undaunted Courage*, 41.
33 Alexander Lee, "Beethoven and Napoleon," *History Today*, March 3, 2018, https://www.historytoday.com/archive/music-time/beethoven-and-napoleon.
34 "The Chemical Revolution of Antoine-Laurent Lavoisier," American Chemical Society, June 8, 1999, http://www.acs.org/content/acs/en/education/whatischemistry/landmarks/lavoisier.html.

Chapter 2. Family Background and Biography of Meriwether Lewis

1 Ambrose, *Undaunted Courage*, 21.
2 Jane Lewis Henley, email to Marti Peck, December 5, 2016.
3 Brown and Harpole, *Warner Hall*, 58.
4 Arend Flick, emails to Marti Peck, June 6 and June 15, 2021. Ambrose cited the article in *Undaunted Courage* as follows: Rochonne Abrams, "The Colonial Childhood of Meriwether Lewis," *Bulletin of the Missouri Historical Society* 34, no. 4, pt. 1 (July 1978): 218.
5 Jane Lewis Henley, email to Marti Peck, December 5, 2016.
6 Jane Lewis Henley, email to Marti Peck, December 5, 2016.
7 Jane Lewis Henley, email to Marti Peck, December 5, 2016.
8 Ambrose, *Undaunted Courage*, 22.
9 Arend Flick, email to Marti and David Peck, June 15, 2021.
10 Ambrose, *Undaunted Courage*," 21.
11 Flick, "The Gilmer Daybook," 15–16.
12 Arend Flick, email to Marti Peck, July 31, 2021.
13 Arend Flick, email to Marti Peck, July 31, 2021.
14 Sarah Travers Lewis Scott Anderson, *Lewises, Meriwethers and Their Kin* (Baltimore, MD: Genealogical Publishing Co., 2008), 115.
15 Flick, "The Gilmer Daybook," 17.
16 Flick, "The Gilmer Daybook," 21.
17 Dillon, *Meriwether Lewis*, 13. More recent research by Arend Flick, Ph.D., presented at a Lewis and Clark Trail Heritage Foundation online meeting on August 15, 2021, suggests that Lucy and Captain Marks were more likely married in the spring of 1782 when Meriwether Lewis was seven years old. Flick's findings are based on documentation that Jefferson wrote a letter on April 16, 1781, to David Jameson stating that Jefferson would not recommend John Marks for a governmental position of county lieutenant based on his lack of owning any property. In 1782, Flick notes, there is documentation that Marks's financial situation had

improved and that he now owned slaves and some property, which may have come to him through the dowager rights of his then wife, Lucy, who had inherited a portion of the Locust Hill plantation upon the death of her husband William Lewis.

18 Ambrose, *Undaunted Courage*, 22.
19 Ambrose, *Undaunted Courage*, 28.
20 Cassandra Pybus, "Jefferson's Faulty Math: The Question of Slave Defections in the American Revolution," *William and Mary Quarterly* 62, no. 2 (April 2005), 243.
21 Long, "British Lieutenant Colonel Banastre Tarleton."
22 Hendrix and Benson, "Did Meriwether Lewis Ever Live in Georgia?"
23 Patricia L. Zontine, "Lucy Thornton Meriwether (February 4, 1752–September 8, 1837)," Monticello, April 2009, https://www.monticello.org/sites/library/exhibits/lucymarks/lucymarks/bios/lucytmeriwether.html.
24 Ambrose, *Undaunted Courage*, 26, 27.
25 Ambrose, *Undaunted Courage*, 27.
26 Ambrose, *Undaunted Courage*, 27.
27 Dillon, *Meriwether Lewis*, 15.
28 Ambrose, U*ndaunted Courage*, 28.
29 Meriwether Lewis to Lucy Lewis, November 24, 1794, as cited in Dillon, *Meriwether Lewis*, 20. In this letter, Meriwether declared to his mother, "I am quite delighted with the soldier's life."
30 Flick, "William Diven, the Jay Treaty." Flick's excellent article notes that Elliott entered the Continental army in 1777 and rose to the rank of captain only to be reduced in rank to lieutenant in 1792. Elliott had been shot in a previous duel with another officer shortly after the Battle of Fallen Timbers in 1794. According to Flick, "Elliott's time in Wayne's army was volatile" (p. 13).

   Special thanks to Jim Holmberg, curator of the Filson Historical Society, Louisville, Kentucky, for providing us copies of Lieutenant Elliott's biographical information in Francis B. Heitman, *Historical Register and Dictionary of the United States Army*, vol. 1 (Washington, DC: Government Printing Office, 1903).

   Special thanks also are extended to Thomas Danisi, whose extensive research for his 2012 book *Uncovering the Truth about Meriwether Lewis* led to his discovery of the entire original court-martial proceedings in the archives of the Historical Society of Pennsylvania. Prior to this, biographers writing about this event had based their conclusions on a summary of the proceedings found in the National Archives. The transcript demonstrated how remarkably well Lewis served as his own defense attorney. He was firm and resolute. Given how highly Lewis prided himself on his integrity and good reputation, he must have felt significant anger and fear due to this challenge to his honor.

31 Flick, "William Diven," 11–18 (quote is on p. 13).
32 Arend Flick, email to David Peck, June 15, 2021; Danisi, *Uncovering the Truth about Meriwether Lewis*, 28.
33 Ambrose, *Undaunted Courage*, 49–50.
34 Ambrose, *Undaunted Courage*, 47.
35 Ambrose, *Undaunted Courage*, 47.
36 Dillon, *Meriwether Lewis*, 24
37 Bakeless, *Lewis and Clark: Partners in Discovery*, 70.
38 Ambrose, *Undaunted Courage*, 59–60 (quote is on p. 60).
39 Ambrose, *Undaunted Courage*, 63.
40 Flick, "William Diven."
41 Ambrose, *Undaunted Courage*, 64.
42 Ambrose, *Undaunted Courage*, 84–87.
43 Ambrose, *Undaunted Courage*, 80–81.
44 Ambrose, *Undaunted Courage*, 87.
45 Peck, *Or Perish in the Attempt*, 43–47.
46 Ambrose, *Undaunted Courage*, 91.
47 Ambrose, *Undaunted Courage*, 93.
48 Ambrose, *Undaunted Courage*, 101.
49 *Encyclopedia Virginia*, s.v. "Jefferson's Instructions to Meriwether Lewis (June 20, 1803)," /encyclopediavirginia.org/entries/thomas-jeffersons-instructions-to-meriwether-lewis-june-20-1803/.
50 For an unmatched analysis of Lewis and Clark's dealings with Native Americans, see James P. Ronda's *Lewis and Clark among the Indians*.
51 Ronda, *Lewis and Clark among the Indians*, 22.
52 Ronda, *Lewis and Clark among the Indians*, 21.
53 Thomas Jefferson to Meriwether Lewis, January 22, 1804, as cited in Jackson, *Letters of the Lewis and Clark Expedition*, 1:165–66.
54 Ronda, *Lewis and Clark among the Indians*, 26.
55 Ronda, *James, Lewis and Clark among the Indians*, 28.

56   Ronda, *Lewis and Clark among the Indians*, 41. It is interesting to note that during the Lewis and Clark bicentennial in 2003–06, a group of reenactors making their way up the Missouri River was confronted by a group of Sioux. For many reasons, in the eyes of some Native Americans, the bicentennial was not something to "celebrate" because it represented the beginning of the end of their ancient way of life.

57   The spelling of this Shoshone woman's name continues to be a point of controversy in the Lewis and Clark world. The generally accepted spelling by most scholars is Sacagawea. However, there are many people in her homeland area of Idaho and western Montana who continue to spell it Sacajawea. In this text we spell her name Sacagawea.

58   Moulton, *Journals*, 4:9–10.

59   Moulton, *Journals*, 4:225–26. Canoe trips are available for modern-day explorers who desire to see the White Cliffs. Adventurers can experience the beauty of this area on guided and catered three-day trips. I (David) have done this trip three times. The river is mostly slow and calm, flowing along at about four to five knots. You need not row if you choose to spend your time in a canoe gazing on the "scenes of visionary enchantment." You can even camp at the same sites where the Corps camped, in established campgrounds.

60   Moulton, *Journals*, 4:262–63. The mud in this area is made of a very finely divided particulate clay. When it gets wet, it is known as "gumbo." I (David) have slipped on this soil, and it is beyond just slippery. I have gone from a standing position to flat on the ground in a moment without sensing any instability prior to falling—it happened that quick!

61   Moulton, *Journals*, 4:284.

62   Moulton, *Journals*, 4:292. It is believed that this site is in modern-day Great Falls, Montana, near a power plant on the north side of the Missouri River.

63   Moulton, *Journals*, 4:298.

64   Moulton, *Journals*, 5:70.

65   Moulton, *The Lewis and Clark Expedition Day by Day*, 243.

66   Moulton, *Journals*, 5:74.

67   Moulton, *Journals*, 5:197–218.

68   Moulton, *Journals*, 6:33.

69 The Corps had by this time nearly depleted their trade goods. Their medical practice supplied them with both food items, usually dogs, and the good will of the tribes, who supplied them with both horses and dogs as menu items. Moulton, *Journals*, 7:54, 56, 115, 210, 217–18 (horses); 7:88, 90, 92, 115, 149, 152–54 203–4, 212–13 (dogs).
70 MacGregor, *The Journals of Patrick Gass*, 130.
71 Moulton, *Journals*, 8:88.
72 Moulton, *Journals*, 7:105.
73 Moulton, *Journals*, 7:142–43.
74 Moulton, *Journals*, 7:151–52.
75 Moulton, *Journals*, 7:210.
76 Moulton, *Journals*, 8:113.
77 Moulton, *Journals*, 8:133.
78 Moulton, *Journals*, 8:133–135.
79 Moulton, *Journals*, 8:135
80 Ambrose, *Undaunted Courage*, 383.
81 Moulton, *Journals*, 8:136, 138.
82 Ambrose, *Undaunted Courage*, 425.
83 Ambrose, *Undaunted Courage*, 433.
84 Stroud, *Bitterroot*, 222–23.
85 Ambrose, *Undaunted Courage*, 439.
86 Ambrose, *Undaunted Courage*, 439.
87 Ambrose, *Undaunted Courage*, 443.
88 Danisi and Jackson, *Meriwether Lewis*, 260.
89 One reason government officials gave for not reimbursing Lewis was that he had not received prior authorization for the expenditures. It also seems that Lewis had not supplied the War Department with sufficient "papers and documents" regarding the payments he was seeking reimbursement for. Ambrose, *Undaunted Courage*, 456.
90 Danisi, *Uncovering the Truth about Meriwether Lewis*, 226.
91 Danisi and Jackson, *Meriwether Lewis*, 277.
92 Danisi and Jackson, *Meriwether Lewis*, 286.
93 Stroud, *Bitterroot*, 265–66.
94 "Part 1: Summer of 1809, Part 2: Lewis's Last Journey," Discovering Lewis & Clark, lewis-clark.org/article/3173, pt. 2 of 6.
95 Ambrose, *Undaunted Courage*, 472.
96 Ambrose, *Undaunted Courage*, 471.
97 Ambrose, *Undaunted Courage*, 472.

98 Ambrose, *Undaunted Courage*, 471–72.
99 Turnbow, "The Man Who Abandoned Meriwether Lewis," 20–31.
100 Gilbert C. Russell to Thomas Jefferson, Chickasaw Bluffs, 31 January 1810, in the Thomas Jefferson Papers, Founders Online, National Archives, as cited in Stroud, *Bitterroot*, 279–80.
101 Donald Jackson, *Letters of the Lewis and Clark Expedition* (Urbana: University of Illinois Press, 1978), 2:748, as cited in Ambrose, *Undaunted Courage*, 473.
102 Ambrose, *Undaunted Courage*, 473.
103 Ambrose, *Undaunted Courage*, 473.
104 Ambrose, *Undaunted Courage*, 473.
105 Ambrose, *Undaunted Courage*, 473.
106 Danisi, *Uncovering the Truth about Meriwether Lewis*, 243–44.
107 Ambrose, *Undaunted Courage*, 475.
108 Gilbert Russell's Statement for the Record, November 26, 1811, as cited in Danisi, *Uncovering the Truth about Meriwether Lewis*, 245.

Chapter 3. Philosophical Influences on Meriwether Lewis: Thomas Jefferson and the Enlightenment

1 Principe, *The Scientific Revolution*.
2 Schouls, "Descartes and the Idea of Progress," 423.
3 Kenny, *The Rise of Modern Philosophy*, 39.
4 Meacham, *Thomas Jefferson*, 18.
5 Meacham, *Thomas Jefferson*, 193, 208.
6 Lepore, "The Sharpened Quill."
7 Meacham, *Thomas Jefferson*, 181.
8 "Slavery FAQs—Property," The Jefferson Monticello, https://www.monticello.org/slavery/slavery-faqs/property/.
9 *Stanford Encyclopedia of Philosophy*, s.v. "Francis Bacon," https://plato.stanford.edu/entries/francis-bacon/.
10 "*Stanford Encyclopedia of Philosophy*, s.v. "John Locke," https://plato.stanford.edu/entries/plato/locke/.
11 *Stanford Encyclopedia of Philosophy*, s.v. "Voltaire," https://plato.stanford.edu/entries/voltaire.
12 Mitsis, *The Oxford Handbook of Epicurus and Epicureanism*, 730.
13 Principe, *The Scientific Revolution*.

Chapter 4. Intoxication Nation: Meriwether Lewis and Alcohol

1. Starrs and Gale, *The Death of Meriwether Lewis*, 45, 343.
2. Starrs and Gale, *The Death of Meriwether Lewis*, 56.
3. "Alcohol and Public Health," "Excessive Alcohol Use Is a Risk to Men's Health," and "Binge Drinking," Centers for Disease Control and Prevention, cdc.gov, accessed January 3, 2018.
4. Blood alcohol content table, section 26, *California Driver Handbook*, 2021, https://www.dmv.ca.gov/portal/handbook/california-driver-handbook/alcohol-and-drugs/.
5. Kumar, Abbas, and Aster, *Robbins and Cotran Pathologic Basis of Disease*, 417.
6. Blum, *The Poisoner's Handbook*, 36, 197.
7. Blum, *The Poisoner's Handbook*, 107.
8. Blum, *The Poisoner's Handbook*, 209, 210.
9. "Alcohol Poisoning Deaths," Centers for Disease Control and Prevention, January 2015, https://www.cdc.gov/vitalsigns/alcohol-poisoning-deaths/index.html.
10. Kumar, Abbas, and Aster, *Robbins and Cotran Pathologic Basis of Disease*, 1305.
11. "Delirum tremens," MedlinePlus, https://medlineplus.gov/ency/article/000766.htm, last updated June 9, 2021.
12. Rorabaugh, *The Alcoholic Republic: An American Tradition*, 7.
13. Lender and Martin, *Drinking in America*, 2, 9.
14. Increase Mather, "Wo to Drunkards," Evans Early American Imprint Collection, ps://quod.lib.umich.edu/e/evans/N00124.0001.001/1:3?rgn=div1;view=fulltext.
15. Rorabaugh, *The Alcoholic Republic*, 95–96.
16. Meacham, *Every Home a Distillery*, 14.
17. Meacham, *Every Home a Distillery*, 13.
18. Meacham, *Every Home a Distillery*, 7.
19. Andrew Barr, *A Social History of America* (New York: Carroll & Garf, 1999), 34, as cited in Meacham, *Every Home a Distillery*, 13–14.
20. Meacham, *Every Home a Distillery*, 6.
21. Rorabaugh, *The Alcoholic Republic*, 138.
22. Wikipedia, s.v. "Colonial Molasses Trade," https://en.wikipedia.org/wiki/Colonial_molasses_trade.
23. Rorabaugh, *The Alcoholic Republic*, 18–19.
24. Rorabaugh, *The Alcoholic Republic*, 19.

25 Harold Titus, "Thomas Nelson—Jefferson Escapes," U.S. Historical Fiction [blog], Oct. 26, 2015, authorharoldtitus.blogspot.com.
26 Rorabaugh, *The Alcoholic Republic*, 19.
27 Rorabaugh, *The Alcoholic Republic*, 19.
28 Rorabaugh, *The Alcoholic Republic*, 20.
29 Rorabaugh, *The Alcoholic Republic*, 151.
30 Rorabaugh, *The Alcoholic Republic*, 15.
31 Meacham, *Thomas Jefferson*, 123.
32 Jane O'Brien, "The Time When Americans Drank All Day Long," *BBC News Magazine*, March 9, 2015, https://www.bbc.com/news/magazine-31741615.
33 Jane O'Brien, "The Time When Americans Drank All Day Long," *BBC News Magazine*, March 9, 2015, https://www.bbc.com/news/magazine-31741615.
34 "David Wallace, "Gallons of Alcohol Consumed in the United States Per Capita," *Infographic Journal*, July 20, 2017, https://infographicjournal.com/gallons-of-alcohol-consumed-in-the-us-per-capita/; Rorabaugh, *The Alcoholic Republic*, 8.
35 Rorabaugh, *The Alcoholic Republic*, 11.
36 Rorabaugh, *The Alcoholic Republic*, 6.
37 Rorabaugh, *The Alcoholic Republic*, 18.
38 Rorabaugh, *The Alcoholic Republic*, 87.
39 Rorabaugh, *The Alcoholic Republic*, 14.
40 Rorabaugh, *The Alcoholic Republic*, 34.
41 McCleskey, "Methodists: Drinking Still a Touchy Topic."
42 Lender and Martin, *Drinking in America*, 38.
43 Lender and Martin, *Drinking in America*, 125.
44 Lender and Martin, *Drinking in America*, 125–27.
45 Lender and Martin, *Drinking in America*, 132.
46 Lender and Martin, *Drinking in America*, 132.
47 Noll, *America's God*.
48 Rorabaugh, *The Alcoholic Republic*, 139.
49 Rorabaugh, *The Alcoholic Republic*, 139.
50 Jamison, *Night Falls Fast*, 126.
51 Jamison, *Night Falls Fast*, 145.
52 Jamison, *Night Falls Fast*, 20.
53 Moulton, *Journals*, 4:329.
54 Moulton, *Journals*, 4:329, 330.

55 Moulton, *Journals*, 4:362.
56 Moulton, *Journals*, 8:353.
57 Moulton, *Journals*, 8:360.
58 Moulton, *Journals*, 8:367.
59 Ambrose, *Undaunted Courage*, 403–4.
60 Moulton, *Journals*, 8:372n2. We have great curiosity about the other toasts that were not recorded for history. Suggestions for those toasts would make for a very funny evening around a campfire along the White Cliffs of the Missouri.
61 Starrs and Gale, *The Death of Meriwether Lewis*, 54–55.
62 Rorabaugh, *The Alcoholic Republic*, 142.
63 Rorabaugh, *The Alcoholic Republic*, 143.
64 Edgar Woods, *Albemarle County in Virginia* (Bridgewater, VA: Green Bookman, 1932), 39–40, as cited in Ambrose, *Undaunted Courage*, 31–32.
65 "Meriwether Lewis's Court-Martial Proceedings, November 6–11, 1795," appendix B in Danisi, *Uncovering the Truth about Meriwether Lewis*, 256, 257, 259, 261.
66 See Starrs and Gale, *The Death of Meriwether Lewis*, 245.
67 Danisi, *Uncovering the Truth about Meriwether Lewis*, 333; Vardis Fisher, *Suicide or Murder?*, 71. Thomas Danisi states that this was one of the IOUs generated for payment by William Clark that Lewis listed prior to his journey to Washington in September 1809, but neither Danisi nor Fisher describes this IOU as being for eight barrels of whiskey.
68 Danisi, *Uncovering the Truth about Meriwether Lewis*, 295; Fisher, *Suicide or Murder?*, 71.
69 "History of Barrels," River Drive, https://www.riverdrive.co/history-of-barrels/.
70 Gary Moulton wrote about the challenges Lewis faced in St. Louis "when problems mounted and demons set in." Moulton, *The Lewis and Clark Journals: An American Epic of Discovery*, 454.

Chapter 5. Pleasures and Poisons: Medicine in the World of Meriwether Lewis

1 Genesis 3:19 NLT.
2 Blum, *The Poisoner's Handbook*, 105.
3 Paracelsus was one of the true characters of early medicine. See Peck, *Or Perish in the Attempt*, 315–16.

4   Peck, *Or Perish in the Attempt*, 77.
5   Davis, "Unregulated Potions Still Cause Mercury Poisoning."
6   Dart, *Medical Toxicology*, 1439.
7   Azevedo, "Toxic Effects of Mercury."
8   Chan, "Inorganic Mercury Poisoning."
9   As cited in Peck, *Or Perish in the Attempt*, 45–46.
10 Danisi, *Uncovering the Truth about Meriwether Lewis*, 188–89.
11 Stroud, *Bitterroot*, 264.
12 This handwritten note is described in Danisi, *Uncovering the Truth about Meriwether Lewis*, 326.
13 Stroud, *Bitterroot*, 265.
14 Dr. Streed's testimony is from the transcript of the coroner's jury, as cited in Starrs and Gale, *The Death of Meriwether Lewis*, 98.
15 Rush, *Medical Inquiries and Observations*, vols. 1–4.
16 Armitage, "In Defense of Presentism."
17 For more on these nineteenth-century medical practices, see Peck, *Or Perish in the Attempt*.
18 Rush, *Medical Inquiries and Observations*, 2:142–43.
19 Rush, *Medical Inquiries and Observations*, 2:204 (gout, hydrophobia), 1:229 (sore legs). These citations reflect just a few of the uses of these medications prescribed in the early 1800s. A casual reading of these texts reveals the utter confusion and ignorance of physicians of this era.

Chapter 6. Meriwether Lewis: Mental Derangement and Syphilis

1   Ravenholt, "Triumph Then Despair: The Tragic Death of Meriwether Lewis," *Epidemiology* 5, no. 3 (May 1994): 366–79.
2   For more historical information about this disease, see Peck, *Or Perish in the Attempt*, 112–19.
3   Moulton, *Journals*, 5:232–34.
4   Ravenholt, "Triumph Then Despair, 366–79.
5   Pollard, MacCorquodale, and Ravenholt, "Editorial: Meriwether Lewis' Cause of Death," 97.
6   Pollard MacCorquodale, and Ravenholt, "Editorial: Meriwether Lewis' Cause of Death," 97–98.
7   Ravenholt, "Triumph Then Despair," 375.
8   Moulton, *Journals*, 11:294.
9   Moulton, *Journals*, 7:282–83.
10 Moulton, *Journals*, 7:283.

11 Charles G. Clarke and Dayton Duncan, *The Men of the Lewis and Clark Expedition*, as cited in "William Bratton Biography," Lewis and Clark in Kentucky, https://lewisandclarkinkentucky.org/kentucky-people/the-nine-young-men-from-kentucky/william-bratton/william-bratton-biography/.
12 Response by "Bob" to "Tough Diagnoses: Neurosyphilis, Then and Now," *NEJM-Journal Watch* [blog], Dec. 6, 2010, https://blogs.jwatch.org/hiv-id-observations/index.php/tough-diagnoses-neurosyphilis-then-and-now/2010/12/06/.
13 Tramont, "*Treponema pallidum* (Syphilis)," 2476–77.
14 Rowland, *Merritt's Textbook of Neurology*, 152.
15 Charles Q. Choi, "Case Closed? Columbus Introduced Syphilis to Europe," Live Science, December 27, 2011, htpps://www.livescience.com/17643-columbus-introduced-syphilis-europe.html.
16 Tramont, "*Treponema pallidum* (Syphilis)," 2474.
17 Mouton, *Journals*, 5:215.
18 Moulton, *Journals*, 6:239.
19 Tramont, "*Treponema pallidum* (Syphilis)," 2477.
20 Ahsan and Burrascano, "Neurosyphilis: An Unresolved Case of Meningitis"; Rodrigo Hasbun, "What Is the Presentation of Syphilitic Meningitis?" Medscape, July 16, 2019, https://emedicine.medscape.com/article/232915-clinical#b2.
21 Crozatti et al., "Atypical Behavioral and Psychiatric Symptoms."
22 Klausner, "The Great Imitator Revealed: Syphilis."
23 Crozatti et al., "Atypical Behavioral and Psychiatric Symptoms," 43–47.
24 Moulton, *Journals*, 5:121.

Chapter 7. A Collision of Worldviews: Christianity, the Enlightenment, and Freemasonry

1 J. G. Wilson and J. Fiske, eds. "Waddel, James," in *Appletons' Cyclopaedia of American Biography* (New York: D. Appleton, 1900), as cited in Wikipedia, s.v. "James Waddel," https://en.wikipedia.org/wiki/James_Waddel; Joseph Waddell, *Home Scenes and Family Sketches* (Stoneburner & Prufer, 1900), as cited in Wikipedia, s.v. "James Waddel."
2 Waddell, *Home Scenes*, as cited in Wikipedia, s.v. "James Waddel," https://en.wikipedia.org/wiki/James_Waddel.
3 Moulton, *The Lewis and Clark Journals: An American Epic of Discovery*, 454.

4　Patricia L. Zontine, "Lucy Meriwether Lewis Marks (1752–1837): Her Life and Her World," Monticello, April 2009, www.monticello.org/sites/library/exhibits/lucymarks/lucymarks/lucy.html.

5　Cairns, *Christianity through the Centuries*, 369.

6　"What Is Purgatory?" Catholic Answers, https://www.catholic.com/tract/purgatory.

7　Luther, *Basic Luther*.

8　John Calvin, preface to *Commentary on the Book of Psalms*, trans. James Anderson, vol. 1 (Grand Rapids, MI: Eerdmans, 1948), xi–xii, as cited in Cottret, *John Calvin*, 67.

9　Christine Leigh Heyrman, "Puritanism and Predestination," National Humanities Center, nationalhumanitiescenter.org/tserve/eighteen/ekeyinfo/puritan.htm.

10　"Protestantism: History—Schisms and Sects," Patheos, https://www.patheos.com/library/protestantism/historical-development/schisms-sects.

11　"Religion and the Founding of the American Republic," Library of Congress, https://www.loc.gov/exhibits/religion/rel03.html.

12　"Religion and the Founding of the American Republic," Library of Congress, https://www.loc.gov/exhibits/religion/rel03.html. The philosophical position of the Deists has always intrigued us as it implies that God's existence and purposes are dependent upon our understanding them. As was true with many Enlightenment-era thinkers, the Deists did not understand the mysterious force of gravity, let alone the purposes and ways of God. We think that the position of the school of Deistic thought that a god who had the power to create things such as gravity and life is not able or interested in intervening in human history is irrational.

13　Noll, *America's God*.

14　Rorabaugh, *The Alcoholic Republic*, 138.

15　Rorabaugh, *The Alcoholic Republic*, 138.

16　Wikipedia, s.v. "Religion in Wales," https://en.wikipedia.org/wiki/Religion_in_Wales.

17　Noll, *America's God*, 145.

18　*Encyclopedia Britannica*, s.v. "Arminianism," https://www.britannica.com/topic/Arminianism.

19　*Encyclopedia Britannica*, s.v. "Holy Club," britannica.com/topic/Holy-Club; Wikipedia, s.v. "Holy Club," en.wikipedia.org/wiki/Holy_Club.

20 John McGee to Thomas L. Douglass, as cited in John B. McFerrin, *History of Methodism in Tennessee* (Nashville, 1869–1873), 1:297. See also Rorabaugh, *The Alcoholic Republic*, 106.
21 "George Whitefield: Sensational Evangelist of Britain and America," *Christianity Today*, https://www.christianitytoday.com/history/people/evangelistsandapologists/george-whitefield.html.
22 "George Whitefield": Sensational Evangelist of Britain and America," *Christianity Today*, https://www.christianitytoday.com/history/people/evangelistsandapologists/george-whitefield.html.
23 Wikiwand, s.v. "History of Methodism in the United States," https://www.wikiwand.com/en/History_of_Methodism_in_the_United_States.
24 Tennent delivered a sermon on this theme in 1740 at Nottingham, Pennsylvania. Gilbert Tennent, *The Danger of an Unconverted Ministry*, https://college.cengage.com/history/ayers_primary_sources/danger_unconverted_ministry.htm.
25 Rorabaugh, *The Alcoholic Republic*, 208.
26 Rorabaugh, *The Alcoholic Republic*, 207.
27 Noll, *America's God*, 166.
28 Chang, "A Brief History of Anglo-Western Suicide: From Legal Wrong to Civil Right," 164.
29 William Blackstone, "From *Commentaries on the Laws of England*," May 23, 2015, The Ethics of Suicide Digital Archive, https://ethicsofsuicide.lib.utah.edu /selections/blackstone/.
30 Wikipedia, s.v. "Suicide Legislation," https://en.wikipedia.org/wiki/Suicide_legislation.
31 John Wesley, "Thoughts on Suicide," May 23, 2015, The Ethics of Suicide Digital Archive, https://ethicsofsuicide.lib.utah.edu/selections/john-wesley/.
32 John Wesley, "Thoughts on Suicide," May 23, 2015, The Ethics of Suicide Digital Archive, https://ethicsofsuicide.lib.utah.edu/selections/john-wesley/.
33 Caleb Fleming, "From *A Dissertation upon the Unnatural Crime of Self-Murder*," May 23, 2015, The Ethics of Suicide Digital Archive, https://ethicsofsuicide.lib.utah.edu /selections/caleb-fleming/.
34 Isaac Watts, *A Defense against the Temptation to Self-Murder* (London: Printed for J. Clark, R. Hett, E. Matthews and R. Ford, 1726), May 23, 2015, The Ethics of Suicide Digital Archive, https://ethicsofsuicide.lib.utah.edu /selections/isaac-watts/.

35 Increase Mather, *A Call to the Tempted: A Sermon on the Horrid Crime of Self Murder* (Boston: printed by B. Green, 1682), May 23, 2015, The Ethics of Suicide Digital Archive, https://ethicsofsuicide.lib.utah.edu /selections/increase-mather/.

36 Immanuel Kant, "From *Grounding for the Metaphysics of Morals* . . . ," 23, 2015, The Ethics of Suicide Digital Archive, May https://ethicsofsuicide.lib.utah.edu /selections/kant/.

37 John Locke, "From *The Second Treatise of Government* . . . ," May 23, 2015, The Ethics of Suicide Digital Archive, https://ethicsofsuicide.lib.utah.edu /selections/.

38 Thomas Jefferson to Dr. Samuel Brown, in Bergh, *The Writings of Thomas Jefferson*, 13:310–11.

39 David Hume, "From *Of Suicide*," May 23, 2015, The Ethics of Suicide Digital Archive, https://ethicsofsuicide.lib.utah.edu /selections/david-hume/.

40 Voltaire, "From *Philosophical Dictionary*," May 23, 2015, The Ethics of Suicide Digital Archive, https://ethicsofsuicide.lib.utah.edu /selections/voltaire/.

41 "Meriwether Lewis, Master Mason," Discovering Lewis & Clark, www.lewis-clark.org/article/2091.

42 Mark Tabbert, "Freemasonry in Colonial America," George Washington's Mount Vernon, https://www.mountvernon.org/george-washington/freemasonry/freemasonry-in-colonial-america/.

43 Noll, *America's God*, 205.

44 "Meriwether Lewis, Master Mason," Discovering Lewis & Clark, www.lewis-clark.org/article/2091.

45 "Different Types of Masonic Regalia and Their Significance," Bricks Masons, https://medium.com/@bricksmasonsseo/different-types-of-masonic-regalia-and-their-significance-d4d7d0d516d9.

46 Tabbert, "Freemasonry in Colonial America," George Washington's Mount Vernon, https://www.mountvernon.org/george-washington/freemasonry/freemasonry-in-colonial-america/.
Noll, *America's God*,

47 *A Dictionary of Methodism in Britain and Ireland*, s.v. "Freemasonry," https://dmbi.online/index.php?do=app.entry&id=1061#:~:text=In%20his%20Journal%20for%2018,so%20many%20concur%20to%20keep!.

48 Finney, *The Character, Claims, and Practical Workings of Freemasonry*, 266–67.

49 "Guidance to Methodists on Freemasonry" (The Methodist Church of Great Britain, 1985), 495, https://www.methodist.org.uk/media/2019/fo-statement-guidance-to-methodists-on-freemasonry-1985.pdf.
50 "Guidance to Methodists on Freemasonry," 496.
51 "Guidance to Methodists on Freemasonry," 496.
52 "Guidance to Methodists on Freemasonry," 497.
53 Randolph, *Memoirs, Correspondence and Private Papers of Thomas Jefferson*, 366.
54 Patricia L. Zontine, "Lucy Meriwether Lewis Marks (1752–1837): Her Life and Her World," Monticello, April 2009, www.monticello.org/sites/library/exhibits/lucymarks/lucymarks/lucy.html. We contacted Jane Lewis Henley regarding this issue, and she wrote the following to us in an email: This is the common belief of members of the family, probably passed on in some letters written by my great aunt Sarah Travers Scott Anderson who was my grandfather Dr. Meriwether Lewis Anderson's sister and second born to Charles Harper Anderson, Jr. She married George Loyall Gordon at age 39 at Locust Hill. Aunt Sadie Gordon later lived in Stafford Courthouse, VA. Her husband was the County Surveyor. She lived into her 90's and wrote many letters to her kinfolk about life at Locust Hill where she was born in 1874 and died in her late 90's. She was the historian of the family and assisted her mother in the publication of the family genealogy *The Lewises, Meriwethers, and Their Kin* by Sarah Travers Lewis Scott Anderson. She is the person who probably passed on this belief. I knew her and received letters regularly. She is the person who looked after the family papers and had ones of historical note put into various libraries in Virginia.
55 Thomas Jefferson to Gilbert C. Russell, April 18, 1810, as cited in Danisi, *Uncovering the Truth about Meriwether Lewis*, 243.
56 John Wesley, "On Public Diversions," as cited in Wikipedia, s.v. "Christian Views on Alcohol," https://wikipedia.org/wiki/Christian_views_on_alcohol#cite_note-142.
57 Cherrington, *The Evolution of Prohibition*, 37–38.
58 As our philosopher nephew Benjamin Peck succinctly stated, Enlightenment naturalism and Deism are intrinsically hopeless. After accomplishing all Lewis had, what was it all worth? What did it matter? In Deism and naturalism, the answer is that it does not matter—we all die and that's it. There is no personal God in Deism and in naturalism one is simply the product of chance. Despite the prevailing idea of progress, progress

is ultimately an ambiguous, relative concept in this worldview. Having made such great efforts on behalf of humanity in hopes of progress, it is not difficult to see how Lewis would fall into disillusionment and despair. Benjamin L. Peck, personal communication to David Peck, October 15, 2020.
59 Frances Hunter, "The War of the Poets," Frances Hunter's American Heroes Blog, November 3, 2011, https://franceshunter.wordpress.com/2011/11/03/the-war-of-the-poets/.

Chapter 8. Meriwether Lewis and Malaria: Truth and Fiction

1   Jenkinson, *The Character of Meriwether Lewis: Explorer in the Wilderness*, 282–83.
2   "The 'World Malaria Report 2019' at a Glance," World Health Organization, Dec. 4, 2019, https://www.who.int/news-room/feature-stories/detail/world-malaria-report-2019.
3   "Causes: Malaria," National Health Service, https://www.nhs.uk/conditions/malaria/causes/.
4   Thomas Jefferson to Paul Allen, August 18, 1813, as cited in Danisi, *Uncovering the Truth about Meriwether Lewis*, 247–50.
5   Danisi and Danisi, "Uncovering Jefferson's Account of Lewis's Mysterious Death," 19.
6   Danisi and Danisi, "Uncovering Jefferson's Account," 19.
7   Danisi and Danisi, "Uncovering Jefferson's Account," 20.
8   Danisi and Jackson, *Meriwether Lewis*, 308.
9   Thomas Jefferson to Biddle and Allen, as cited in Crosby, "Hypochondriac Affections," 8.
10 John Mason Goode et al., *Pantologia: A New Cylopaedia* (London: 1814), as cited in Crosby, "Hypochondriac Affections," 8.
11 Crosby, "Hypochondriac Affections," 10.
12 As cited in Crosby, "Hypochondriac Affections," 10. In my (David's) opinion, this article is the most carefully researched, documented, and well-written article regarding this issue.
13 Crosby, "Hypochondriac Affections," 10.
14 Rush, *Medical Inquiries and Observations*, 3:35.
15 Rush, *Medical Inquiries and Observations* 3:12.
16 Rush, *Medical Inquiries and Observations* 3:19.
17 Robert Hooper and Samuel Akerly, *Lexicon Medicum*, 13th ed. (New York: Harper & Brothers, 1841), 443, as cited in Danisi, *Uncovering the Truth about Meriwether Lewis*, 201.

18 Danisi and Danisi, "Uncovering Jefferson's Account of Lewis's Mysterious Death," 22.
19 Danisi and Danisi, "Uncovering Jefferson's Account," 25.
20 Danisi, *Uncovering the Truth about Meriwether Lewis*, 178.
21 Danisi, *Uncovering the Truth about Meriwether Lewis*, 181.
22 John Breck Treat to the Secretary of War, September 18, 1808, RG75, M271, Roll 1, frame 0488, National Archives and Records Administration, as cited in Danisi, *Uncovering the Truth about Meriwether Lewis*, 182.
23 Danisi, *Uncovering the Truth about Meriwether Lewis*, 185.
24 "Malaria Parasite, Mosquito, and Human Host," National Institute of Allergy and Infectious Diseases, https://www.niaid.nih.gov /diseases-conditions/malaria-parasite.
25 "NIH Study Supports New Approach for Treating Cerebral Malaria," National Institutes of Health, Feb. 18, 2020, https://www.nih.gov/news-events/news-releases/nih-study-supports-new-approach-treating-cerebral-malaria/.
26 "Immunity to Malaria," immunopaedia.org.za, https://www.immunopaedia.org.za/immunology/special-focus-area/4-immunity-to-malaria/. The detailed immunology of the mosquito-host interaction is quite complicated. See this website and others cited in this chapter for more information.
27 Adhikari et al., "Perceptions of Asymptomatic Malaria Infection."
28 Ganguly et al., "High Prevalence of Asymptomatic Malaria," 1439–44.
29 Thomas Jefferson to Gilbert C. Russell, April 18, 1810 as cited in Danisi, *Uncovering the Truth about Meriwether Lewis*, 243.
30 Danisi, *Uncovering the Truth about Meriwether Lewis*, 202–3, 401n89.
31 Idro et al., "Cerebral Malaria."

Chapter 9. Bullets and How They Kill
1 As cited in Starrs and Gale, *The Death of Meriwether Lewis*, 111–21.
2 Di Maio, *Gunshot Wounds*, 53–54.
3 For more information on Lewis's 1806 gunshot wound, see Peck, *Or Perish in the Attempt*, 275–78.
4 As cited in Starrs and Gale, *The Death of Meriwether Lewis*, 59.
5 As cited in Starrs and Gale, *The Death of Meriwether Lewis*, 59.
6 Chuinard, "How Did Meriwether Lewis Die?" [part 2], 8.

7   Dale Carrison, D.O., personal communication to David Peck, March 6, 2021.
8   Glenn Wagner, D.O., personal communication (recorded on video) to Marti and David Peck, February 2020.
9   Starrs and Gale, *The Death of Meriwether Lewis*, 106.
10   Dale Mortenson, M.D., personal communication to David Peck, September 2020.
11   Dale Mortenson, M.D., personal communication to David Peck, September 2020.
12   Dale Mortenson, M.D., personal communication to David Peck, September 2020.
13   Dale Mortenson, M.D., personal communication to David Peck, September 2020.
14   Dale Carrison, D.O., email to David Peck, March 10, 2021.
15   Anthony Leo, M.D., personal communication to David Peck, May 21, 2021.
16   John Brahan to the Secretary of War, October, 18, 1809, as cited in Danisi, *Uncovering the Truth about Meriwether Lewis*, 234; *Democratic Clarion* (Nashville, Tennessee), October, 20, 1809, as cited in Danisi, *Uncovering the Truth about Meriwether Lewis*, 235; *Missouri Gazette*, November 2, 1809, as cited in Danisi, *Uncovering the Truth about Meriwether Lewis*, 237.
17   Alexander Wilson to Alexander Lawson, May 18, 1810, as cited in Danisi, *Uncovering the Truth about Meriwether Lewis*, 243–44.
18   Dale Carrison, D.O. personal communication to David Peck, March 10, 2021.
19   Glenn Wagner, D.O. personal communication to David Peck, February 2020, emphasis added.
20   Glenn Wagner, D.O. personal communication to David Peck, February 2020.
21   Di Maio, *Gunshot Wounds*, 65–76.
22   Glenn Wagner, D.O. personal communication to David Peck, February 2020.

Chapter 10. Understanding Mental Health and Meriwether Lewis
1   Kushner, *American Suicide*, 120–32.
2   American Psychological Association, *Ethical Principles of Psychologists and Code of Conduct* (2017), sec. 9.01(b), https://www.apa.org/ethics/code.

3   Millon, *Masters of the Mind*, 15.
4   *Encyclopedia Britannica*, s.v. "Philippe Pinel: French Physician," britannica.com/biography/Philippe-Pinel.
5   Becky Little, "The 1840 U.S. Census Was Overly Interested in Americans' Mental Health," History.com, May 15, 2019, https://www.history.com/news/census-change-mental-illness-controversy; Rhonda C. McClure, "What Is an 'Idiot' in the Census?" Genealogy.com, April 26, 2001, https://www.genealogy.com/articles/over/heard042601.html; "Targeting the 'Unfit,'" Facing History and Ourselves, https://www.facinghistory.org/resource-library/targeting-unfit.
6   Garrett, *Psychotherapy for Psychosis*.
7   Dillon, *Meriwether Lewis*, 344.
8   Lingiardi and McWilliams, *Psychodynamic Diagnostic Manual*, 2.
9   American Psychiatric Association, *Diagnostic and Statistical Manual of Mental Disorders*, 160–61.
10 American Psychiatric Association, *Diagnostic and Statistical Manual*, 160–62.
11 McWilliams, *Psychoanalytic Diagnosis*.
12 McWilliams, *Psychoanalytic Diagnosis*, 101.
13 Colarusso, *Child and Adult Development*.
14 Nicandri, *River of Promise*, 265–66.

Chapter 11. A Psychological Interview of Meriwether Lewis
1   Danisi, *Uncovering the Truth about Meriwether Lewis*, 224.
2   Danisi, *Uncovering the Truth about Meriwether Lewis*, 224.
3   Danisi and Jackson, *Meriwether Lewis*, 275.
4   Stroud, *Bitterroot*, 260.
5   Frederick Bates to his brother, mid-April 1809, as cited in Danisi and Jackson, *Meriwether Lewis*, 259–60.
6   Danisi and Jackson, *Meriwether Lewis*, 260–61.
7   Transcript of the court-martial of Meriwether Lewis, as cited in Danisi, *Uncovering the Truth about Meriwether Lewis*, 24–34.
8   Transcript of the court-martial of Meriwether Lewis, as cited in Danisi, *Uncovering the Truth about Meriwether Lewis*, 268.
9   Moulton, *Journals*, 7:104.
10 Moulton, *Journals*, 7:210.
11 Moulton, *Journals*, 8:113.
12 Moulton, *Journals*, 8:133.

13 Moulton, *Journals*, 8:135.
14 Letter from Meriwether Lewis to William Simmons, August 18, 1809, as cited in Danisi, *Uncovering the Truth about Meriwether Lewis*, 225.
15 Danisi and Jackson, *Meriwether Lewis*, 277.
16 Danisi and Jackson, *Meriwether Lewis*, 284–85.
17 Ambrose, *Undaunted Courage*, 42.
18 Betts and Bear, *The Family Letters of Thomas Jefferson*, 202.
19 Ambrose, *Undaunted Courage*, 429–30.
20 Lewis wrote in 1807, "[W]hat may be my next adventure god knows, but on this I am determined to get a wife." Meriwether Lewis to Mahlon Dickerson, Nov. 3, 1807, as cited in Danisi, *Uncovering the Truth about Meriwether Lewis*, 216.
21 Ambrose, *Undaunted Courage*, 430.
22 Meriwether Lewis to William Preston, July 25, 1808, as cited in Danisi, *Uncovering the Truth about Meriwether Lewis*, 220.
23 Ambrose, *Undaunted Courage*, 438.
24 Lewis wrote to his mother: "My life is still one continued press of business which scarcely allows me leisure to write to you. I have consequently not written to you as often as I could have wished." Meriwether Lewis to Lucy Meriwether Marks, December 1, 1808, as cited in Jenkinson, *The Character of Meriwether Lewis* (2011), 263.
25 Meriwether Lewis to Lucy Meriwether Marks, December 1, 1808, as cited in Stroud, *Bitterroot*, 254.
26 Ambrose, *Undaunted Courage*, 444.
27 Lewis wrote to his mother:
    I'm anxious to know if John Marks has returned to Phila. or not, and if he has gone on [to study medicine], what prospect he has for the means of supplying himself with money, or whether he is sufficiently supplied already. I am also anxious to know whether Mary [Polly] is married or not, and where she is. If she is married and has moved to Georgia [where she was born and grew up].
    Meriwether Lewis to Lucy Meriwether Marks, December 1, 1808, as cited in Stroud, *Bitterroot*, 254.
28 Hendrix and Benson, "Did Meriwether Lewis Ever Live in Georgia?," 12–13.
29 Long, "British Lieutenant Colonel Banastre Tarleton."
30 Vardis Fisher, *Suicide or Murder?*, 23–25.
31 Moulton, *Journals*, 4:9–10.

32 Danisi and Jackson, *Meriwether Lewis*, 32. Lewis's cousin Peachy Gilmer Jr. wrote that Lewis was "always remarkable for perseverance, which in the early period of his life seemed nothing more than obstinacy in pursuing the trifles that employ that age; a martial temper, great steadiness of purpose, self-possession, and undaunted courage."
33 Moulton, *Journals*, 4:292.
34 Rush, *Medical Inquiries and Observations*, 1:4.
35 Rush, *Medical Inquiries and Observations*, 1:17.
36 Rush, *Medical Inquiries and Observations*, 1:236.
37 Rush, *Medical Inquiries and Observations*, vols. 1 and 2. Chapters in these volumes discuss Rush's preferred treatments for these diseases.
38 Rush, *Medical Inquiries and Observations*, 1:229.
39 Jenkinson, *The Character of Meriwether Lewis* (2011), 363.
40 Rush, *Medical Inquiries and Observations*, 1:165.
41 Danisi and Jackson, *Meriwether Lewis*, 277–78.
42 After Lewis's death, Clark wrote to his brother Jonathan, "I fear O! I fear the waight of his mind has over come him, what will be the Consequence?" Holmberg, *Dear Brother*, 218.
43 Holmberg, *Dear Brother*, 207.
44 Jenkinson, *The Character of Meriwether Lewis* (2011), 281.
45 Jenkinson, *The Character of Meriwether Lewis* (2011), 282.
46 This imagined report from Lewis concerning his drinking prior to arriving at Fort Pickering is taken from Gilbert Russell's statement to Thomas Jefferson in 1810:

The fact is which you may yet be ignorant of that his untimely death may be attributed solely to the free use he made of liquor which he acknowledged very candidly after he recovered & expressed a firm determination never to drink any more spirits or use snuff again both of which I deprived him of for several days & confined him to claret & a little white wine. But after leaving this place by some means or other his resolution left him & this agent [Neely] being extremely fond of liquor, instead of preventing the Govr from drinking or putting him under any restraint advised him to it & from every thing I can learn gave the man every chance to seek an opportunity to destroy himself.

Gilbert Russell to Thomas Jefferson, January 31, 1810, as cited in Starrs and Gale, *The Death of Meriwether Lewis*, 248.

Chapter 12. A Psychological Profile of Meriwether Lewis

1. Lingiardi and McWilliams, *Psychodynamic Diagnostic Manual*, 38.
2. Lingiardi and McWilliams, *Psychodynamic Diagnostic Manual*, 6.
3. Lingiardi and McWilliams, *Psychodynamic Diagnostic Manual*, 6.
4. Lingiardi and McWilliams, *Psychodynamic Diagnostic Manual*, 134–35.
5. Lingiardi and McWilliams, *Psychodynamic Diagnostic Manual*, 29–54.
6. Lingiardi and McWilliams, *Psychodynamic Diagnostic Manual*, 39.
7. Lingiardi and McWilliams, *Psychodynamic Diagnostic Manual*, 40.
8. Ambrose, *Undaunted Courage*, 41.
9. American Psychiatric Association, *Diagnostic and Statistical Manual of Mental Disorders*, 237.
10. Jenkinson, *The Character of Meriwether Lewis* (2011), 211.
11. Jenkinson, *The Character of Meriwether Lewis* (2011), 253.
12. "Thomas Jefferson to Meriwether Lewis, 16 August 1809," in the Thomas Jefferson Papers, Founders Online, National Archives, https://founders.archives.gov/documents/Jefferson/03-01-02-0345.
13. Clarence E. Carter, ed., *The Territorial Papers of the United States*, vol. 14, *The Territory of Louisiana-Missouri 1806–1814* (Washington, DC: Government Printing Office, 1949), 222, as cited in Ambrose, *Undaunted Courage*, 446.
14. Jenkinson, *The Character of Meriwether Lewis* (2011), 262–63, 266.
15. Jenkinson, *The Character of Meriwether Lewis* (2011), 263.
16. Ambrose, *Undaunted Courage*, 454.
17. Nicandri, *River of Promise*, 265.
18. Ambrose, *Undaunted Courage*, 27.
19. Levi Lincoln to Thomas Jefferson, April 17, 1803, in the Thomas Jefferson Papers, Founders Online, National Archives, https://founders.archives.gov/documents/Jefferson/01-40-02-0136-0004.
20. Levi Lincoln to Thomas Jefferson, April 17, 1803, in the Thomas Jefferson Papers, Founders Online, National Archives, https://founders.archives.gov/documents/Jefferson/01-40-02-0136-0004.
21. Lingiardi and McWilliams, *Psychodynamic Diagnostic Manual*, 39.
22. Moulton, *Journals*, 4:141.
23. Danisi, *Uncovering the Truth about Meriwether Lewis*, 242.
24. Lingiardi and McWilliams, *Psychodynamic Diagnostic Manual*, 39.
25. Lingiardi and McWilliams, *Psychodynamic Diagnostic Manual*, 29.
26. Moulton, *Journals*, 5:118.
27. Ambrose, *Undaunted Courage*, 467.

28 Ambrose, *Undaunted Courage*, 467.
29 Ambrose, *Undaunted Courage*, 467.
30 Danisi, *Uncovering the Truth About Meriwether Lewis*, 228.
31 Dillon, *Meriwether Lewis*, 325.
32 Lingiardi and McWilliams, *Psychodynamic Diagnostic Manual*, 75.
33 Lingiardi and McWilliams, *Psychodynamic Diagnostic Manual*, 118–19.
34 Lingiardi and McWilliams, *Psychodynamic Diagnostic Manual*, 81.
35 Peck, *Or Perish in the Attempt*, 158, 164–65.
36 Allen, Fonagy, and Bateman, *Mentalizing in Clinical Practice*, 3.
37 Moulton, *Journals*, 4:10.
38 Lingiardi and McWilliams, *Psychodynamic Diagnostic Manual*, 95.
39 Danisi and Jackson, *Meriwether Lewis*, 279.
40 Ambrose-Tubbs, *Why Sacagawea Deserves the Day Off*, 71–88.
41 Lingiardi and McWilliams, *Psychodynamic Diagnostic Manual*, 99.
42 As cited in Ambrose, *Undaunted Courage*, 416–18.
43 Ambrose, *Undaunted Courage*, 418.
44 Lingiardi and McWilliams, *Psychodynamic Diagnostic Manual*, 100–101.
45 Moulton, *Journals*, 8:135.
46 Lingiardi and McWilliams, *Psychodynamic Diagnostic Manual*, 103.
47 Lingiardi and McWilliams, *Psychodynamic Diagnostic Manual*, 107–8.
48 Lingiardi and McWilliams, *Psychodynamic Diagnostic Manual*, 107.
49 Moulton, *The Lewis and Clark Journals: An American Epic of Discovery*, 454.
50 Frances Hunter, "Meet the Parents: William Lewis & Lucy Meriwether, "Frances Hunter's American Heroes Blog, January 14, 2021, https://franceshunter.wordpress.com/2010/01/14/meet-the-parents-william-lewis-lucy-meriwether/.
51 Moulton, *The Lewis and Clark Journals: An American Epic of Discovery*, 110–13.
52 Moulton, *The Lewis and Clark Journals: An American Epic of Discovery*, 113–16.
53 Moulton, *Journals*, 6:190, 6:436, 8:113.
54 Lingiardi and McWilliams, *Psychodynamic Diagnostic Manual*, 114.
55 Lingiardi and McWilliams, *Psychodynamic Diagnostic Manual*, 116.
56 James Neelly to Thomas Jefferson, October 18, 1809, as cited in Ambrose, *Undaunted Courage*, 473.

57 Gilbert Russell's statement, November 26, 1811, as cited in Danisi, *Uncovering the Truth about Meriwether Lewis*, 245.
58 Lingiardi and McWilliams, *Psychodynamic Diagnostic Manual*, 134–259.

Chapter 13. Meriwether Lewis and the Second Man on the Moon
1 Oregon Public Broadcasting, *Unfinished Journey*.
2 Aldrin, *Magnificent Desolation*.
3 Moulton, *The Lewis and Clark Expedition Day by Day*, 121–22.
4 Aldrin, *Magnificent Desolation*, 42.
5 Jenkinson, *The Character of Meriwether Lewis* (2011), 363.
6 Aldrin, *Magnificent Desolation*, 132.
7 Aldrin, *Magnificent Desolation*, 100.
8 Moulton, *Journals*, 5:79. After establishing contact with the Shoshone tribe on August 13, 1805, Lewis noted that the Shoshone made physical contact with them in a display of affection and that "we wer all caressed and besmeared with their grease and paint till I was heartily tired of the national hug."
9 Tom Horvath, personal communication to David Peck, April 23, 2020.
10 Aldrin, *Magnificent Desolation*, 119–20.
11 Aldrin, *Magnificent Desolation*, 126.
12 Aldrin, *Magnificent Desolation*, 145–46.
13 Dillon, *Meriwether Lewis*, 341.
14 Dillon, *Meriwether Lewis*, 342.
15 Holmberg, *Dear Brother*, 218.
16 For a detailed discussion of Jefferson's comment on Lewis's "hypochondriac affections," see Crosby, "Hypochondriac Affections."
17 Ambrose, *Undaunted Courage*, 441.
18 Jamison, *Night Falls Fast*, 88.
19 Jamison, *Night Falls Fast*, 189.
20 Stroud, *Bitterroot*, 273.
21 Holmberg, *Dear Brother*, 243
22 Holmberg, *Dear Brother*, 243. See pp. 248–49 for the full text of Clark's letter.
23 Holmberg, *Dear Brother*, 210.
24 Dillon, *Meriwether Lewis*, 323–24.
25 Danisi, *Uncovering the Truth about Meriwether Lewis*, 268.

26 Thomas Jefferson to Gilbert C. Russell, April 18, 1810, as cited in Stroud, *Bitterroot*, 180.
27 Danisi, *Uncovering the Truth about Meriwether Lewis*, 197.
28 Jenkinson, *The Character of Meriwether Lewis* (2011), 363.
29 Jenkinson, *The Character of Meriwether Lewis* (2011), 364.
30 Jenkinson, *The Character of Meriwether Lewis* (2011), 373.
31 Jackson, *Letters*, 2:575n.
32 Holmberg, *Dear Brother*, 207.
33 Aldrin, *Magnificent Desolation*, 165–66.

Chapter 14. Murder or Suicide?

1 Guice, *By His Own Hand?*, 76.
2 Starrs and Gale, *The Death of Meriwether Lewis*, 46–65.
3 Jenkinson, *The Character of Meriwether Lewis* (2011), 434–35.
4 Wheeler, *The Trial of Lewis and Clark 1804–1904*, 193.
5 Dillon, *Meriwether Lewis*, 344, 350.
6 Chuinard, "How Did Meriwether Lewis Die?" [part 3], 4.
7 Tony Turnbow, personal communication to David Peck, July 27, 2021.
8 Danisi, *Uncovering the Truth about Meriwether Lewis*, 192–210.
9 Clay Jenkinson, *The Thomas Jefferson Hour*, radio broadcast #1420, Dec. 8, 2020, https://jeffersonhour.com/blog/1420.
10 Starrs and Gale, *The Death of Meriwether Lewis*, 58.
11 Dillon, *Meriwether Lewis*, 344.
12 Tom Horvath, personal communication to David and Marti Peck, April 23, 2020.
13 Dillon, *Meriwether Lewis*, 344.
14 Starrs and Gale, *The Death of Meriwether Lewis*, 200.
15 Al Álvarez, *"A Suicide's Excuses": The Savage God: A Study of Suicide* (London: Weidenfeld and Nicolson, 1971), 97, as cited in Jamison, *Night Falls Fast*, 86.
16 Starrs and Gale, *The Death of Meriwether Lewis*, 53.
17 Fisher, *Suicide or Murder?*, 197.
18 "Is Depression Genetic?," Healthline, https://www.healthline.com/health/depression/genetic; 'Mood Disorders," Johns Hopkins, https://www.hopkinsmedicine.org/health/conditions-and-diseases/mood-disorders; "Major Depression and Genetics," Stanford Medicine, https://med.stanford.edu/depressiongenetics/mddandgenes.html; Berrettini, "Genetics of Major Mood Disorders."

19 Guice, "'It Seems to Be More Probable,'" 77–78.
20 Guice, "'It Seems to Be More Probable,'" 78.
21 Gilbert C. Russell to Thomas Jefferson, January 31, 1810 as published in Starrs and Gale, *The Death of Meriwether Lewis*, 248–49.
22 Guice, "'It Seems to Be More Probable,'" 78.
23 Starrs and Gale, *The Death of Meriwether Lewis*, 96.
24 Starrs and Gale, *The Death of Meriwether Lewis*, 96.
25 Starrs and Gale, *The Death of Meriwether Lewis*, 96.
26 Starrs and Gale, *The Death of Meriwether Lewis*, 64.
27 Starrs and Gale, *The Death of Meriwether Lewis*, 96.
28 Fried, *Rush*, 266.
29 Fried, *Rush*, 115.
30 Starrs and Gale, *The Death of Meriwether Lewis*, 98.
31 Holmberg, *Dear* Brother, 206.
32 Holmberg, *Dear Brother*, 210.
33 Holmberg, *Dear Brother*, 213n7.
34 Levi Lincoln to Thomas Jefferson, April 17, 1803, in the Thomas Jefferson Papers, Founders Online, National Archives, https://founders.archives.gov/documents/Jefferson/01-40-02-0136-0004.
35 Holmberg, *Dear Brother*, 217–18.
36 Stroud, *Bitterroot*, 282.
37 James J. Holmberg, personal communication to David Peck, October 1, 2020. Holmberg first saw the original Clark letter when he opened a trunk that contained multiple original letters from William Clark that were donated to the Filson Historical Society in 1998 by descendants of Clark. Imagine Holmberg's surprise and delight upon seeing these contents and finding the original! See Holmberg, *Dear Brother*, 217, for a photocopy of the disputed William Clark letter dated Oct. 28, 1809.
38 Stroud, *The Life and Death of Meriwether Lewis*, 7.
39 Christopher Klein, "A Brief History of Presidential Drinking, History.com, February 13, 2015 (updated September 3, 2018), https://www.history.com/news/a-brief-history-of-presidential-drinking.
40 Meriwether Lewis to Lucy Marks, December 24, 1794, Lewis Papers, as cited in Ambrose, *Undaunted Courage*, 42.
41 Danisi and Jackson, *Meriwether Lewis*, 279.
42 Stroud, *Bitterroot*, 278.
43 Glenn Wagner, D.O., personal communication to David Peck, October 5, 2019.

44 Starrs and Gale, "Coroner's Inquest: The Death of Meriwether Lewis," *The Death of Meriwether Lewis*, 56.
45 Jenkinson, *The Character of Meriwether Lewis* (2011), 330.
46 Jenkinson, *The Character of Meriwether Lewis* (2011), 330.
47 Jenkinson, *The Character of Meriwether Lewis* (2011), 331.
48 Jenkinson, *The Character of Meriwether Lewis* (2011), 331.
49 James R. Bentley, ed., "Two Letters of Meriwether Lewis to Major William Preston," *Filson Club History Quarterly* 44 (1970): 171.
50 Jenkinson, *The Character of Meriwether Lewis* (2011), 332.
51 Jenkinson, *The Character of Meriwether Lewis* (2011), 332.
52 Cutright, "'Rest, Rest, Perturbed Spirit.'"
53 Benemann, "My Friend and Companion" [parts 1 and 2].
54 Wikipedia, s.v. "Meriwether Lewis," https://en.wikipedia.org/wiki/Meriwether_Lewis.
55 Ellen Baumler, "The Death of Meriwether Lewis: Murder or Suicide?" *Great Falls Tribune*, August 30, 2017, https://www.greatfallstribune.com/story/life/2017/08/30/death-meriwether-lewis-murder-suicide/618083001/.
56 Anthony Leo, M.D., medical examiner of Fayette County, Iowa, personal communication to David Peck, July 31, 2021.
57 Starrs and Gale, *The Death of Meriwether Lewis*, 52.
58 A medical examiner in a death investigation addresses various categories when conducting a death investigation. The first consideration is the manner of death (which is different than the cause of death).
59 Anthony Leo, M.D., personal communication to David Peck, July 31, 2021.
60 Clay Jenkinson, "Part 5: Weighing Evidence," Lewis & Clark Trail Heritage Foundation, www.lewis-clark.org/article/3176.
61 "Part 1: Summer of 1809, Part 2: Lewis's Last Journey," Discovering Lewis & Clark, lewis-clark.org/article/3173, p. 2 of 6.
62 Peck, *Or Perish in the Attempt*, 285–86.
63 Two hundred members of the Lewis family requested that the reported remains of Meriwether Lewis be exhumed and forensically examined. A concerted effort was made with the help of James Starrs, an internationally recognized forensic scientist and professor of law. Permission for the exhumation of the remains of Meriwether Lewis was granted by the Department of the Interior on January 11, 2008, and the permit process was started. The Department of the Interior reversed itself and turned down the family's request for exhumation, stopping the permit process

on April 2, 2010. Jane Lewis Sale Henley, letter to Dave and Marti Peck, October 18, 2019.

The Lewis family renewed their efforts for an exhumation in order to bury Lewis's body in Arlington National Cemetery, but this request was rejected with the reasoning that his remains are being well cared for by the National Park Service. As of the summer of 2021, according to Andy Sale, the Lewis family has set aside efforts to exhume Meriwether's remains. Andy Sale, four-times-great-grandnephew of Meriwether Lewis, email to Marti Peck, May 14, 2021.

Index

alcohol. *See also* Jefferson, Thomas; Lewis, Lucy Meriwether; Neelly, James; opium; personality of Meriwether Lewis; Russell, Gilbert; Wesley, John
- adolescents' use of, 19, 103, 104, 107
- American military's use of, 94, 107, 110–11, 348
- Benjamin Rush on, 100, 104, 110–11
- condemnation of by Methodists and Quakers, 102–3, 104, 170
- distilleries in early America, 91, 100, 104
- early Americans' use of, 19, 98–107, 182, 282
- effects of alcohol on the human body, 90, 92–98, 108–9, 305, 309, 366
- Gettler's formula for levels of intoxication, 93–94
- how alcohol-containing drinks are made, 90–91
- Lewis and Clark Expedition's use of, 111–13, 334
- Meriwether Lewis's purchase of whiskey in 1809, 115–17, 119, 243, 334, 346, 347, 352, 357–58, 364, 366
- Meriwether Lewis's comment on "oceans of whiskey," 29, 107, 182–83, 321, 358

alcohol *(cont.)*
- Meriwether Lewis's death and, 184–85, 203, 204–5, 219, 223–24, 307–8, 313–14, 334, 344–45, 346–47, 360
- Meriwether Lewis's use of before 1809, 89–90, 107, 109–15, 118–19, 333–34, 344, 358, 364, 370
- Meriwether Lewis's use of during 1809, 75–76, 95, 108, 113, 115–19, 136, 236, 307, 308, 313–15, 346, 352, 356, 359, 364
- postmortem exams and, 379–80, 381
- Thomas Jefferson's reference to Meriwether Lewis's "habit," 119, 192, 203, 314, 334, 352
- twenty-first-century Americans' use of, 8, 90, 95, 383–84
- whiskey, 48, 57, 91, 99, 100–02, 104, 110–13, 115–17, 345, 349
- withdrawal from, 348–50, 352, 359

Aldrin, Buzz
- life of, 318–28
- similarities to Meriwether Lewis, 318–28, 330, 333–35, 339, 341, 357

Allen, Paul, 193, 294

Álvarez, Al, 342

Ambrose, Stephen
- David and Marti Peck's friendship with, 2–3

Ambrose, Stephen *(cont.)*
  on Meriwether Lewis's psychology, 69, 77, 193, 223, 289
  on Meriwether Lewis's work as governor, 27, 330, 375
  on the family history of Meriwether Lewis, 32, 33
  on the Lewis and Clark Expedition, 23, 372
Ambrose-Tubbs, Stephenie, 223, 302
Anglicanism, 103, 106, 159, 160, 161, 164–70
Apollo 11. *See* Aldrin, Buzz
Aquinas, Thomas, 80
Arikara tribe, 24, 58–59
Asbury, Francis, 170–71

Bacon, Francis, 80, 82, 84–85
barks. *See* Peruvian bark
Bates, Frederik
  as secretary of Upper Louisiana Territory, 71, 72–73, 175, 236–37, 335, 355
  conflict with Meriwether Lewis, 72–73, 183, 289, 305, 331–33, 342, 353
  on Meriwether Lewis's alcohol abuse, 90, 108, 118, 325, 347
  interaction with Meriwether Lewis at Masonic Ball, 73, 236–37, 296, 306, 310
  William Clark's opinion of, 331–32
Benson, Guy Meriwether, 9–10, 32, 44, 110
Biddle, Nicholas, 194
bipolar disorder. *See* personality of Meriwether Lewis
Blackfeet tribe
  killing of two Blackfeet by Corps of Discovery, 67–69, 234, 235, 242, 290–91, 306
  Meriwether Lewis's description of, 311
  relations with other tribes, 24, 66, 155

borderline personality organization, 229–30
Brahan, John, 185
Bratton, William, 145–47, 149
Breckenridge, Letitia, 362, 363
bullets, 207–22. *See also* death of Meriwether Lewis; forensics
  effects on human tissue, 208–9, 210–13
  in the early 1800s, 209–10
Burr, Aaron, 71

calomel. *See* mercury
Calvin, John, 163–64, 167
Calvinism, 163–65, 166–67, 169
Carr, William, 75, 295, 302, 330, 358, 371
Carrison, Dale, 212, 214, 217, 219–20, 222
character organization in personality, 232–33
Charcot, Jean-Martin, 227
Chouteau, Auguste, 112
Christianity, history of, 161–70. *See also* Anglicanism; Calvinism; Deism; Lewis, Meriwether; life in early America; Methodism; Protestant Revolution; Puritanism
Christy, William, 112
Chuinard, Eldon, 207, 213–14, 216, 218, 222, 338, 339, 369
cinchona. *See* Peruvian bark
Clark, Julia, 71, 72
Clark, William
  as co-leader of the Corps of Discovery, 24, 27, 55–66, 69–70, 112–13, 138, 144, 146, 286
  career after the Lewis and Clark Expedition, 70, 72
  effects of mercury on, 127–28
  fictional interview with Marti Peck, 275–77
  Frederick Bates and, 73, 237, 310, 331–32

Clark, William *(cont.)*
   friendship with Meriwether Lewis, 50, 116, 292, 302, 314, 315, 334–35, 363–65
   invitation to join the Corps of Discovery, 55–56
   on Meriwether Lewis's mental state in 1809, 185, 192, 295, 321, 329, 332, 334, 343, 352–56, 358, 359–60, 370, 371
class, social. *See* life in early America
Colarusso, Calvin, 234
Collins, John, 111
Colter, John, 111
coroner's jury of 1996 (concerning Meriwether Lewis's death)
   on Meriwether Lewis's alcohol use, 90, 346–48, 358
   on Meriwether Lewis's death, 209, 213–14, 337–38, 361, 368–69
   on Meriwether Lewis's opium use, 138
   overview of, 4, 346, 368
Corps of Discovery. *See* Lewis and Clark Expedition
Covid-19, 140–41, 189, 339–40
Crosby, Michael, 194–96, 205
Cruzatte, Pierre, 58, 69, 210, 212, 235
Cutright, Paul Russell, 364

Danisi, John, 197–99
Danisi, Thomas, 32, 115, 187–88, 192–205, 338, 366–67
Dearborn, Henry, 330
death of Meriwether Lewis. *See also* alcohol; bullets; Clark, William; coroner's jury of 1996; forensics; Grinder, Pricilla; Jefferson, Thomas; Lewis, Lucy Meriwether; Neelly, James; personality of Meriwether Lewis; Russell, Gilbert
   anti-suicide (murder) theories, 77–78, 179–80, 213–14, 219, 337–39, 357–61, 367
   debate over murder vs. suicide, 3–7, 77–78, 207, 337–73

death of Meriwether Lewis *(cont.)*
   facts of, 76–77, 207–8
   final days of, 74–78, 312–14, 352–54, 356–61
   malaria and, 192, 204–5
   suicide theories, 77–78, 192, 369–73
   two-hour survival of gunshot wounds, 207, 213–18, 222, 379
Deism, 82, 87, 165, 174, 183, 184, 185
delirium tremens, 95–96, 348–50
depression. *See* personality of Meriwether Lewis
Descartes, René, 80
Di Maio, Vincent, 211
diagnosis of disease based on treatment, 135, 138, 140, 198, 202–3
Diagnostic and Statistical Manual of Mental Illnesses (DSM), 90, 231–32, 302
Dickerson, Mahlon
   friendship with Meriwether Lewis, 53, 71, 302, 345, 362–63, 364, 371
   on Meriwether Lewis, 315, 334
Dillon, Richard, 230, 328–29, 338, 341, 342
Drouillard, Joseph, 58, 63–64, 65, 67–68, 329
DSM. *See Diagnostic and Statistical Manual of Mental Illnesses*

early America. *See* life in early America
Elliott, Joseph
   conflict with Meriwether Lewis, 49–50, 114–15, 233, 235, 299–300, 321–22, 332–33
   service in military, 49–50, 53
emotional conflicts (interpersonal vs. intrapsychic). *See* personality of Meriwether Lewis
emotional defenses. *See* personality of Meriwether Lewis
Enlightenment philosophy
   history of, 7, 29, 79–81, 100, 159, 163, 165, 226

Enlightenment philosophy *(cont.)*
   influence on Meriwether Lewis, 83–88, 158–59, 180, 183–84, 185, 315, 335
   influence on Thomas Jefferson, 25, 26–28, 81–88
   suicide and, 171, 173–174
Epstein, Larry, 68
erethism. *See* mercury
Eustis, William, 28, 73–74, 295, 296, 332, 353
exhumation of Meriwether Lewis's body. *See* forensics

Fields, Joseph, 67–69
Fields, Reuben, 67–69
Fisher, Vardis, 115, 338–39, 343–44, 360
Flick, Arend, 33, 34, 39, 40–41, 50, 403n17, 404n30
forensics. *See also* Wagner, Glenn
   determination of a suicide, 368–69, 381–83, 384–86
   past examinations of Meriwether Lewis's body, 367–68
   proposed examination of Meriwether Lewis's body, 154, 220–22, 374–75, 377–88
Fort Clatsop (Oregon), 64–65
Fort Mandan (North Dakota), 42, 59–60, 320, 333
Fort Pickering (Tennessee), 51. *See also* Russell, Gilbert
Francisco, Jerry, 215–16
Freemasonry (Masonic Lodge). *See also* Bates, Frederick
   history of, 175–76
   Meriwether Lewis's membership in, 51, 117, 174–76, 185, 305, 335, 365
   Methodism on, 176–79, 181–82
   on suicide, 176
Freud, Sigmund, 227–28

Gale, Kira, 89–90, 115

Gass, Patrick, 15, 65, 111, 145–46, 304, 327
Gettler, Alexander, 93–94
Gilmer, George, 40–41
Gilmer, Peachy, 45–46, 289, 423n32
Great Falls of the Missouri (Montana), 61–62, 241, 318
Grinder, Pricilla, 76–77, 119, 185, 213, 219, 358–59, 370, 371
Grinder's Stand (Tennessee), 76, 209–210, 307, 314, 338, 350, 386
grizzly bears. *See* Lewis and Clark expedition
Guice, John
   anti-suicide theory of, 3–4, 213–14, 337–38, 339, 343, 361, 368–69, 371
   on Meriwether Lewis's alcohol use, 90, 345–46, 347, 364
   on Meriwether Lewis's suicide attempt, 113
gunshot wounds. *See* bullets

Hall, Hugh, 111
Hein, HannaLore, 339
Hemingway, Ernest, 308
Henley, Jane Lewis, 9, 32, 33–35, 166, 239, 240, 417n54
Hidatsa tribe, 24, 58–59, 63, 64
histeria. *See* mental illness
Holmberg, James, 5, 331–32, 352–55
Hooper, Robert, 196–97
Horvath, Tom, 326, 341
Hume, David, 79, 81, 173–74
"hypochondriac affections"
   Benjamin Rush on, 195–96
   depression and, 193, 295
   hypochondriasis, 182, 193, 196, 203, 205
   malaria and, 187–88, 193, 195, 199
   Thomas Jefferson's use of the term, 41, 192–98, 203, 205, 294–95, 328–29, 343–44, 352
"hypocondriac affections." *See* "hypochondriac affections"
hysteria. *See* mental illness

International Classification of Diseases (ICD), 230–31
interviews (fictional) with Meriwether Lewis and William Clark, 249–79

Jackson, John, 187–88, 192–97, 204–5, 366–67
Jamison, Kay Redfield, 108, 224, 330, 340, 342
Jefferson, Thomas. *See also* alcohol; Deism; Enlightenment philosophy; "hypochondriac affections"; Lewis, Meriwether; Peruvian bark
    appointment of Meriwether Lewis to governorship, 27, 70, 326, 375
    as a slave owner, 18, 43, 83
    as U.S. president, 25–27, 71, 73
    during the American Revolution, 102
    family connections to Meriwether Lewis, 33, 39, 46
    Freemasons and, 176
    influence on Meriwether Lewis, 47, 52–54, 83–84, 88, 158, 180, 302, 332–33
    Lewis and Clark Expedition and, 27–28, 53–55, 57–58, 63, 70, 112, 118–19, 319, 347–48
    Lewis and Clark Expedition journals and, 27, 236, 287–88, 326, 330, 353
    life in France, 82–83
    on Meriwether Lewis's personality, 194, 203, 205, 223, 294–95, 315, 328–29, 334, 343–44
    on Meriwether Lewis's death, 184, 192–93, 203, 295, 338, 339, 344–45, 358, 368–69, 371
    on suicide, 173–74
    political naiveté of, 27–28, 375
    religion of, 87–88, 165, 180–81, 183
    use of alcohol by, 99–100, 324–25, 348, 356–57
Jenkinson, Clay
    on Meriwether Lewis's alcoholism, 334

Jenkinson, Clay *(cont.)*
    on Meriwether Lewis's appointment as governor, 27
    on Meriwether Lewis's failure to publish the expedition journals, 286–87
    on Meriwether Lewis's final days and death, 5–6, 187–88
    on the murder/suicide debate, 5, 337, 339, 370–71
    on similarities between Buzz Aldrin and Meriwether Lewis, 318, 334
    radio programs on the Lewis and Clark Expedition, 317, 339
Johnson, Paul, 26, 28

Kushner, Howard, 223–24

laudanum. *See* opium
Leo, Anthony, 218, 368
Lewis, Elizabeth (great-grandmother of Meriwether Lewis), 34–35, 36, 38
Lewis, John (the Councilor), 34–35, 38
Lewis, John (the Immigrant), 32, 33–34, 38
Lewis, Lucy Meriwether (Meriwether Lewis's mother). *See also* Locust Hill plantation; Methodism
    family history of, 15–16, 35–37, 38, 39, 42, 43, 46, 47
    marriage to John Marks, 41–42
    marriage to William Lewis, 35, 36–37, 38
    on alcohol, 107, 182–83
    reaction to Meriwether Lewis's death, 171, 179–80, 182–85, 359, 372
    religious faith of, 160–61, 169–71, 176, 180–84, 365
    use of medicinal plants by, 44
Lewis, Meriwether. *See also* alcohol; Aldrin, Buzz; Ambrose, Stephen; Bates, Frederick; Blackfeet tribe; coroner's jury of 1996; death of Meriwether Lewis; Deism; Dickerson, Mahlon; Elliott, Joseph; Enlightenment

Lewis, Meriwether *(cont.)*
  philosophy; forensics; Freemasonry; Guide, John; Jefferson, Thomas; Jenkinson, Clay; Lewis and Clark Expedition; Locust Hill plantation; malaria; medicine; mercury; Moulton, Gary; Neelly, James; Nicandri, David; opium; Peruvian bark; personality of Meriwether Lewis; Philadelphia; *Psychodynamic Diagnostic Manual*; Rush, Benjamin; Russell, Gilbert; slavery; syphilis; Wagner, Glenn
  adolescence of, 45–47
  as army officer, 48–52
  as co-leader of the Corps of Discovery, 54–70
  as governor of Upper Louisiana Territory, 27–28, 70–76, 117–18, 137, 174–75, 183, 236–37, 286–87, 295, 297, 310, 325–26, 38, 331, 358, 375, 382
  as Jefferson's personal secretary, 47, 52–53
  as plantation owner, 47–48
  childhood, 39–44
  court-martial, 50, 114–15, 233, 235, 289, 290, 291, 308, 321–22, 332, 353, 354, 358, 382
  debt, 73–74, 75, 332–33, 352–53
  education, 45–46, 54–55, 160
  encounter with grizzly bear, 60, 62, 234, 290–91, 298
  family history, 32–39
  family tree, 38
  fictional interviews with Marti Peck, 249–75, 277–79
  friendship with William Clark, 50, 116, 292, 302, 314, 315, 334–35, 363–65
  legacy, 10–11, 373–76
  relationships, 301–3, 361–65
  racism, 9
  religion, 158, 166–67, 174, 180–81, 183–84
  residence in Georgia, 43–44, 46–47, 110

Lewis, Meriwether *(cont.)*
  similarities to Buzz Aldrin, 318–35, 341, 357
  social class, 19, 37, 39, 303
Lewis, Reuben, 37, 38, 42, 43, 44, 46, 71, 363
Lewis, Robert "of Belvoir" (grandfather of Meriwether Lewis), 34–35, 36, 37, 38
Lewis, William (father of Meriwether Lewis)
  death, 15, 16, 40–42, 47
  marriage to Lucy Meriwether, 35, 36–37, 38
  military service, 37, 39, 40
Lewis and Clark Expedition, 56–70, 372. *See also* alcohol; Ambrose, Stephen; Blackfeet tribe; Clark, William; Jefferson, Thomas; medicine; mercury; Native Americans; opium; Peruvian barks; syphilis; names of individual members of the Corps of Discovery
  grizzly bears and, 60, 62, 210, 234, 290–91, 298
  journals of, 27, 70–71, 74–75, 236, 285–87, 288, 295, 298, 304, 326, 330, 353, 375
  maps of route, 241
  Meriwether Lewis's preparations for, 53–56
life in early America, 14–30, 158–59. *See also* alcohol; Christianity; Enlightenment philosophy; Freemasonry; malaria; medicine; mercury; Methodism; Native Americans; opium; Philadelphia; Rorabaugh, W. J.; slavery
  childhood, 16, 18
  communications, 23–24
  education, 21–23
  entertainment, 23
  food, 16–17
  industrialization, 29
  marriage, 15–16
  physical demands, 14

life in early America *(cont.)*
  politics, 25–26, 28
  religion, 17, 82, 159, 164–71
  science, 29–30
  sexuality, 17–18
  social class, 16, 19, 25, 37, 39, 103, 106, 158, 166
  travel, 23–24
Lincoln, Levi, 55, 290, 354
Locke, John, 82, 84, 85–86, 173, 174
Locust Hill plantation (Virginia)
  Lucy Lewis Marks and, 46–67, 161, 182
  Meriwether Lewis and, 31–32, 44, 51, 71
  William Lewis's inheritance of, 35
"Louis Veneri." *See* syphilis
Luther, Martin, 162–63, 166, 174

M axis (Profile of Mental Functioning). *See* personality of Meriwether Lewis; *Psychodynamic Diagnostic Manual* (PDM-2)
MacCorquodale, Donald, 145–46
Madison, James
  Meriwether Lewis and, 53, 75, 83, 296, 353
  on James Waddell, 160
  political policies of, 25, 26, 28, 55
  river named after, 63
malaria, 187–205. *See also* Peruvian bark
  cause of, 133, 188–89
  diagnosis of, 198–99
  "hypochondriac affections" and, 187–88, 192–99
  Meriwether Lewis and, 135, 138, 140, 154, 187–88, 192–205, 313–14, 334, 338, 351, 352, 366–67
  postmortem exam and, 380, 381
  "severe intermittent paroxysm" and, 197–98
  symptoms of, 153, 189–92, 199–202
  treatment of, 133, 137–38, 189, 198–203

Mandan tribe, 24, 58–59, 248, 287–88
manic-depressive illness. *See* personality of Meriwether Lewis, bipolar disorder
Marks, John (father of Meriwether Lewis), 38, 42, 43, 44, 46, 47, 169
Marks, John Hastings (half brother of Meriwether Lewis), 38, 42, 43, 44, 288, 344, 422n27
Marks, Lucy. *See* Lewis, Lucy Meriwether
Masonic Lodge. *See* Freemasonry
McNeal, Hugh, 63–64
McWilliams, Nancy, 232–33
Meacham, Jon, 18, 82
Meacham, Sara, 99
medicine. *See also* Lewis and Clark Expedition; malaria; mercury; opium; Peruvian bark; Rush, Benjamin; Saugrain, Antoine; syphilis
  in early America, 14, 18, 21, 22–23, 122–40
  philosophy-based vs. science-based, 7–9, 81, 86
  used by Meriwether Lewis prior to his death, 139–40
mental health. *See* mental illness; personality of Meriwether Lewis
mental illness. *See also* personality of Meriwether Lewis
  categorized as insane, idiotic, or feeble-minded, 226
  history of Western understanding of, 226–28
  hysteria and, 195–96, 227, 284
  modern assessment and diagnosis of, 228–33
mercury, 123–32. *See also* syphilis
  Benjamin Rush's use of, 125, 126–28, 132, 140, 367
  effects on the human body, 125–32, 149, 151, 271, 367
  erethism caused by, 129–32
  Lewis and Clark Expedition use of, 127–29, 130–32, 144, 150
  Meriwether Lewis's use of, 131–32, 139–40, 145, 151, 154, 366–67

mercury *(cont.)*
   postmortem exam and, 154, 381
   salivation caused by, 149, 271
   use of in early America, 14, 125
   William Clark's use of, 127–28
Meriwether, Jane (grandmother of Meriwether Lewis), 34, 35, 36, 38
Meriwether, Lucy. *See* Lewis, Lucy Meriwether
Meriwether, Nicholas II, 34, 36, 38
Meriwether, William, 38, 44, 45
Methodism. *See also* Lewis, Lucy Meriwether
   egalitarian views of, 161
   growth of in early America, 168–71
   history of, 164, 165, 167–71
   on alcohol, 102–3, 104, 169–70
   on Freemasonry, 176–79
   on suicide, 171–73
Miller, Isaac, 74, 115–16, 352
Moore, Samuel, 367
Mortenson, Dale, 216
Moulton, Gary
   Lewis and Clark journals and, 5, 56, 63
   on Meriwether Lewis's demons, 160, 183, 185, 308
   on Meriwether Lewis's psychology in general, 5, 174, 193, 344

Napoleon (Bonaparte), 25–26, 28, 29
narcissism, 228–29, 295–96. *See also* personality of Meriwether Lewis
National Park Service, 128, 367, 386, 430n63
Native Americans. *See also* Arikara tribe; Blackfeet tribe; Hidatsa tribe; Mandan tribe; Nez Perce tribe; Sacagawea; Shoshone tribe; syphilis; Teton tribe; Wah-clel-lar tribe; Yankton tribe
   and the Lewis and Clark Expedition, 9, 27–28, 57–58, 60, 65, 66–68, 300, 311, 374
   in early America, 24, 71–72

Neelly, James
   accompaniment of Meriwether Lewis on Natchez Trace, 75–77, 209, 292–93, 313–14, 358–59
   account of Meriwether Lewis's suicide, 76, 77, 119, 185, 357, 358, 359, 370
   use of alcohol by, 76, 292, 358
neurosyphilis. *See* syphilis
neurotic personality organization, 230, 296, 306, 341. *See also* personality of Meriwether Lewis
neurotransmitters, 228–29
Newman, John, 111
Newton, Isaac, 29, 80, 82, 84, 86
Nez Perce tribe, 65–66, 101, 138, 147, 151, 299–300
Nicandri, David
   on Meriwether Lewis's psychology, 77, 223, 234–35, 289, 291, 300, 354
   on the murder/suicide debate, 3–4
Noll, Mark, 106, 167, 175

obsessive-compulsive personality style and disorder. *See* personality of Meriwether Lewis
opium
   Benjamin Rush's use of, 101, 136–37, 138, 140
   forensic exam and, 380, 384
   in early America, 106
   laudanum, 100, 101, 351
   Lewis and Clark Expedition's use of, 101, 135, 138
   Meriwether Lewis's use of, 134, 136–39, 204, 351, 352, 385

P axis (Personality Syndromes). *See* personality of Meriwether Lewis; *Psychodynamic Diagnostic Manual* (PDM-2)
Pahkee tribe. *See* Blackfeet tribe
Paine, Thomas, 82, 106–7
PDM-2. *See Psychodynamic Diagnostic Manual* (PDM-2)

Peale, Charles Wilson, 71
Pernier, John, 75, 76, 77, 182, 185, 209, 358, 359
personality of Meriwether Lewis. *See also* alcohol; Lewis, Meriwether
   acting out, 307–8, 315
   adaptation, resiliency, and strength capacity, 308
   affective range, communication, and understanding capacity, 298–99
   Asperger's syndrome/autism spectrum disorder and, 223, 302
   bipolar disorder and, 223, 224, 341
   defensive functioning capacity, 232–35, 306–8, 315
   depressive tendencies, 193, 194, 197, 223–24, 232, 293–95, 234, 236, 284, 292–95, 296, 308, 314–15, 321, 328–30, 333–34, 341–44, 353–56, 360–61, 371–72
   differentiation and integration (identity) capacity, 300–01
   ego strength, 315
   emotional conflicts, internal and interpersonal, 223–24, 235–37
   fictional interviews with Marti Peck, 245–75, 277–79
   impulse control and regulation capacity, 305–6
   loss and grief, 224, 288–89, 303–4
   M axis (Profile of Mental Functioning), 283, 296–314
   meaning and purpose capacity, 312–13
   mentalization and reflective functioning capacity, 299–300
   modern view of personality, 228–30
   narcissistic tendencies, 295–96, 315, 331, 333
   neurotic level of personality organization, 230, 296–314, 315, 328, 341
   obsessive-compulsive personality style, 284–93, 302, 315

personality of Meriwether Lewis *(cont.)*
   other authors' theories about, 4–5, 223–24, 282–83
   P axis (Personality Syndromes), 283–96
   posttraumatic stress disorder, 77, 223, 234–35, 289–91
   psychological profile of Meriwether Lewis, 223–37, 281–315
   regulation, attention, and learning capacity, 297
   relationships and intimacy capacity, 301–3, 361–65
   S axis (Symptom Patterns: The Subjective Experience), 283, 314–15
   self-confidence, 66, 234–35, 282, 290, 303–5, 319–20, 331, 375
   self-esteem regulation and quality of internal experience capacity, 303–5
   self-observing capacities, 309–312
   sense of honor, 10, 16, 37, 63, 185, 233–34, 235–37, 296, 298, 306, 328, 329, 331–33, 353–54, 356, 357
   sexual orientation, 303
   suicide attempts, 75, 108, 113, 307
personality organization, levels of, 232
Peruvian bark, 132–35. *See also* malaria
   as treatment for malaria, 137, 195, 198–200, 202–3
   Benjamin Rush's use of, 138, 140, 202–3
   Jefferson's use of, 197–98
   Lewis and Clark Expedition's use of, 132–34
   Meriwether Lewis's use of, 134–35, 138, 139–40, 154, 202–3
   side effects of, 134
Philadelphia (Pennsylvania)
   in early America, 21–23, 104, 141
   Meriwether Lewis's studies in, 54–55, 297, 382
   Meriwether Lewis's visits to, 70–71, 74–75, 115, 345, 363, 364

philosophy. *See* Enlightenment philosophy
Pinel, Philippe, 226
Pollard, Joseph, 145
postmortem exam. *See* forensics
posttraumatic stress disorder. *See* personality of Meriwether Lewis
Potts, John, 111
presentism, historical, 138–39
Preston, William, 363
Protestant Reformation. *See* Calvin, John; Calvinism; Luther, Martin
Pryor, Nathaniel, 111
psychoanalysis, 224–25. *See also* mental illness; personality of Meriwether Lewis
psychological profile of Meriwether Lewis. *See* personality of Meriwether Lewis
Psychodynamic Diagnostic Manual (PDM-2). *See also* personality of Meriwether Lewis
    dimensions of levels of personality organization, 232, 282–83
    P axis, M axis, and S axis and their application to Meriwether Lewis, 283–315
    purpose of and differences from the DSM, 231–32
psychotic personality organization, 229
PTSD. *See* posttraumatic stress disorder
Puritanism, 17, 98–99, 159, 164–65, 167, 173

quina quina. *See* Peruvian bark

Ravenholt, Reimert, 143–52, 154–56, 337, 369
religion. *See* Anglicanism; Calvin, John; Christianity; Jefferson, Thomas; Lewis, Lucy Meriwether; Lewis, Meriwether; life in early America; Luther, Martin; Methodism; Puritanism; Quakerism

Rice, Delong, 367
Rorabaugh, W. J.
    on alcohol use in early America, 98, 102, 105, 107, 113–14, 170
    on rapid cultural change in early America, 109–110, 166, 169
Rush, Benjamin. *See also* alcohol; "hypochondriac affections"; mercury; opium, Peruvian bark
    as father of American psychiatry, 226, 350
    medical training of Meriwether Lewis by, 20–21, 54, 122
    medical education of, 16, 21, 160, 382
    medical theory of, 8–9, 87, 132, 140, 197, 198–99
    on mental illness, 226, 292, 313, 350
    on treatment of alcohol withdrawal, 348–49
Rush's pills, 54, 125, 127–28, 130, 132, 367
Russell, Gilbert
    account of Meriwether Lewis's death, 89, 185, 221, 313–14, 343, 352, 423n46
    comments on James Neelly, 76, 292, 313–14
    treatment of Meriwether Lewis at Fort Pickering, 75, 77, 78, 151, 205, 292, 307, 313, 338–39, 346, 348–50, 358–59

S axis (Symptom Patterns: The Subjective Experience). *See* personality of Meriwether Lewis; *Psychodynamic Diagnostic Manual* (PDM-2)
Sacagawea, 59, 63, 64, 101, 134
Sale, Andy, 32, 430n63
salivation. *See* mercury
Saugrain, Antoine, 74, 134, 137, 139, 140, 198–99
science. *See* life in early America
Scientific Revolution, 80–81, 84–85, 86–88

Shields, John, 63–64, 147, 329
Shoshone tribe. *See also* Sacagawea
    as possible source of syphilis, 131, 147, 150, 151, 154–55
    Lewis's first encounter with, 63–64, 323, 329
Simmons, William, 73, 296
Sioux tribe (Teton). *See* Teton tribe
Sioux tribe (Yankton). *See* Yankton tribe
slavery
    anti-slavery movement, 171, 180
    in early America, 19, 22, 26, 43, 100
    in Haiti, 29
    Meriwether Lewis and, 47–48, 234, 304
    sexual relations between slaves and owners, 18
    Thomas Jefferson and, 18, 83
Small, William, 81–82
smallpox, 24, 58–59, 141
social class. *See* life in early America
Starrs, James, 89–90, 115
Stoddard, Amos, 302, 359
Streed, Thomas, 138, 346–49, 351
Stroud, Patricia, 136–37, 338, 355–56, 360, 364
Sturdevant, Dan, 343
suicide. *See also* death of Meriwether Lewis; forensics; personality of Meriwether Lewis
    hesitation before pulling the trigger, 360–61
    motivation to die by, 340
    religious and secular views on, 171–74
syphilis, 143–56. *See also* mercury
    Lewis and Clark expedition members and, 143–47
    Meriwether Lewis and, 131–32, 143, 147–56, 366, 387–88
    Native Americans and, 131, 144, 147, 150, 151, 154–55
    neurosyphilis, 147–53, 337, 366, 387–88

syphilis *(cont.)*
    treatment with mercury, 126–27
    William Lewis and, 40
Tarleton, Banastre, 42–43, 102
Teton tribe, 24, 28, 58, 59, 235
Thompson, J. B., 111
Three Forks of the Missouri (Montana), 62–63, 66, 127
Traveler's Rest (Montana), 66, 128, 241
Two Medicine Fight Site (Montana), 67–69, 241, 242, 306
Turnbow, Tony, 76, 338, 358

University of Virginia Library, Special Collections, 115–16

Voltaire, 84, 86–88, 173–74

Waddell, James, 16, 46, 160
Wagner, Glenn. *See also* forensics
    interview with, 377–88
    on forensic study of Meriwether Lewis's remains, 154, 221–22, 374, 378–83, 385–88
    on Meriwether Lewis's gunshot wounds, 209, 214–16, 221–22, 360–61, 379–80
    on deaths by suicide, 219, 360–61, 381–82, 384–85
Wah-clel-lar tribe, 66
War Department. *See* Eustice, William
Warner Hall (Gloucester County, Virginia), 34–35, 37, 38, 240
Wayne, Anthony, 49, 51
Wernicke-Korsakoff's syndrome, 95
Wesley, Charles, 167–69, 171
Wesley, John
    as founder of Methodism, 167–69, 170
    on alcohol, 171, 183
    on Freemasonry, 176–77
    on suicide, 171–72, 174, 183
Wheeler, Olin, 338
whiskey. *See* alcohol
Whiskey Rebellion, 48–49

White Cliffs (Montana), 60–61, 241, 406n59
Whitefield, George, 169, 171
Wilson, Alexander, 77, 185, 219
Windsor, Richard, 61, 235, 298

Yankton tribe, 58
York, 145–47, 150

www.ingramcontent.com/pod-product-compliance
Lightning Source LLC
Chambersburg PA
CBHW071801080526
44589CB00012B/637